D0221722

MORNING REPORT

INTERNAL MEDICINE

NOTICE

Medicine is an ever-changing science. As new research and clinical experience broaden our knowledge, changes in treatment and drug therapy are required. The editors and the publisher of this work have checked with sources believed to be reliable in their efforts to provide information that is complete and generally in accord with the standards accepted at the time of publication. However, in view of the possibility of human error or changes in medical sciences, neither the editors nor the publisher nor any other party who has been involved in the preparation or publication of this work warrants that the information contained herein is in every respect accurate or complete. Readers are encouraged to confirm the information contained herein with other sources. For example and in particular, readers are advised to check the product information sheet included in the package of each drug they plan to administer to be certain that the information contained in this book is accurate and that changes have not been made in the recommended dose or in the contraindications for administration. This recommendation is of particular importance in connection with new or infrequently used drugs. Readers should also consult their own laboratories for normal values.

MORNING REPORT

INTERNAL MEDICINE

THOMAS P. ARCHER, M.D.
Senior Cardiology Fellow, Division of Cardiology
Former Chief Resident in Internal Medicine
The Ohio State University College of Medicine and Public Health
Columbus, Ohio

JOHN J. YOUNG, M.D.
Senior Cardiology and Critical Care Fellow, Division of Cardiology
Former Chief Resident in Internal Medicine
The Ohio State University College of Medicine and Public Health
Columbus, Ohio

ERNEST L. MAZZAFERRI, M.D.
Professor and Chairman, Division of Internal Medicine
The Ohio State University College of Medicine and Public Health
Columbus, Ohio

McGraw-Hill

HEALTH PROFESSIONS DIVISION

New York St. Louis San Francisco Auckland Bogotá Caracas Lisbon London Madrid
Mexico City Milan Montreal New Delhi San Juan Singapore Sydney Tokyo Toronto

McGraw-Hill

A Division of The **McGraw·Hill** Companies

Morning Report: Internal Medicine

Copyright © 2000 by the McGraw-Hill Companies, Inc. All rights reserved. Printed in the United States of America. Except as permitted under the United States Copyright Act of 1976, no part of this publication may be reproduced or distributed in any form or by any means, or stored in a data base or retrieval system, without the prior written permission of the publisher.

1 2 3 4 5 6 7 8 9 0   QPKQPK   9 9

ISBN 0-07-006692-2

This book was set in Bembo by Better Graphics, Inc.
The editors were Joseph A. Hefta, Martin J. Wonsiewicz, and Peter J. Boyle; the production supervisor was Catherine Saggese; the cover and text designer was Patrice Fodero Sheridan; the indexer was Edwin Durbin. Quebecor Printing/Kingsport was printer and binder.

This book is printed on acid-free paper.

Library of Congress Cataloging-in-Publication Data

Archer, Thomas P.
    Morning report, internal medicine / Thomas P. Archer, John J.
Young, Ernest L. Mazzaferri.
        p.   cm.
    A collection of challenging clinical cases of patients of the Ohio
State University Medical Center, presented by an internal medicine
resident at a daily conference known as the "morning report."
    Includes bibliographical references and index.
    ISBN: 0-07-006692-2
    1. Internal medicine case studies.   I. Young, John J.
II. Mazzaferri, Ernest L., 1936–   .   III. Ohio State University.
College of Medicine.   IV. Title.   V. Title: Internal medicine.
    [DNLM: 1. Internal Medicine Case Report.   WB 115 A672m 1999]
RC66.A69   1999
616'.09--dc21
DNLM/DLC
for Library of Congress   99-33659
                                                                          CIP

To Diane, for her love and support,
and our three wonderful children,
Michael, David, and Jennifer.
—TPA

In loving memory of my father,
and to my family for their love, support, and understanding.
—JJY

To my grandchildren,
who are the joy of my life.
—ELM

CONTENTS

PREFACE

What follows is a collection of interesting and challenging clinical problems of patients of The Ohio State University Medical Center. Each of these cases was presented by an internal medicine resident at a daily conference known as "morning report." The format of this conference involves a resident presenting an "unknown case" to fellow residents and the department chairman or other expert faculty member. The internal medicine chief resident and faculty member lead the group in an interactive exchange to formulate a differential diagnosis of the presenting problem. Once the diagnosis is established, the important diagnostic, pathophysiologic, and therapeutic features of the disease are discussed. This daily interaction reinforces the essential skills of history taking and physical examination required of all physicians in the day-to-day care of patients.

The 50 clinical cases presented in this book follow the format of a morning report. Each case begins with a brief history followed by the pertinent physical examination findings, laboratory tests, and diagnostic studies. The reader can then review the information and test his or her diagnostic skill. The correct diagnosis is then revealed, followed by a discussion (supplemented by tables and pictures) of the important features of the disease process. As further reinforcement, each case is followed by a list of 5 to 7 concise clinical pearls. Finally, each case is concluded with a list of excellent references.

We hope that students and residents will find this book useful, and that the practicing internist will learn from its pages as well.

The authors gratefully acknowledge the following persons in contributing to this book: Drs. Stephen Burgun, Dan Barbero, Brian Bowyer, David Bromet, Lou Chorich, Edward Copelan, Michael Deucher, Curt Daniels, Miriam Freimer, Thomas Keeling, Peter Kourlas, Kenneth Knox, Sean Malone, Julie Mangino, Subha Raman, Nancy Reau, and Stephen Schaal.

The authors would also like to recognize Sharon Ledford for her administrative assistance, and Dennis Mathias and Ben Hawksworth for their technical support.

Thomas P. Archer, M.D.
John J. Young, M.D.
Ernest L. Mazzaferri, M.D.

71-YEAR-OLD MALE WITH FATIGUE

A 71-year-old male with a history of hypertension, coronary artery disease (status-post coronary artery bypass graft × 2, 12 years ago), and benign prostatic hypertrophy presented with a complaint of fatigue. He reported good exercise tolerance; however, over the past 2 months he had noticed increased difficulty walking nine holes of golf. He denied chest discomfort, palpitations, or syncope, but had noted occasional lightheadedness and shortness of breath when walking the longer holes. He was last hospitalized approximately 1 year ago for chest discomfort; a stress echocardiogram at that time revealed no inducible wall motion abnormalities. His regular medications were aspirin, metoprolol, and hydrochlorothiazide. He had not smoked for 12 years and drank one beer a week.

PHYSICAL EXAMINATION

VITAL SIGNS: Temperature, 98.4°F (approx. 36.9°C); pulse, 72; respiration 20; blood pressure, 122/78 mmHg

GENERAL: Appeared younger than stated age

HEENT: Normal

NECK: No thyromegaly

LUNGS: Clear

CARDIAC: Irregularly irregular rhythm; no gallops, grade I/VI systolic murmur at the apex without radiation; mild left ventricular enlargement; jugular venous pulse normal; no carotid bruits

ABDOMEN: Normoactive bowel sounds, soft, nontender; no hepatosplenomegaly

EXTREMITIES: No cyanosis or edema

NEUROLOGIC: Nonfocal

RECTAL: Diffusely enlarged prostate; guaiac negative

LABORATORY FINDINGS

WBC 8.9 K/μL (normal differential); Hb 14.1 g/dL, platelets 288 K/μL. Electrolytes, glucose, urea nitrogen, and creatinine normal. Thyroxine, thyroid-stimulating hormone normal. Urinalysis normal. Electrocardiogram shown (Fig. 1-1).

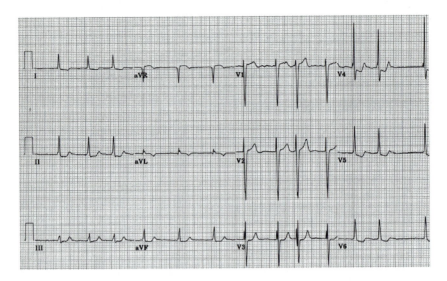

Figure 1-1.
Patient's electrocardiogram.

What is the likely cause of this patient's symptoms and how should they be treated?

This patient has atrial fibrillation (AF). Before leaving the office, treatment with warfarin was started, metoprolol was increased to 50 mg twice daily, and the options were discussed, which included cardioversion or anticoagulation and rate control.

AF is the most common supraventricular arrhythmia. It is believed to affect between 1 and 1.5 million individuals in the United States, accounting for over 1 million hospital days. The prevalence of AF increases with age and is slightly more common in men than women. In those aged 50 to 59 years, the prevalence of AF is 0.5 percent, whereas in those aged 80 to 89 years it is 8.8 percent. Importantly, the presence of AF heralds considerable morbidity, with a mortality rate that is double that of age-matched controls. A great deal of the morbidity and a portion of the mortality are owing to the increased rate of stroke; in fact, AF is the leading cause of embolic strokes (about 75,000/year).

Risk factors for the development of AF include: a history of congestive heart failure, valvular heart disease and stroke, left atrial enlargement, abnormal mitral or aortic valve function, hypertension, and age. AF presents in three distinct clinical circumstances: (1) as a primary arrhythmia in the absence of definable structural heart disease; (2) as a secondary arrhythmia owing to systemic abnormality; and (3) as a secondary arrhythmia associated with structural heart disease. The pathophysiologic distinction between these categories is important. In the presence of structural cardiac disease, the atria are often dilated and fibrotic (focal or diffuse). In systemic disorders, such as thyrotoxicosis, the atria are usually normal but may have scattered fibrosis. As a result, patients with structural disease will often have persistent or *chronic AF*, whereas those with noncardiac disorders will have *paroxysmal AF*. However, patients with structural disease may present with paroxysmal AF, which becomes chronic over time. Recent observations suggest that AF may induce electrical changes in the atria that may predispose to its persistence or recurrence, giving truth to the adage: Atrial fibrillation begets atrial fibrillation. *Lone or primary AF* refers to a subgroup of patients with persistent AF but no evidence of heart disease.

AF is believed to be the result of multiple reentrant impulses wandering throughout the atria, creating continuous electrical activity and reduced mechanical activity. The ability to maintain this chaotic process is determined by conduction and refractory properties of the atrial tissue, and autonomic influences. In addition to the potential for a rapid inappropriate heart rate, patients with AF have loss of normal atrioventricular synchrony and an irregular ventricular rhythm. This may result in a marked decrease in cardiac output, particularly in those individuals who are dependent on effective atrial contraction to overcome impaired diastolic filling (e.g., left ventricular hypertrophy, mitral stenosis, and hypertrophic cardiomyopathy). Variation in the RR interval also results in a constantly changing diastolic filling period, irrespective of atrial contraction. These phenomena likely account for the majority of patient symptoms. Persistent rapid tachycardia for a period of several months may result in a reversible form of left ventricular dysfunction, termed tachycardia-induced cardiomyopathy.

The symptoms of AF are extremely variable and are dependent on a number of factors, including ventricular rate and function, presence of valvular disease, coexisting medical conditions, and patient perceptions. Although some patients will not experience symptoms, most will report palpitations, lightheadedness, fatigue, or dyspnea. On physical examination, the cardiac rhythm is irregularly irregular, with variation in the intensity of heart sounds and absence of atrial activity in the jugular venous pulsations. Individuals dependent on effective atrial contraction (see the preceding) may present in congestive heart failure. In patients with an accessory pathway (Wolff-Parkinson-White syndrome), anterograde conduction of AF over the accessory pathway may cause ventricular fibrillation and sudden cardiac death.

Therapeutic goals to consider in the management of patients with AF include rate control, prevention of thromboembolism, and restoration of sinus rhythm. Controlling the ventricular rate may cause a dramatic diminution of the patient's symptoms. Therefore, agents that depress conduction and prolong refractoriness of the AV node are often required to improve hemodynamics and control symptoms. Commonly used agents include digitalis, beta-blockers, and calcium channel blockers. Digoxin, although a longtime favorite, should be considered first-line treatment *only in patients with congestive heart failure from impaired left ventricular systolic function*. Acute rate control can best be achieved with intravenous verapamil, diltiazem, or beta-blockers in patients with normal left ventricular function. In patients with impaired left ventricular systolic function, intravenous diltiazem may be helpful. Beta-blockers are especially efficacious in patients with thyrotoxicosis or increased sympathetic states. Individuals with an accessory pathway, in the setting of AF, may demonstrate acceleration of conduction over the pathway in the presence of verapamil or diltiazem; therefore, these drugs should be avoided. Instead, the patient should receive prompt cardioversion for severe symptoms, or if stable, treatment with intravenous procainamide. Radiofrequency catheter ablation of the AV node with pacemaker insertion is an alternative for those patients whose rate is not controlled with drugs or who are drug intolerant. Importantly, this therapy does not change the risk of systemic emboli or the need for chronic anticoagulation since the patient remains in atrial fibrillation. A recently initiated National Institutes of Health-sponsored clinical trial (Atrial Fibrillation Follow-up Investigation of Rhythm Management [AFFIRM]) will help evaluate the advantages and disadvantages of rate control versus maintenance of sinus rhythm.

Prevention of thromboembolism is a most important aspect of management in patients with AF. The rate of ischemic stroke among the elderly with AF is 5 percent per year, approximately six times that of age-matched controls. Although most of the strokes related to AF are embolic from the left atrium or left atrial appendage, up to 25 percent of the strokes in the setting of AF are owing to associated vascular and cardiac diseases. Characterization of subpopulations of AF patients into high- and low-risk groups of stroke based on coexisting illnesses, helps to determine those patients who would gain the greatest benefit from anticoagulant therapy. Five clinical variables are independently predictive of thromboembolic risk: history of hypertension, prior stroke or transient ischemic attack, diabetes, age more than 65 years, and recent heart failure. Echocardiographic predictors include left atrial enlargement and impaired left ventricular function. Five randomized trials have convincingly demonstrated the benefit of anticoagulation with warfarin in the reduction of stroke in AF patients. The mean reduction in ischemic stroke was 70 percent, with an incremental risk of serious bleeding of less than 1 percent per year. In another study, the risk of major bleeding was significantly higher in patients older than 75 years; therefore, these patients should have closer monitoring of INR levels. All high-risk patients who can safely tolerate anticoagulation should be treated with warfarin, with a target INR of 2.0 to 3.0. AF patients who cannot tolerate anticoagulation should take daily aspirin. Regarding low-risk patients, that is, patients less than 65 years old with no evidence of structural heart disease, current American College of Cardiology recommendations suggest 325 mg of aspirin daily with close follow-up for the development of risk criteria.

Restoration of sinus rhythm may further improve symptoms and hemodynamics. It is recommended that at least one attempt should be made to restore sinus rhythm if the patient is symptomatic and success is likely. Statistically, the highest likelihood of cardioversion or drug conversion occurs within the first 12 months after onset. A wide variety of antiarrhythmic drugs are available with diverse electrophysiologic effects on atrial tissue (e.g., procainamide, disopyramide, quinidine, propafenone, flecanide, sotalol, and amiodarone). Selection of the most appropriate agent is dependent on a number of clinical variables. Proarrhythmia is the most serious risk associated with these agents and is of particular concern in patients with a history of congestive heart failure. Inpatient initiation and dose titration is warranted in these patients. Nonpharmacologic alternatives include electrical cardioversion (often useful in combination with pharmacologic therapy), the surgical maze procedure, and catheter ablation techniques. The utility of implantable atrial defibrillators awaits the results of clinical trials.

Pharmacologic and electrical cardioversion can be complicated by systemic embolism. Therefore, therapeutic anticoagulation should be given for 3 weeks prior to cardioversion and continued for 4 weeks following cardioversion in patients with AF of unknown duration or longer than 48 hours. An alternative approach involves anticoagulation with heparin and tranesophageal echocardiography for evaluation of atrial or atrial appendage thrombi. If thrombus is present, the patient is treated with coumadin and cardioversion is deferred. If no thrombus is identified, the patient is cardioverted and warfarin is continued for 4 weeks. This approach may be helpful in those patients in whom prompt restoration of sinus rhythm is desirable.

Our patient returned after 4 weeks of therapeutic anticoagulation and a higher dose of metoprolol. Although he felt somewhat better, he still noted "heavy breathing" with exertion. He subsequently underwent electrical cardioversion to normal sinus rhythm with resolution of his exertional dyspnea. He has remained in normal sinus rhythm for 3 months.

 CLINICAL PEARLS

- AF is the most common supraventricular tachycardia.
- The prevalence of AF increases with age.
- AF heralds considerable morbidity and mortality, some of which is accounted for by an increased rate of stroke.
- The symptoms of AF are extremely variable and are dependent on the presence of underlying heart disease and any coexisting medical conditions.
- The 3 therapeutic goals in the management of AF are rate control, prevention of thromboembolism, and restoration of sinus rhythm.
- Prevention of thromboembolism is very important to avoid the devastating complication of stroke.
- Attempts at restoration of sinus rhythm are most likely to be successful within 12 months after onset in selected patients.

REFERENCES

1. Prystowsky EN, Benson DW Jr, Fuster V, et al. Management of patients with atrial fibrillation: A statement for healthcare professionals from the subcommittee on electrocardiography and electrophysiology, American Heart Association. *Circulation* 93:1262–1277, 1996.
2. Pritchett EL. Management of atrial fibrillation. *N Engl J Med* 326: 1264–1271, 1992.
3. Risk factors for stroke and efficacy of antithrombotic therapy in atrial fibrillation: Analysis of pooled data from five randomized controlled trials. *Arch Intern Med* 154:1449–1457, 1994.

34-YEAR-OLD MALE WITH PROGRESSIVE FATIGUE AND WEIGHT LOSS

A 34-year-old male with a history of transposition of the great vessels and a single ventricle (status-post–Blalock-Taussig shunt at age 16 and modified Fontan procedure at age 27), and atrial tachyarrhythmias presented in follow-up with a 4-month history of increasing fatigue and weight loss. He reported good exercise tolerance during this time period, but had felt increasingly tired and weak, particularly at the end of the day. He denied chest pain, shortness of breath, lightheadedness, or recent difficulty with palpitations. He had remained in normal sinus rhythm for the past 2 years since he was started on amiodarone. Prior to that time, he had been treated with multiple antiarrhythmics with little success. At one point, he was considered for atrioventricular (AV) node ablation and pacemaker insertion, but another thoracotomy procedure was required because of his cardiac anatomy. His other medications included digoxin and propranolol. He did not smoke and drank alcohol sparingly.

PHYSICAL EXAMINATION

VITAL SIGNS: Temperature, 98.9°F (approx 37°C); pulse, 68; respiration, 20; blood pressure, 132/88 mmHg
GENERAL: Pleasant, normal-appearing male
HEENT: Normal
NECK: Goiter, no nodules; no cervical lymph node enlargement
LUNGS: Clear

CARDIAC: Regular rate and rhythm; accentuated S_2, grade III/VI systolic ejection murmur at the left upper sternal border without radiation; jugular venous pulse normal

ABDOMEN: Normoactive bowel sounds, soft, nontender; no hepatosplenomegaly

EXTREMITIES: No clubbing or edema

NEUROLOGIC: Nonfocal

LABORATORY FINDINGS

WBC 8.0 K/µL (normal differential); Hb 15.3 g/dL; electrolytes, glucose, urea nitrogen, and creatinine normal; alanine aminotransferase 99 U/L (normal: 0–60); aspartate aminotransferase 72 U/L (normal: 0–60); serum total thyroxine 19.0 µg/dL (normal 4.5–12.0); free thyroxine index 22 (normal: 4.5–12.0); thyroid-stimulating hormone <0.04 IU/mL (normal: 0.2–5.0). Pulmonary function tests: moderate decrease in diffusing capacity, no change from previous study. Chest x-ray: post-thoracotomy changes, no new interstitial infiltrates or pleural disease.

What is the likely cause of this patient's symptoms and how should they be treated?

This patient has amiodarone-induced thyrotoxicosis. This is a complication of treatment with amiodarone that occurs in up to 5 percent of patients and may be manifest at any time during treatment with the drug.

Amiodarone is a Vaughn-Williams class III antiarrhythmic agent that was approved by the Food and Drug Administration in 1985 for the treatment of serious ventricular tachyarrhythmias. In August 1995, the intravenous formulation was approved for the treatment of life-threatening arrhythmias. Amiodarone is also efficacious in the treatment of supraventricular tachyarrhythmias and may provide mortality benefit in patients with idiopathic (nonischemic) cardiomyopathy. Discovered in 1961, it was originally marketed as an antianginal agent because it is a potent vasodilator and beta-blocker.

In the systemic circulation, amiodarone is highly protein- and lipid-bound, and distributes extensively throughout the body, including in adipose, hepatic, myocardial, pulmonary, kidney, thyroid, skin, ocular, splenic, and pancreatic tissues. It is metabolized by the liver to one principal metabolite, desethyl-amiodarone (DEA), which has antiarrhythmic and pharmacokinetic properties comparable to the parent drug. Because of the unique pharmacokinetic properties of amiodarone, a loading period is usually required when it is administered orally. Although a serum concentration of 1 to 2 μg/mL is considered therapeutic in most patients, blood levels generally have little clinical utility.

The side effects of amiodarone are numerous and occur in up to 80 percent of patients. However, only 10 to 15 percent of patients require withdrawal of the drug because of toxicity. The side effects are often related to the daily or cumulative dose of the drug and the duration of treatment. The most common side effects include pulmonary toxicity, hepatotoxicity, peripheral neuropathy, drug interactions, corneal micro deposits, blue-gray skin (Fig. 2-1), photosensitivity, and thyroid dysfunction.

More than half of the patients chronically treated with amiodarone have abnormal thyroid function studies, although most are clinically euthyroid. This is because about 40 percent of the drug by weight is organic iodine, 10 percent of which may be converted to free iodine. A normal maintenance dose of 200 to 600 mg of amiodarone results into a daily intake of 7.5 to 22.5 mg/day of iodine. The usual daily iodine intake in the United States ranges from 0.2 to 0.8 mg, whereas the minimum daily requirement is only about 0.1 mg. Thus, the amount of iodine in amiodarone causes a tremendous increase in the body's iodide pool with a concomitant increase in its thyroidal uptake. In addition, amiodarone interferes with the peripheral conversion of thyroxine (T_4) to triiodothyronine (T_3), causing an increase in serum reverse T_3, and a decrease in serum T_3 concentrations. It also inhibits the entry of T_4 and T_3 into peripheral tissues, which raises serum T_4 levels without causing thyrotoxicosis. This results in about a 40 percent increase in serum T_4 concentrations, often above the normal range, 1 to 4 months after starting the drug. However, this is an expected change that, in itself without symptoms, does not signify hyperthyroidism. The high iodine levels may conversely inhibit the conversion of T_4 to T_3 in the pituitary, increasing serum thyroid-stimulating hormone (TSH) concentrations, which after about 3 months return to normal. Despite these changes in thyroid function tests, most patients are clinically euthyroid, have normal serum TSH

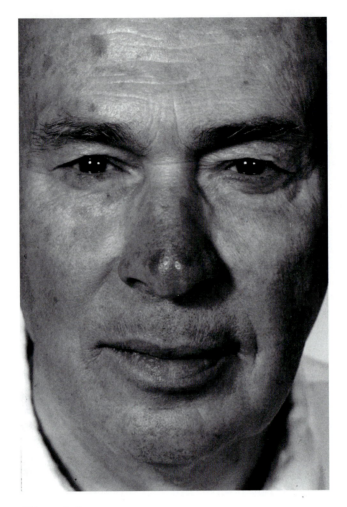

Figure 2-1.
Blue-gray skin pigmentation. (See Plate 1.)

concentrations, and do not require therapy. Unfortunately, serum levels of amiodarone or DEA are not predictive of thyroid dysfunction.

Clinically important thyroid dysfunction is manifest in about 10 to 15 percent of patients receiving amiodarone. Hyperthyroidism or amiodarone-induced thyrotoxicosis, which occurs in 2 percent of patients in the United States, is more common in geographic areas with low dietary iodine intake, whereas hypothyroidism, which occurs in 8 to 10 percent of patients in the United States, is more prevalent in areas with a high dietary iodine intake and where Hashimoto's disease is also more common.

The development of amiodarone-induced thyrotoxicosis is not completely understood. It occurs in patients with and without underlying thyroid disease, and has a slight predilection for males. Aside from iodine-induced overproduction of thyroid hormone, three other pathogenetic mechanisms have been proposed: (1) impaired thyroid iodine autoregulation; (2) amiodarone-induced antithyroid antibodies; and (3) a direct, dose-dependent cytotoxic effect on thyroid follicles. Impaired handling of iodine by the thyroid is suggested by its high iodine content during amiodarone-induced thyrotoxicosis, which returns to normal after resolution of the hyperthyroidism despite continuing the drug. This phenomenon cannot be owing to excessive iodine intake alone. Amiodarone may induce thyroid antibodies according to some, but not all studies. Some believe this occurs only in the presence of pre-existing thyroid disease and that its incidence is similar to that of spontaneously occurring hyperthyroidism. In one series, surgically resected thyroid glands from patients with amiodarone-induced thyrotoxicosis revealed groups of involuted follicles surrounded by a parenchyma showing mild degeneration to total destruction. Although the follicular changes are similar to those occurring in other forms of thyroiditis, the surrounding parenchymal damage is not. Similar cytoplasmic abnormalities can be seen in other organs that are targets of amiodarone toxicity, for example, pneumocytes and hepatocytes. In addition, the elevations in serum interleukin-6 concentrations that occur in amiodarone-induced thyrotoxicosis are similar to those seen in subacute thyroiditis, but are significantly higher than occur in spontaneous hyperthyroidism. Although thyroiditis may be self-limiting, the more destructive lesions are not.

The classic symptoms of thyrotoxicosis (weight loss, weakness, goiter, tremor) may not be present in amiodarone-induced hyperthyroidism, which simply may be manifest by a recurrence of the tachyarrhythmia. Importantly, although hypothyroidism rarely develops after the first 18 months of therapy, thyrotoxicosis may occur at any time during treatment with amiodarone. Interpretation of thyroid function studies can be confusing in this setting. However, the combination of clinical features suggesting thyrotoxicosis (often somewhat vague), with elevated serum thyroxine and suppressed serum TSH concentrations confirm the diagnosis.

The treatment of amiodarone-induced thyrotoxicosis is the most challenging aspect of the disorder. It prompts the clinician to address several questions: (1) Can amiodarone be stopped? (2) Is antithyroid therapy needed? and (3) What is the best form of antithyroid therapy? Stopping

amiodarone therapy may be difficult to impossible in patients with refractory tachyarrhythmias that have been controlled only with this drug.
Moreover, despite stopping the drug, its extensive distribution and long
half-life (22–55 days) may prolong the thyrotoxicosis for up to 8 months.
Some patients, particularly those with large nodular or diffuse goiters,
may be resistant to antithyroid drug therapy. Potassium perchlorate may
be used with thionamides to purge the high intrathyroidal iodine stores,
but it is associated with serious side effects, such as aplastic anemia and the
nephrotic syndrome. Prednisone used in combination with thionamides
may produce salutary effects after only 10 days, but the high doses of
steroids that are required are often a deterrent. One recent study by Dickstein and coworkers found that lithium bicarbonate used in combination
with propylthiouracil was beneficial. Radioactive iodine is not an option
because the high iodide concentration in plasma suppresses the uptake of
thyroidal radioactive iodine. Regardless of the medical therapy chosen,
controlling amiodarone-induced thyrotoxicosis may take weeks because
of the large amount of thyroid hormone in the gland. When discontinuing amiodarone is not an option and medical therapy is impractical or has
failed, total or near-total thyroidectomy provides rapid control of thyrotoxicosis while allowing amiodarone therapy to be continued.

The development of amiodarone-induced hypothyroidism may be related to a failure of the thyroid to escape from the Wolff–Chaikoff effect
(impaired thyroid hormone biosynthesis caused by high intrathyroidal iodide concentrations). However, this is uncommon in the normal thyroid
gland. Hypothyroidism is more likely owing to pre-existing subclinical
thyroid disease, marked by elevated antithyroid antibody titers that predispose the thyroid to the inhibitory effects of iodine excess. In support
of this concept, some studies find that women with pre-existing microsomal or thyroglobulin antibodies have a much higher likelihood of developing amiodarone-induced hypothyroidism than men without
anti-thyroid antibodies. Transient hypothyroidism can occur in patients
with or without underlying thyroid disease, whereas persistent hypothyroidism (despite amiodarone withdrawal) is almost always seen in patients
with underlying thyroid disorders. Amiodarone might accelerate the natural history of the thyroid disorders. As typically occurs with all forms of
hypothyroidism, the clinical presentation may be subtle. Dry skin, fatigue, cold intolerance, low energy, and mental sluggishness are some of
the suggestive symptoms. The diagnosis is established by a low serum-free
thyroxine level and an elevated serum TSH concentration. Patients at

high risk for amiodarone-induced hypothyroidism, for example, women with pre-existing thyroid antibodies, should have thyroid function tests done about every 6 months during the first 2 years of amiodarone therapy.

The treatment options for amiodarone-induced hypothyroidism include discontinuing or decreasing the dose of amiodarone, administering replacement therapy with levothyroxine, or both. The goal of replacement therapy, in contrast to other forms of hypothyroidism, is to bring the serum thyroxine level to the upper end of normal or slightly above, as opposed to titrating the dose of levothyroxine to the level of serum TSH (which may remain high because of pituitary changes in thyroid hormone deiodination induced by amiodarone). Reducing the TSH level to normal may make the patient thyrotoxic and exacerbate the arrhythmia. Therapy should be started with 25 to 50 μg per day and increased by 12- to 25-μg increments every 4 to 6 weeks.

Patients should have baseline free thyroxine and TSH concentrations measured prior to starting amiodarone, at 3 months, and every few months thereafter.

Because of the refractory nature of our patient's atrial tachyarrhythmias, despite multiple different antiarrhythmic agents, he was advised to have total thyroidectomy. The surgery was performed without difficulty and he has remained asymptomatic on amiodarone therapy. His dose of levothyroxine has been titrated to his level of serum thyroxine.

 ## CLINICAL PEARLS

- Amiodarone is a class III antiarrhythmic that is efficacious in the treatment of atrial and ventricular arrhythmias.
- Side effects may develop in up to 80 percent of patients receiving amiodarone.
- More than half of the patients treated with long-term amiodarone develop abnormal thyroid function tests; however, most remain clinically euthyroid.
- Clinically significant thyroid dysfunction occurs in about 10 to 15 percent of patients taking amiodarone.
- The proposed mechanisms of amiodarone-induced thyrotoxicosis include: (1) impaired thyroid iodine autoregulation; (2) amiodarone-induced antithyroid antibodies; and (3) a direct cytotoxic effect on the thyroid follicles.

The treatment of amiodarone-induced thyrotoxicosis is dependent on the importance of continuing the drug. Medical therapy may be successful but may take weeks to work, whereas surgery allows rapid control of the hyperthyroid state and continued use of amiodarone.

REFERENCES

1   Harjai KJ, Licata AA. Effects of amiodarone on thyroid function. *Ann Intern Med* 126:63–73, 1997.
2.   Amiodarone product insert. Philadelphia, Wyeth Laboratories, Inc., March 21, 1997.
3.   Podrid PJ. Amiodarone: Reevaluation of an old drug. *Ann Intern Med* 122:689–700, 1995.
4.   Dickstein G, Shechner C, Adawl F, et al. Lithium treatment in amiodarone-induced thyrotoxicosis. *Am J Med* 102:454–458, 1997.

56-YEAR-OLD MAN WITH FATIGUE AND JOINT PAIN

A 56-year-old exterminator presented with a 2-week history of diffuse arthralgia, fatigue, and a dry nonproductive cough. He also reported night sweats, intermittent low-grade fevers, and a 10-pound weight loss over the same time period. Ten days prior to presentation he was seen at an urgent care center, where, after a normal chest x-ray, he was prescribed a 10-day course of antibiotics. Despite this, his symptoms persisted. He denied chest pain, shortness of breath, hemoptysis, nausea, vomiting, diarrhea, or pruritus.

His past medical history was notable only for hypertension and resection of a benign retro-orbital mass as a child. His only medications were nifedipine and an antibiotic of unknown type. Family history was remarkable for hypertension, type 2 diabetes mellitus, and coronary artery disease. He was happily married and had three healthy adult children. He smoked a pack of cigarettes daily for the past 25 years, but rarely drank alcohol. There was no recent travel, new chemical exposures, or tuberculosis exposure.

PHYSICAL EXAMINATION

VITAL SIGNS: Temperature, 99.7°F (37.5°C); pulse, 100; respiration 20; blood pressure, 109/60 mmHg
GENERAL: Ill-appearing
HEENT: Gingiva, see Figure 3-1
NECK: No thyromegaly, 1-cm lymph node in right supraclavicular fossa
LUNGS: Clear
CARDIAC: Normal

ABDOMEN: Normoactive bowel sounds, soft, diffusely tender; palpable spleen tip; liver palpable 2 cm below the costal margin
RECTAL: Normal sphincter tone, no masses, guaiac negative
EXTREMITIES: No edema
SKIN: No lesions

LABORATORY FINDINGS

WBC, 196.4 K/µL (93% blasts, 3% segmented neutrophils, 4% lymphocytes); Hb, 12.4 g/dL (MCV, 81 fl); platelets, 103 K/µL; electrolytes: sodium, 137 mmol/L, potassium, 3.0 mmol/L, chloride, 95 mmol/L, bicarbonate, 32 mmol/L; blood urea nitrogen, 6 mg/dL; creatinine, 0.8 mg/dL; calcium, 3.9 meq/L (normal, 4.3–5.2); phosphorus, 4.0 (normal, 2.5–4.5); lactate dehydrogenase 3,650 U/L (normal, 0–625); albumin, 3.0 g/dL (normal, 3.8–5.1); lactate, 2.5 mmol/L (normal, 0.3–1.1).

What is the most likely diagnosis and how should this patient be treated?

This patient has acute myelogenous leukemia (AML). Figure 3-1 demonstrates gingival hyperplasia as a consequence of infiltration by leukemic cells, most commonly seen with myelomonocytic (M4) and monocytic (M5) subtypes of AML, which is a disease of immature hematopoetic cells. It is characterized by a defect in maturation beyond the myeloblast (or promyelocyte) stage. The proliferating cells predominate in the bone marrow, eventually replacing other hematopoietic elements. As a result, patients often present with anemia, infections, or bleeding complications.

AML is accountable for 80 percent of the acute leukemias in adults and is slightly more common in men than women. Its incidence increases with age, peaking in the sixth and seventh decades. Although its etiology remains unknown, both genetic and environmental factors appear to be important in this regard. Several congenital disorders, including Down syndrome, Wiskott-Aldrich syndrome, Bloom syndrome, and Fanconi anemia, appear to predispose individuals to the development of AML. In

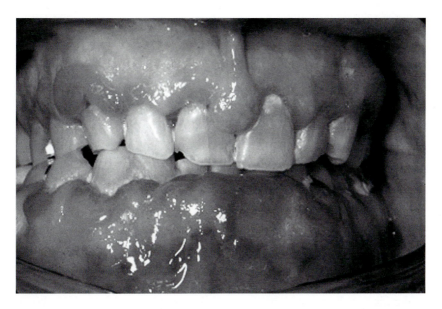

Figure 3-1.
Gingival hyperplasia. (See Plate 2.)

addition, AML may develop from other clonal hematopoietic stem cell disorders, such as polycythemia rubra vera, idiopathic myelofibrosis, and the preleukemic syndromes. A number of proto-oncogenes have been identified in patients with AML, which are likely responsible for leuke-mogenesis. The most common abnormality in AML is mutation of the *ras* gene. Although a number of environmental factors have been sug-gested, only three have been well established in the literature: high-dose radiation exposure, chronic benzene exposure, and alkylating agents.

To establish a diagnosis of acute leukemia, either the bone marrow, peripheral blood, or extramedullary tissues must contain leukemic cells. Typically, the bone marrow is infiltrated by a monomorphic population of leukemic blasts with a substantial reduction in other marrow elements. It is crucial to distinguish between AML and acute lymphatic leukemia (ALL), because of marked differences in the natural history, prognosis, and response to chemotherapeutic agents of the two. The cells in AML are larger than lymphoblasts and have a lower nucleus:cytoplasm ratio. Auer rods, which are stick-like cytoplasmic inclusions, are diagnostic of AML and are seen in up to 20 percent of patients, particularly those with the M3 subtype. Cytochemical stains (i.e., myeloperoxidase) are also frequently helpful in confirming the diagnosis. Sophisticated molecular and cytogenetic diagnostic techniques are available for use in difficult cases or when a cytogenetic abnormality is suspected.

Once the diagnosis is established, AML can be further classified into one of eight different pathologic subtypes (M0–M7) based on cell morphology, histochemical stains, and cell surface markers. Aside from the pathologic significance of this classification scheme, specific clinical features are associated with some subtypes. For example, the acute promyelocytic subtype (M3) is often associated with the development of disseminated intravascular coagulation (DIC), whereas acute myelomonocytic (M4) and acute monocytic (M5) subtypes commonly involve extramedullary tissues—skin, gingiva, and the nervous system.

Only 25 percent of patients with AML have an identifiable preleukemic syndrome. The others experience symptoms of less than 3 months duration, that are often nonspecific, such as fatigue, weakness, palpitations, and dyspnea associated with anemia. More explicit signs of leukemia may be present, however, including bleeding from thrombocytopenia, and infection from neutropenia and breakdown of mucosal barriers. Because the neutrophil population that remains is often quite immature and functionally impaired, septicemia without an identifiable source occurs frequently. Hepatomegaly and splenomegaly are much more common in ALL, but can occur in up to 30 percent of patients with AML (typically, M4, M5 early, and any subtype at end stage). Lymphadenopathy is very uncommon in AML except in the monocytic subtype (M5). Bone pain or arthralgia, at times localized to the sternum, occur in about half the patients as the result of an expanding leukemic cell mass. Although central or peripheral nervous system involvement is much less common in AML than ALL, the M5 subtype bears consideration if meningeal symptoms are present. The skin may show nonspecific lesions (Sweet syndrome) or leukemia cutis (painless, tan or violaceous, palpable infiltrates), or may be involved with granulocytic sarcoma. The gastrointestinal manifestations of AML most often involve the mouth, colon, and anal canal. Gingival or periodontal infiltration or a dental abscess may prompt a visit to the dentist. In others, renal impairment may develop from leukemic infiltration, ureteral obstruction (uric acid stones), urate nephropathy, or from complications of infections and bleeding.

Nonspecific but important laboratory manifestations include a rise in serum uric acid and lactate dehydrogenase as a consequence of rapid cell turnover, especially with myelomonocytic (M4) and monocytic (M5) subtypes. In the absence of a "tumor lysis" syndrome mentioned in the following, electrolyte abnormalities are infrequent and mild except for hypokalemia, which is common, owing to proximal renal tubular dysfunction. Approximately 5 percent of patients with AML present with peripheral blood blast cell counts over $100,000/\mu L$. This poses a high risk of leukostasis, a syndrome in which the microcirculation—especially of the lungs, brain, and penis—is occluded by leukemic blast cells. Patients with this syndrome present with dyspnea, headache, confusion, or priapism. Prompt treatment with hydroxyurea, sometimes with leukopheresis, is necessary to prevent intracranial hemorrhage, the most serious complication of leukostasis.

It is generally recommended that patients with AML undergo treatment within 24 to 36 hours of establishing the diagnosis. Therapy with a combination of drugs—cytarabine and an anthracycline antibiotic (daunorubicin, demethoxydaunorubicin)—typically results in complete remission in 60 to 80 percent of the patients under age 60 who do not have an underlying myelodysplastic or preleukemic state. Once remission is achieved, two to three cycles of so-called consolidation chemotherapy may produce favorable results. Nonetheless, most of those who achieve complete remission relapse within the first 24 months and with each subsequent remission, the disease becomes progressively less responsive to therapy. In most series, only between 10 to 30 percent of patients have a 5-year disease-free survival. Allogeneic bone marrow transplantation (BMT) is an effective treatment option in AML. Unfortunately, half of the patients presenting with AML are over 60 years of age, and most centers limit the use of BMT to younger patients. Allogeneic transplantation for younger patients in first remission is often recommended, but the results are not consistently superior to intensive chemotherapy. In contrast, young patients in second remission or early first relapse are likely to derive significant survival benefit from allogeneic BMT compared with conventional chemotherapy. Autologous transplantation for patients in their first remission is also commonly explored; however, its effectiveness and role have not been adequately studied. As with AML itself, the best results with BMT have been reported in children and young adults.

Our patient was promptly treated with leukopheresis with successful diminution in his leukocyte count. Histochemical staining and immunophenotyping of the bone marrow aspiration and biopsy specimen were consistent with acute myelomonocytic leukemia (M4). Treatment with daunorubicin and cytarabine resulted in remission. His hospital course was complicated by pneumonia and gram-negative sepsis while he was neutropenic. He was eventually discharged to home with plans to receive consolidation chemotherapy at his local hospital.

 # CLINICAL PEARLS

- AML is a clonal malignant disease of immature hematopoetic cells.
- Although the etiology of AML remains unknown, both genetic and enviromental factors appear to be important.
- AML is responsible for 80 percent of acute leukemias in adults and is more common in men than women.
- The majority of patients with AML present with signs and symptoms of less than 3 months' duration.
- Auer rods, which are stick-like cytoplasmic inclusions, are diagnostic of AML, are seen about 20 percent of patients.
- Peripheral blood blast cell counts over $100,000/\mu L$ may obstruct the microcirculation and cause the leukostasis syndrome, resulting in intracranial hemorrhage, severe hypoxia, and priapism.
- Leukostasis requires immediate treatment with hydroxyurea or leukopheresis.
- Allogeneic bone marrow transplantation is an effective therapy in young patients.

REFERENCES

1. Lichtman MA. Acute myelogenous leukemia. *Williams Hematology*, 5th ed. Beutler E, Lichtman MA, Coller BS, Kipps TJ (eds). New York, McGraw-Hill, 1995.
2. Minden M, Imrie K, Keating A. Acute leukemia in adults. *Curr Opin Hematol* 3(4):259–265, 1996.
3. Lowenberg B. Treatment of acute myelogenous leukaemia. *J Intern Med* 740(suppl):17–22, 1997.
4. Bishop JF. The treatment of adult acute myeloid leukemia. *Semin Oncol* 24(1):57–69, 1997.
5. Burnett AK, Eden OB. The treatment of acute leukaemia. *Lancet* 349(9047):270–275, 1997.

33-YEAR-OLD MALE WITH CHRONIC DIARRHEA

A 33-year-old married automobile mechanic presented with a 6-month history of diarrhea associated with intermittent crampy abdominal pain and nausea, a skin rash, and a 40-pound weight loss. He reported up to seven loose bowel movements per day that were typically associated with crampy mid-epigastric abdominal pain. Aside from an unusually foul odor, he was unable to further characterize his stools, and denied fevers, chills, night sweats, hematemesis, hematochezia, melena, or HIV risk factors. Just before the diarrhea had begun, he developed a pruritic skin rash over his elbows and forearms that persisted. During a hospitalization 3 months ago for this problem, multiple stool cultures, colonoscopy, and an abdominal CT scan were negative and he received no specific therapy. He had no family history of chronic diarrhea or inflammatory bowel disease, but his father died of lymphoma. His regular medications included megestrol, prochlorperazine, and diphenoxylate. He took no over-the-counter medications, denied illicit drug use, and reported drinking only an occasional beer. He recently had stopped smoking. There was no recent travel history or change in dietary habits.

PHYSICAL EXAMINATION

VITAL SIGNS: Temperature, 98.7°F (37°C); pulse, 96; respiration, 18; blood pressure, 122/80 mmHg
GENERAL: Cachectic
HEENT: Oropharynx: dry mucous membranes
NECK: No thyromegaly or lymphadenopathy
LUNGS: Clear

CARDIAC: Normal

ABDOMEN: Normoactive bowel sounds, soft, diffusely tender; no hepatosplenomegaly

RECTAL: Normal sphincter tone, no masses, guaiac negative

EXTREMITIES: No edema

SKIN: See Figure 4-1

LABORATORY FINDINGS

WBC, 14.4 K/μL (87% segmented neutrophils, 6% lymphocytes); Hb, 16.5 g/dL (MCV 94 fl); platelets, 386 K/μL; electrolytes: sodium, 136 mmol/L, potassium, 5.1 mmol/L, chloride, 94 mmol/L, bicarbonate, 25 mmol/L; blood urea nitrogen, 21 mg/dL; creatinine, 0.9 mg/dL; calcium, 3.9 mEq/L (normal, 4.3–5.2); phosphorus, 4.0 mg/dL (normal, 2.5–4.5); amylase, <30 U/L (normal, 0–140); lipase, <10 U/L (normal, 0–200); lactate dehydrogenase, 1373 U/L (normal, 0–625); alkaline phosphatase, 129 U/L (normal, 0–105); albumin, 3.0 g/dL (normal, 3.8–5.1); stool cultures negative; no fecal leukocytes detected

What is the likely diagnosis and how should this patient be treated?

This patient has celiac sprue, also termed celiac disease, non-tropical sprue, or gluten-sensitive enteropathy. The skin lesions shown in Figure 4-1 are dermatitis herpetiformis. They are intensely pruritic papulovesicular lesions that typically appear in a symmetric distribution on extensor areas—elbows, knees, buttocks, scapulae, the sacrum, or the scalp. Their presence is virtually pathognomonic in the appropriate clinical setting. Skin biopsy reveals granular immunoglobulin A (IgA) deposits at the dermal–epidermal junction. Intestinal involvement from celiac disease in patients with dermatitis herpetiformis is typically mild and may be asymptomatic. Withdrawal of gluten from the diet often reverses not only the intestinal but also the skin lesions. Dermatitis herpetiformis and celiac disease share the HLA-DQ2 haplotype, and both diseases may occur as a familial trait.

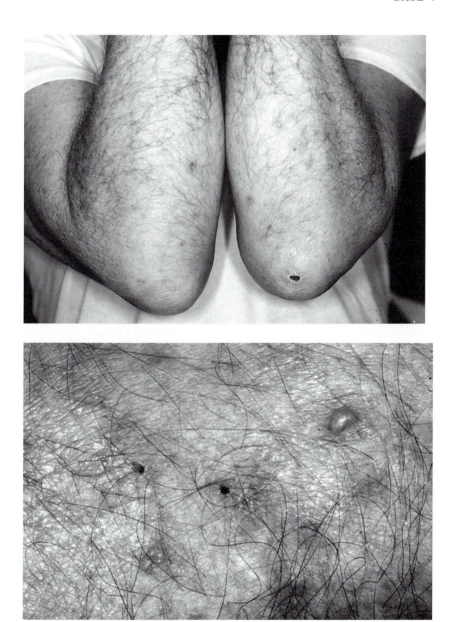

Figure 4-1.
Dermatitis herpetiformis. (See Plate 3.)

Celiac disease is believed to afflict about one in 1000 individuals. In some European countries, recent screening studies reported prevalence rates as high as one in 100 individuals. In fact, most investigators believe the disease is underdiagnosed. This is most likely a consequence of the changing clinical features of the disease, with a shift toward milder symptoms and even asymptomatic presentations. In addition, the advent of genetic testing and increased availability of serologic testing has allowed for the identification of individuals with latent disease. As a result, it appears that symptomatic celiac sprue constitutes only a small fraction of the spectrum of gluten sensitivity.

Celiac sprue is a chronic disease characterized by malabsorption of nutrients as a result of mucosal injury to the small intestine caused by specific protein constituents of some cereal grains. Although the mechanisms responsible for the injury remain unclear, removal of gluten (wheat) and prolamin (rye, barley, oats) from the diet results in prompt resolution of the intestinal lesions and malabsorption. Four major mechanisms have been implicated in the pathophysiology of this disorder: an enzyme deficiency, an immunological disorder, a membrane glycoprotein defect, and a mucosal permeability defect. Although each of these four may play a role in the pathogenesis of this disease, many believe that it is primarily an immunological disorder. Nonetheless, there is accumulating evidence that both immune mechanisms and genetic factors are important in this regard.

The familial predisposition of celiac disease is well known: Its prevalence in healthy first-degree relatives is reported to be as high as 20 percent. Concordance in identical twins is approximately 70 percent, compared with only 30 percent in HLA–identical siblings. In addition, a strong association exists for certain class II HLA antigens, most importantly HLA-DR3 and HLA-DQw2. As a consequence, other autoimmune diseases that share these haplotypes are often associated with celiac disease. For example, up to 4 percent of patients with insulin–dependent diabetes mellitus or autoimmune thyroid diseases have celiac disease.

Patients may present with celiac disease at any age, but the incidence (which is bimodal) is highest in early childhood and in the fourth and fifth decades. The clinical manifestations vary tremendously from patient to patient and appear to correlate closely with the length of small intestine that is affected. With extensive mucosal involvement, symptoms are typically severe and include diarrhea, flatulence, weight loss, fatigue, and generalized malabsorption. In contrast, patients with disease limited to the proximal small intestine may be asymptomatic and have only anemia (microcytic, macrocytic, or dimorphic) or unexplained osteopenia—a scenario that appears to be more common in recent years.

The cornerstone of the diagnosis is a small-bowel biopsy. This should be the first test performed when there is a strong clinical suspicion of this disease. The characteristic histologic findings include shortening of villi, damaged absorptive cells, crypt hyperplasia with increased mitoses, and an increased number of lymphocytes in the lamina propria and epithelium (Fig. 4-2). Although these findings in the appropriate clinical setting are highly suggestive of the diagnosis, they may be caused by several other intestinal disorders. Therefore, clinical remission—or in the case of asymptomatic patients biopsy-proven mucosal recovery—on a gluten-free diet is required to establish the diagnosis. Other findings that support the diagnosis are the presence of malabsorption (steatorrhea, positive xylose-tolerance test), luminal dilation, and distortion of mucosal folds on small-bowel barium contrast studies, and positive serologies. These alternative studies are suggested when clinical suspicion for the disease is low or for screening individuals who are at increased risk (associated diseases, heredity, extra-intestinal symptoms). Serum gliadin antibodies are commonly used in screening for celiac disease. IgA and IgG antibodies have

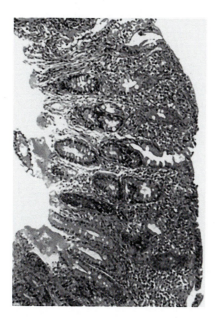 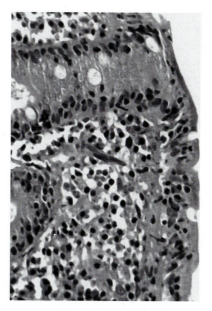

Figure 4-2.
Small bowel biopsy.

sensitivities and specificities for this diagnosis in the range of 70 to 100 percent. Serum reticulin and endomysial antibodies may also be helpful, depending on the population to be screened and laboratory availability. The best sensitivity can be achieved by combining the gliadin antibody test with either the reticulin or endomysial antibody tests. However, a positive serologic test should never replace a biopsy to establish the diagnosis or commit a patient to lifelong gluten restriction.

Symptomatic patients typically respond to gluten restriction, often within a matter of days to weeks. However, compliance with a gluten-free diet is very difficult, because of the ubiquity of wheat products in processed foods. Long-term follow-up studies suggest that only about 50 percent of patients are able to adhere to such a diet, and poor compliance or inadvertent ingestion is the most common cause for persistent symptoms. Consultation with a dietician or other knowledgeable health professional is often helpful. Lack of improvement after 4 to 6 weeks or a recurrence of symptoms despite strict dietary compliance suggests an alternative diagnosis or refractory sprue (Table 4–1). The latter may require a short course of corticosteroids or other immunosuppressant drugs.

Most patients with celiac disease fare well and die of unrelated causes. However, there is a 50- to 100-fold greater risk of small-bowel lymphoma in patients with celiac disease and dermatitis herpetiformis. Interestingly, the risk appears greatest when celiac disease is diagnosed in the elderly. There also is evidence that a gluten-free diet reduces the risk of lymphoma.

Our patient underwent a confirmatory small-bowel biopsy. Gluten withdrawal was subsequently initiated under the guidance of a registered

TABLE 4–1   Alternative Diagnoses Refractory to Gluten Restriction

Tropical sprue
Lymphoma-associated enteropathy
Eosinophilic enteritis
Viral gastroenteritis
Gastrinoma-associated acid hypersecretion
Duodenojejunal Crohn's disease

dietician. Approximately 3 weeks after initiating the diet, he noted resolution of his gastrointestinal complaints and healing of the skin lesions. Nine months after his initial presentation he was within 10 pounds of his baseline weight.

 CLINICAL PEARLS

- Celiac disease is underdiagnosed.
- It is a chronic disease characterized by malabsorption owing to mucosal injury to the small intestine by specific protein constituents (gluten, prolamine) of some cereal grains.
- Genetic and immunologic factors play an important role in celiac disease.
- The peak incidence is bimodal, occurring in early childhood and in the fourth and fifth decades.
- Clinical manifestations of the disease vary tremendously from individual to individual.
- Dermatitis herpetiformis is virtually pathognomonic for the celiac sprue syndrome.
- The cornerstone to the diagnosis of celiac disease is a small-bowel biopsy.
- Gluten restriction is usually successful, but fraught with difficulties of compliance.

REFERENCES

1. Maki M, Collin P. Coeliac disease. *Lancet* 349:1755–1759, 1997.
2. Trier JS. Diagnosis and treatment of celiac sprue. *Hosp Pract* 28(4A): 41–48, 1993.
3. Trier JS. Celiac sprue. *N Engl J Med* 325:1709–1719, 1991.

●

59-YEAR-OLD MALE WITH SYNCOPE

A 59-year-old man with a history of hypertension presented to the emergency department after experiencing an episode of lightheadedness and syncope while walking a short distance. According to several witnesses, he was unconscious for about 10 seconds, during which there was no seizure activity or bowel or bladder incontinence. On regaining consciousness, he reported no confusion and denied chest pain. However, for several months he had been experiencing exertional substernal chest tightness associated with pain radiating to his left arm that abated with rest. He denied other cardiac symptoms but noted progressive fatigue over the past 3 months. He was taking a calcium-channel blocker and an H_2 receptor antagonist.

PHYSICAL EXAMINATION

GENERAL APPEARANCE: A thin man resting comfortably who did not appear chronically ill
VITAL SIGNS: Temperature, 98.6°F (37°C); pulse, 64; blood pressure, 100/64 mm-Hg without orthostatic change; respiratory rate, 18
NECK: No thyromegaly
LUNGS: Clear
HEART: PMI laterally displaced, prominent; thrill palpable at the left upper sternal border; S_1 normal, S_2 single, S_4 present; grade IV/VI harsh systolic crescendo-decrescendo murmur heard best in the right second interspace radiating to the carotids bilaterally; jugular venous pressure normal
CAROTID ARTERIES: Pulses diminished and delayed
LEGS: No edema
RECTAL: Guaiac positive stool

LABORATORY FINDINGS

Electrolytes, normal; hemoglobin, 9.0 mg/dL; mean corpuscular volume, 75 fl; serial creatine kinases, normal; electrocardiogram, sinus rhythm, prominent precordial voltage and ST–strain changes; chest x-ray is shown (Fig. 5-1A & B).

What is the diagnosis and how should it be treated?

This patient has aortic stenosis (AS). The electrocardiogram suggests left ventricular hypertrophy. The chest x-ray reveals calcification of the aortic valve, dilatation of the ascending aorta, and a prominent left ventricle. A transthoracic echocardiogram showed left ventricular hypertrophy and a severely calcified and thickened aortic valve with an area of 0.8 cm^2. At cardiac catheterization he was found to have a high transvalvular pressure

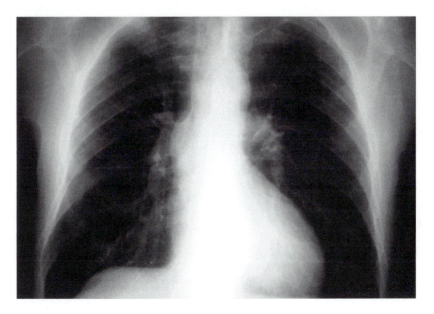

Figure 5-1A.
PA chest x-ray.

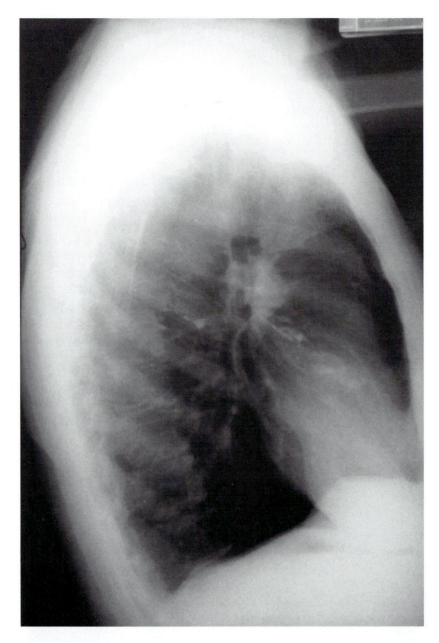

Figure 5-1B.
Lateral Chest x-ray.

gradient (93 mmHg), a stenotic aortic valve (0.7 cm^2), normal left ventricular function, and triple-vessel coronary artery disease. Duodenal and cecal arteriovenous malformations (AVMs) were found on upper and lower endoscopy.

AS is caused by rheumatic, congenital, or degenerative (senile) calcific changes; the latter two are the most common. Congenital AS typically causes symptoms before age 50 years. However, degenerative calcific AS, which is the most frequent form of AS that requires valve replacement, typically becomes manifest later in life as gradual degenerative thickening and calcification of normal valve leaflets occurs. Believed to be a consequence of longstanding mechanical stress on the valve, degenerative thickening also occurs with higher frequency in diabetics and patients with hypercholesterolemia.

Most symptomatic adults with AS are males. There usually is a long latency period, during which the obstruction gradually progresses, increasing the pressure load on the left ventricle. This results in the cardinal symptoms: angina pectoris, syncope, and dyspnea, which have serious prognostic implications when they occur with fixed obstruction. Angina develops in two-thirds of those with critical AS only half of whom have significant coronary artery disease which forecasts a survival of about 5 years. When syncope and dyspnea occur survival is even shorter. Sudden death typically occurs only in previously symptomatic patients and has been much less common since the advent of valve replacement surgery.

The characteristic murmur of AS is a loud, late-peaking, systolic crescendo–decrescendo murmur heard best at the right upper sternal border with radiation to both carotid arteries. With calcific AS, the murmur may have a "rasping" quality at the base with high-frequency sounds at the apex, indistinguishable from the murmur of mitral regurgitation. S$_2$ may be single, paradoxically split, or accentuated and an S$_4$ is usually present. The carotid arterial pulse typically rises slowly, peaks late, is small and sustained, and may contain a palpable thrill radiating from the second intercostal space or the suprasternal notch.

The electrocardiogram usually shows LVH. The chest x-ray typically reveals only a mildly dilated ascending aorta. Echocardiography is the best noninvasive test. Used in conjunction with continuous-wave Doppler ultrasonography, it can identify critical AS (peak systolic pressure gradient > 50 mmHg or aortic valve area of < 0.8 cm^2). Cardiac catheterization will confirm the hemodynamic findings as well as identify other valvular involvement and coronary artery disease.

Gastrointestinal bleeding owing to angiodysplasia, arteriovenous malformations, or idiopathic causes appears to occur more commonly in patients with calcific AS and may remit with valve replacement.

Valve replacement should be considered in only symptomatic patients with severe obstruction. Heart failure is treated with digitalis, sodium restriction, and the judicious use of diuretics to avoid volume depletion. Our patient underwent successful prosthetic aortic valve replacement and two-vessel aortocoronary bypass grafting. The excised valve was a trileaflet valve with degenerative (senile) calcific changes.

 CLINICAL PEARLS

The most common causes of AS are congenital and degenerative (calcific) changes.

The three cardinal symptoms of AS are angina pectoris, syncope, and dyspnea.

AS causes a harsh systolic crescendo–decrescendo murmur and a delayed, low-amplitude carotid pulse.

Echocardiography and Doppler ultrasonography are the best first-line tests.

Gastrointestinal vascular malformations are often associated with calcific AS.

Aortic valve replacement is indicated in symptomatic patients with critical AS, whereas asymptomatic patients must be followed clinically and with serial echocardiography.

REFERENCES

1. Selzer A. Changing aspects of the natural history of valvular aortic stenosis. *N Engl J Med* 317:91–98, 1987.
2. Deutscher S, Rockette HE, Krishnaswami V. Diabetes and hypercholesterolemia among patients with calcific aortic stenosis. *J Chron Dis* 37:407–415, 1984.
3. Carabello BA. Aortic stenosis: How to recognize and assess severity. *Cardiol Rev* 1:59–66, 1993.

4. Galan A, Zoghbi WA, Quinones MA. Determination of severity of valvular aortic stenosis by doppler echocardiography and relation of findings to clinical outcome and agreement with hemodynamic measurements determined at cardiac catheterization. *Am J Cardiol* 67: 1007–1012, 1991.

5. Love JW. The syndrome of calcific aortic stenosis and gastrointestinal bleeding: Resolution following aortic valve replacement. *J Thorac Cardiovasc Surg* 83:779–783, 1982.

64-YEAR-OLD FEMALE WITH SEVERE NECK PAIN

A 64-year-old African-American woman with non-insulin dependent diabetes mellitus presented to the emergency department with a 2-day history of severe neck pain that she attributed to physical exertion during a family vacation the previous week. She denied a history of trauma. After undergoing an examination and a cervical spine series, it was felt that this was musculoskeletal strain and she was sent home with muscle relaxants and Percocet. However, the following night, she returned still complaining of the neck pain, but now had a fever of 103°F (39.4°C) and was intermittently confused. She denied numbness, weakness, or radiation of the pain. In addition to the Percocet and muscle relaxant prescribed the previous evening, medications that she took regularly were a beta-blocker, a loop diuretic, levothyroxine, and a sulfonylurea drug. Seven years ago she had had breast cancer but was considered to be free of disease after being treated with surgery and external radiation. She also had a history of hypothyroidism and idiopathic thrombocytopenia.

PHYSICAL EXAMINATION

VITAL SIGNS: Temperature, 103°F (approx 39.4°C); pulse 98; respiration 24; blood pressure, 161/98 mmHg
GENERAL: Moderately obese and confused
HEENT: Fundi: poorly visualized secondary to patient non-compliance
NECK: Pain with movement and palpation over the cervical paraspinal and trapezius muscles, no nuchal rigidity; no lymphadenopathy or thyromegaly; Brudzinki's and Kernig's signs negative
LUNGS: Bilateral posterior-basal rales

CARDIAC: Normal

ABDOMEN: Unremarkable

EXTREMITIES: Onychomycosis and multiple excoriations over feet bilaterally

NEUROLOGIC: Intermittent confusion; cranial nerves II–XII intact; deep tendon reflexes, normal and symmetric; light touch perception, decreased over bilateral lower extremities to the knees; muscle strength, uncooperative

LABORATORY FINDINGS

WBC 8.3 K/µL (17% band form neutrophils, 69% segmented neutrophils, 9% lymphocytes, 4% monocytes, 1% basophils); Hb 12.3 g/dL; serum electrolytes, urea nitrogen, and creatinine normal; serum glucose, 281 mg/dL; head CT, normal; cerebrospinal fluid, 3 WBC/µL, 1 RBC/µL, glucose 115 mg/dL and protein 52 mg/dL; chest x-ray, left lower lobe infiltrate

HOSPITAL COURSE

The patient was admitted and treated for presumed left lower lobe pneumonia with intravenous ceftriaxone. On the second hospital day, blood cultures grew *Staphylococcus aureus* and she was started on nafcillin. Despite an improvement in her mentation, she continued to have severe neck pain, which was unabated by large doses of narcotics. A magnetic resonance imaging (MRI) scan of her cervical spine was obtained (Fig. 6-1).

What is the diagnosis and how should it be treated?

This patient has a cervical spine epidural abscess. The MRI demonstrates an extensive fluid collection extending from C3 to the upper thoracic vertebrae.

Simply defined, a spinal epidural abscess is a collection of pus or granulation tissue located between the dura mater and the surrounding sup-

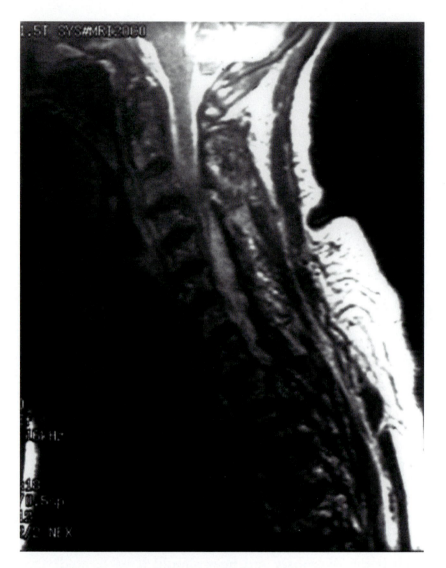

Figure 6-1.
MRI of cervical spine.

porting tissue. The most common location is the thoracic and lumbar spine, whereas abscess in the cervical spine is rare. The abscess cavity is typically in the posterior epidural space and spans four to five vertebral spaces.

Although rare, the importance of early recognition of a spinal epidural abscess is essential because of the potential for a rapid and devastating outcome. Recent series suggest an incidence among hospitalized patients of approximately one to two cases per 10,000. This is slightly increased from previous estimates and is believed to be related to an aging population. Other common risk factors include diabetes mellitus, intravenous drug use, chronic renal failure, degenerative joint disease, cancer, and alcoholism. A history of back trauma is frequently reported.

The characteristic clinical presentation is one of severe "stabbing" back pain. The pain initially is located at the affected level of the spine and percussion tenderness may be elicited. This is followed by nerve root pain and voluntary muscle weakness that may lead to irreversible paralysis within 24 to 36 hours, although some have only pain and weakness for weeks. These manifestations are primarily owing to cord compression; however, localized inflammation may cause thrombosis around the cord with resultant ischemia. Fever is frequently present; however, in many patients where analgesics with antipyretic properties have been used, it may be absent. As expected, patients with an acute epidural abscess often have a peripheral leukocytosis. In addition, the erythrocyte sedimentation rate is very sensitive for the diagnosis, with elevation in nearly all patients, whether acute or chronic.

The diagnosis of an epidural abscess is often difficult in light of its rarity and the array of nonspecific, variable symptoms. As a result, the patient commonly is evaluated on two or three occasions before the diagnosis is established. Plain spine radiographs, although frequently abnormal (degenerative changes, disc space narrowing, etc.), are not diagnostic. As well, cerebrospinal fluid analysis is generally not helpful, showing a nonspecific increase in protein and normal or high white blood cell count. Importantly, lumbar puncture poses a risk of spreading infection to the intrathecal compartment if lumbar involvement is present. In this case, a lateral approach under fluoroscopic guidance may be performed. Although CT-myelography may be used, the gold standard is gadolinium-enhanced magnetic resonance (MR) imaging; it should be quickly obtained in clinically suspicious patients.

Staphylococcus aureus is the most common cause (> 60% of cases), although *Streptococcus* spp., gram-negative rods, anaerobes, and mycobacteria, are ocassionally isolated. Blood cultures are commonly positive: 82 percent for all organisms and 95 percent for *S. aureus*, whereas CSF cultures are positive in less than 25 percent of cases.

The pathophysiology is not completely understoood. Some patients develop an acute metastatic syndrome from an extraspinal infection (hematogenous transmission), whereas in others the abscess arises from a pre-existing osteomyelitis (direct extension). In those cases in which an extraspinal source is determined, skin and soft-tissue infections account for up to 25 percent. Other possible sources include osteomyelitis, previous spinal surgery or trauma, and respiratory and urinary tract infections.

Once the diagnosis is established, emergent surgical debridement of the abscess followed by a 4- to 6-week course of parenteral antibiotics is the mainstay of therapy. There are reports of individuals who are poor surgical candidates who respond to medical management with long-term antibiotics; however, this approach should be used sparingly.

The prognosis in this condition is highly contingent on the clinical and neurologic status at the time of presentation. Morbidity and mortality increases substantially once the patient develops paralysis. Therefore, it is imperative to maintain a high clinical suspicion in those patients who present with suggestive clinical clues, in order that expeditious imaging and treatment be instituted to avoid a potentially devastating outcome.

This patient was taken emergently to surgery for debridement. Cultures grew a penicillinase-positive *S. aureus*. After an extensive evaluation for possible sources of infection, her excoriated feet were believed to be the most likely source. She was considerably improved at the time of discharge and her nafcillin was continued as an outpatient for a total of 6 weeks. At 8-week follow-up she had no recurrence of pain and continues to do well.

CLINICAL PEARLS

- Spinal epidural abscess, usually owing to *Staphylococcus aureus*, is a rare but potentially lethal cause of back pain.
- Common risk factors include diabetes mellitus, chronic renal failure, substance abuse, and cancer.
- Severe back pain is the most common initial complaint.
- A gadolinium-enhanced MRI is the gold standard diagnostic test.
- Treatment is emergent surgical drainage followed by 4 to 6 weeks of parenteral antibiotics.

REFERENCES

1. Baker AS, Ojemann RG, et al. Spinal epidural abscess. *N Engl J Med* 293:463–468, 1975.

2. Maslen DR, Jones SR, et al. Spinal epidural abscess: Optimizing pa-
    tient care. *Arch Intern Med* 153:1713–1721, 1993.
3. Martin RJ, Yuan HA. Neurological care of spinal epidural, subdural,
    and intramedullary abscesses and arachnoiditis. *Orthop Clin North Am*
    27:125–136, 1996.
4. Sapico FL. Microbiology and antimicrobial therapy of spinal infec-
    tions. *Orthop Clin North Am* 27:9–13, 1996.

CASE 7

22-YEAR-OLD WOMAN
WITH ANEMIA

A 22-year-old Caucasian woman was referred for consultation because of a 2-week history of epigastric crampy abdominal pain and anemia. She denied hematemesis, hematochezia, melena, nausea, vomiting, diarrhea, or fatigue. At 7 years of age she underwent a colectomy and ileorectal anastomosis, and had a skin graft of her nasal mucosa for vascular ectasias. Since then, annual colonoscopies have only disclosed rectal polyps. Her only medication was ferrous sulfate. She had normal menses without excessive bleeding. Her father died at 36 years from gastrointestinal bleeding, but no other family member had a similar problem. She did not smoke and reported using alcohol sparingly.

PHYSICAL EXAMINATION

VITAL SIGNS: Temperature, 100.1°F (approx 37.8°C); pulse, 96; respiration, 16; blood pressure, 112/68 mmHg
GENERAL: Age-appropriate and in no apparent distress
HEENT: As in Fig. 7-1, otherwise normal
NECK: No lymphadenopathy or thyromegaly
LUNGS: Clear
CARDIAC: Normal
ABDOMEN: Well-healed midline abdominal scar, normal bowel sounds, soft, nontender, no hepatosplenomegaly
EXTREMITIES: Mild clubbing (Fig. 7-2), no cyanosis or edema
RECTAL: Guaiac positive, no masses
NEUROLOGIC: Nonfocal
SKIN: Multiple punctate telangiectasias on the hands and face

40

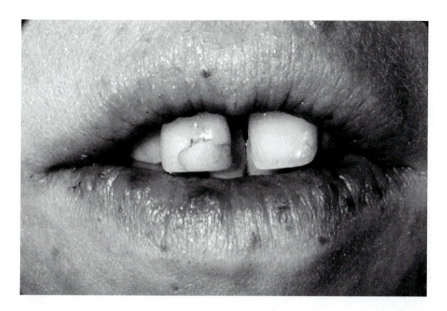

Figure 7-1.
Punctate telangiectasias. (See Plate 4.)

LABORATORY FINDINGS

WBC 6.7 K/μL (normal differential); Hb 8.6 g/dL (MCV 75 fl), platelets 360 K/μL; serum electrolytes, urea nitrogen, creatinine, amylase, and lipase, normal; liver function studies, activated partial thromboplastin time, and prothrombin time, normal; chest x-ray shown (Fig. 7-3).

What is the diagnosis and how should it be treated?

This patient has hereditary hemorrhagic telangiectasia (HHT), also known as Osler-Weber-Rendu disease. Figure 7-1 shows the characteristic punctate telangiectasias on the face and lips. The chest x-ray demonstrates large vessels emanating from multiple pulmonary nodules suggestive of pulmonary arteriovenous malformations (AVMs). Confirmation was obtained by high-resolution chest computed tomography (CT) (Fig. 7-4) and calculation of a right-to-left shunt.

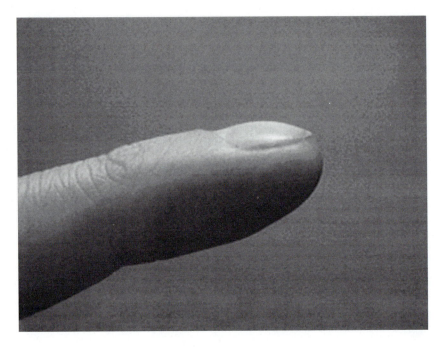

Figure 7-2.
Digital clubbing.

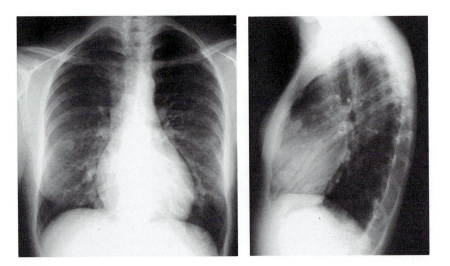

Figure 7-3.
PA and left lateral chest x-ray.

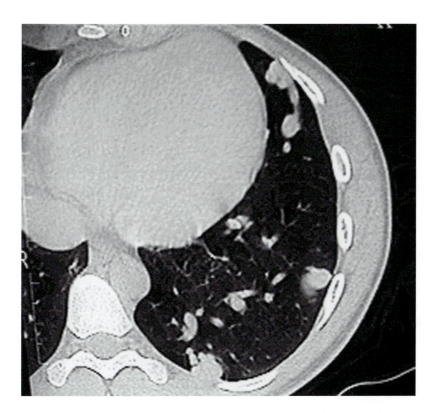

Figure 7-4.
High-resolution chest CT.

HHT is an autosomal dominant disorder characterized by telangiectases on the skin and mucosa, and AVMs in multiple organ systems. It occurs equally in males and females of all races, in a wide geographic distribution. The estimated frequency of this disease is about one to two per 100,000, although recent reports suggest it may be higher in certain populations. Genetic analyses have identified a mutation on chromosome 9 (9q), in some families, which encodes a protein (endoglin) in the receptor for transforming growth factor.

The classic clinical triad comprises telangiectasia, recurrent epistaxis, and a family history of the disorder. The telangiectasias are AVMs consisting of a dilated postcapillary venule connecting directly to a dilated arteriole. They may be punctate (most common), stellate, or linear in shape, up to 3 mm in diameter, and often blanch incompletely with pressure. They typically appear on the face, lips, tip of the tongue, ears, hands, and mucosal surfaces, particularly of the nasopharynx. As a consequence, epistaxis, which is the most common initial symptom occurring in about 96 percent of patients, usually starts around age 12 years. The cutaneous lesions often do not appear until the third decade, but eventually are present in 75 percent of the patients.

The AVMs may appear in any organ, but occur predominantly in the lungs, gastrointestinal (GI) tract, and brain. Pulmonary AVMs are present in up to one-third of the patients, usually in the lower lung fields, and are much more common when there is mutation in the endoglin gene. They cause hypoxemia, from right-to-left shunting, dyspnea, fatigue, cyanosis, and clubbing. Morbidity and mortality are owing to bleeding that causes hemoptysis or hemothorax, and paradoxical emboli that cause cerebral ischemic events (30% of patients). The latter is often the first manifestation of a previously asymptomatic pulmonary AVM. In addition, brain abscesses caused by septic emboli occur in up to 10 percent of patients. Although there is no ideal screening method for pulmonary AVMs, the most useful is arterial blood gas analysis or finger oximetry done in conjunction with a chest x-ray. Suspicious results should be further evaluated with angiography, contrast echocardiography, or high-resolution helical (CT).

The cardinal manifestation of GI involvement is painless bleeding from the upper (the majority) or lower GI tract, which typically does not occur until the fourth or fifth decade. Aspirin and other anti-platelet drugs or anticoagulants are contraindicated in HHT. The liver may show atypical cirrhosis or multiple AVMs, a rare but important complication that should be suspected when there is hepatomegaly or a liver bruit, and can be confirmed with CT and Doppler ultrasound.

The neurologic manifestations mainly occur in the third and fourth decade, two-thirds of which are ascribed to pulmonary AVMs causing ischemia or infection. In others, cerebral or spinal AVMs may cause subarachnoid hemorrhage, headache, seizures, and ischemia caused by shunted blood ("steal"), resulting in neurologic deficits. MRI angiography is the best screening method for this complication. Migraine headaches occur in up to 50 percent of patients, although their cause is unclear.

Once the diagnosis of HHT is established one should screen for pulmonary and cerebral AVMs because of the high risk of serious morbidity or death, particularly when there is a family history of such lesions. Because of the risk of life-threatening pulmonary hemorrhage during pregnancy, affected women should be screened for pulmonary manifestations before conception.

The treatment of HHT is targeted to the affected organ system. Cutaneous lesions can be treated with laser or estrogen therapy. Nasal mucosal lesions causing recurrent epistaxis can be treated with split-skin grafting. Pulmonary AVMs, treated surgically in the past, now may be treated with embolization. Bleeding enteric telangiectases can be treated with hormonal therapy, laser ablation, and amino caproic acid. Iron and possibly folate supplementation are required to avert deficiencies from chronic bleeding. Cerebral AVMs should be considered for resection, irradiation, or embolization.

 ## CLINICAL PEARLS

- HHT is an autosomal dominant disorder manifest by mucocutaneous telangiectasias and visceral arteriovenous malformations (AVMs).
- A mutation (chromosome 9q) that encodes a protein in the receptor for TGF-β may be responsible.
- The classic triad of HHT consists of telangiectasia, recurrent epistaxis, and a family history of the disorder.
- AVMs may appear in any organ, but occur predominantly in the lungs, GI tract, and brain.
- In affected individuals, it is important to screen for pulmonary and cerebral vascular AVMs because of the high risk of morbidity or sudden death.

REFERENCES

1. Haitjema T, Westermann CJJ, et al. Hereditary hemorrhagic telangiectasia (Osler-Weber-Rendu Disease): New insights in pathogenesis, complications, and treatment. *Arch Intern Med* 156:714–719, 1996.
2. Haitjema T, Disch F, Overtoom TTC, et al. Screening family members of patients with hereditary hemorrhagic telangiectasia. *Am J Med* 99:519–524, 1995.
3. Guttmacher AE, Marchuk DA, White RI. Hereditary hemorrhagic telangiectasia. *N Engl J Med* 333:918–924, 1995.
4. Peery WH. Clinical spectrum of hereditary hemorrhagic telangiectasia (Osler-Weber-Rendu Disease). *Am J Med* 82:989–997, 1987.

33-YEAR-OLD WOMAN WITH HIRSUTISM AND WEAKNESS

A 33-year-old married mother of two children was well until about 1 year ago when she stopped exercising because of fatigue and weakness, and began gaining weight. During this time she also developed facial hair and acne. Her menstrual periods became sparse and completely ceased 6 months ago. She consulted her family physician who detected mild hypertension and began treating her with a thiazide diuretic. A short time later, she developed polyuria, nocturia, and mild hypokalemia. Her physician thought she might be developing diabetes mellitus and obtained an early morning cortisol level (21 μg/dL; normal, 4–25) and referred her for further evaluation. Normally a cheerful person, she also admitted to feeling depressed lately.

PHYSICAL EXAMINATION

GENERAL APPEARANCE: Mildly obese with facial hair (Fig. 8-1), thin extremities

VITAL SIGNS: Temperature, 98.4°F (approx 36.9°C); pulse, 78; respiration, 14; blood pressure, 144/94 mmHg; weight, 154 pounds; height, 62 inches

HEENT: Eyes: normal

NECK: No thyromegaly, fullness of the supraclavicular fat pads

CARDIAC: Normal

ABDOMEN: Normal

NEUROLOGIC: Generalized decreased muscle strength—unable to stand from a squatting position without help, difficulty standing from a seated position

SKIN: See Figure 8-2

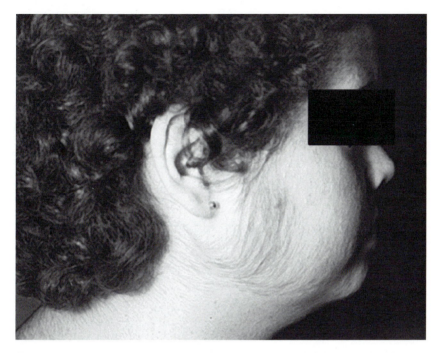

Figure 8-1.
Hirsutism.

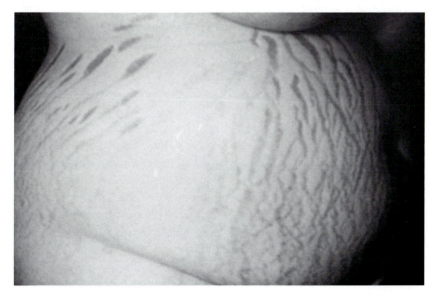

Figure 8-2.
Skin striae. (See Plate 5.)

LABORATORY FINDINGS

WBC, 8.3 K/μL (normal differential); Hb, 15.7 g/dL; platelets, 211 K/μL; serum electrolytes: sodium, 144 mmol/L, potassium, 3.2 mmol/L, chloride, 98 mmol/L, bicarbonate, 34 mmol/L; blood urea nitrogen 22 mg/dL, creatinine, 1.1 mg/dL; fasting serum glucose, 136 mg/dL; arterial blood gas on room air: pH 7.47, P_{CO_2}, 43 mmHg, P_{O_2}, 82 mmHg, H_{CO_3}, 33, O_2 saturation, 99%; serum glycated hemoglobin, 8.1% (normal, 4.8–7.8); urinalysis, normal

What is the likely diagnosis and how should this patient be treated?

This patient has classic Cushing's syndrome. The plasma cortisol value is correct, but should not be measured in a simple early morning specimen to make the diagnosis of Cushing's syndrome. She should have a dexamethasone suppression test and measurement of a 24-hour urine cortisol level (Fig. 8-3).

Although Cushing's syndrome is not a common disorder, it should be considered every day in a primary care practice because its clinical features—obesity, hypertension, and glucose intolerance—are seen daily in primary care practices. In addition, depression is also a common symptom and is an intrinsic feature of endogenous Cushing's syndrome. Several clinical findings help to distinguish Cushing's syndrome from simple obesity. The first in this patient was the distribution of her fat, which was primarily truncal, a finding termed centripetal obesity. Classically the extremities appear thin, rather than obese, because of muscle wasting. Another finding that correlates well with central obesity is fullness of the supraclavicular fossae that is a consequence of fatty deposition, termed supraclavicular fat pads. This finding is not seen with simple obesity. In contrast, the presence of a buffalo hump does not distinguish Cushing's syndrome from obesity because it is regularly seen in both conditions. Proximal muscle weakness, on the other hand, is a key feature of the syndrome, and is usually not seen in simple obesity. Whereas obesity may be accompanied by hirsutism, acne, and menstrual irregularities, the sudden

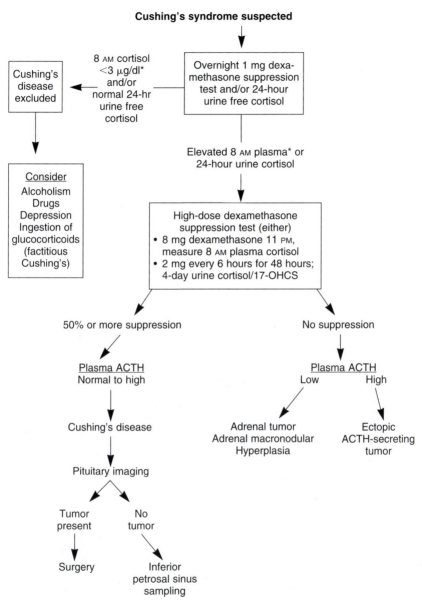

Cushing's syndrome suspected

8 AM cortisol <3 μg/dl* and/or normal 24-hr urine free cortisol

Overnight 1 mg dexamethasone suppression test and/or 24-hour urine free cortisol

Cushing's disease excluded

Consider
Alcoholism
Drugs
Depression
Ingestion of glucocorticoids (factitious Cushing's)

Elevated 8 AM plasma* or 24-hour urine cortisol

High-dose dexamethasone suppression test (either)
• 8 mg dexamethasone 11 PM, measure 8 AM plasma cortisol
• 2 mg every 6 hours for 48 hours; 4-day urine cortisol/17-OHCS

50% or more suppression

No suppression

Plasma ACTH
Normal to high

Plasma ACTH
Low   High

Cushing's disease

Adrenal tumor
Adrenal macronodular
Hyperplasia

Ectopic
ACTH-secreting
tumor

Pituitary imaging

Tumor present

No tumor

Surgery

Inferior petrosal sinus sampling

*See Text

Figure 8-3.
Diagnostic algorithm.

onset of these features in this patient suggests another diagnosis. In addition, the hirsutism shown in Figure 8-1 is usually accompanied by a rounded face—the classic cushingoid facies—(Fig. 8-4)—and the classic skin striae of the disease are shown in Figure 8-2. Other findings may include hypokalemic metabolic alkalosis, hypertension, and glucose intolerance, which further support the clinical diagnosis, as in our patient.

It was a mistake to measure a random plasma cortisol to rule in or rule out the diagnosis. This patient clearly has the disease and further laboratory testing is aimed at finding the source of her Cushing's syndrome. Although aldosterone-secreting adrenal tumors typically produce hypertension and hypokalemic metabolic alkalosis, none of the other clinical features fit with an aldosteronoma.

This patient had a basal serum cortisol level of 24 μg/dL and plasma adrenocorticotrophic hormone (ACTH) of 77 ng/mL (normal, 7–51 ng/mL). After 1 mg of dexamethasone given at 11 PM the evening before, her 8 AM serum cortisol was 26 μg/dL (normal, <5). Her baseline urine free cor-

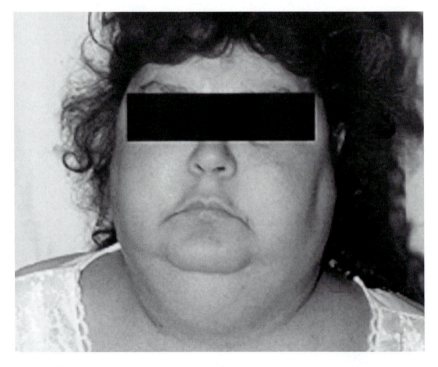

Figure 8-4.
Classic cushingoid facies.

tisol was 485 μg/24 hours (normal, <60). The overnight dexamethasone suppression test is simple, requiring only a serum cortisol level at 8 AM after the patient has taken 1 mg of dexamethasone orally at 11 o'clock the evening before. The test may be falsely positive in obese patients or in those taking any of the following drugs: oral contraceptives (increase corticosteroid binding globulin), phenytoin, rifampin, barbiturates, non-steroidal anti-inflammatory agents, and other drugs that increase the metabolism of dexamethasone or alter its absorption. It may also be falsely positive in patients with depression or under severe stress. However, false positive tests are not a major problem, since the dexamethasone suppression test is only a screening test for Cushing's syndrome. False negative tests are a more serious concern, but can often be eliminated by establishing a normal cortisol level of 3 μg/dL or less (most textbooks recommend a 5 μg/dL cutoff). The most reliable screening test for Cushing's syndrome, although certainly not as easily obtained, is the 24-hour urine measurement of free cortisol. Virtually all patients with Cushing's syndrome have an elevated level of cortisol in their urine.

Once the diagnosis of Cushing's syndrome is established, the cause must be identified. Because most patients have ACTH-secreting tumors, 90 percent of which are in the pituitary gland, there is an almost irresistible urge to visualize the pituitary with an MRI (the best imaging test for the pituitary) and the adrenal glands with an abdominal CT scan. This should not be performed at this point in the evaluation, because many people in the general population have nonfunctional, but radiologically apparent pituitary or adrenal tumors. The differential diagnosis of Cushing's syndrome includes: (1) pituitary hypersecretion of ACTH (pituitary hyperplasia or tumor); (2) autonomous adrenal function (benign or malignant solitary adrenal tumor or macronodular hyperplasia); (3) ectopic production of ACTH; and (4) ingestion of corticosteroids (iatrogenic or factitious).

When biochemical confirmation of the syndrome has been verified by a 24-hour free cortisol measurement, the etiologic diagnosis hinges on the high-dose dexamethasone suppression test, which can be done in several ways. As originally described, the urine is collected on four consecutive days: days 1 and 2 as a baseline (no dexamethasone), and days 3 and 4 while the patient takes 2 mg of dexamethasone every 6 hours. Urine volume and creatinine are measured on each daily urine specimen, because variation in the urine creatinine excretion is normally less than 10 percent, which assures complete collections. Since the pituitary-adrenal axis is intact with ACTH-dependent Cushing's disease (pituitary tumor was originally described by Harvey Cushing) albeit set at a slightly higher ACTH release-point, cortisol production will fall and pituitary ACTH release will drop in response to very high doses of dexamethasone. A positive test was originally described as a 50 percent or greater drop in urinary 17-hydroxycorticosteroid (17-OHCS) excretion; however, now urine free cortisol is usually substituted for the 17-OHCS measurement. Many other modifications of the test have been suggested, mainly because the test is cumbersome and cannot be reliably performed on outpatients. One alternative test is the 8 mg overnight dexamethasone suppression test that substitutes plasma cortisol and ACTH levels for the urine tests. Failure to suppress the urine free cortisol level or plasma cortisol and ACTH after either of the high-dose dexamethasone tests indicates that the pituitary is not involved in the process, and that the hypercortisolemia is owing to an adrenal tumor(s) or to ectopic production of ACTH. This patient underwent an 8-mg dexamethasone suppression in which the drug was given at 11 PM, at 8 AM her plasma cortisol level suppressed to 6 µg/dL and her plasma ACTH level fell to 21 ng/mL. She also underwent a traditional suppression test, during which her 24-hour urine cortisol suppressed to 40 µg/24 hours (92% fall from baseline). These findings were interpreted as positive for a diagnosis of ACTH-dependent Cushing's disease.

Perhaps the most important modifications of high-dose dexamethasone suppression testing relate to the test's interpretation. One study by Flack and associates reported their results with 118 patients who had surgically confirmed Cushing's disease. The diagnostic accuracy of urinary free cortisol and 17-OHCS was about the same; however, neither test was completely reliable, although dexamethasone did lower urine free cortisol more than it did 17-OHCS excretion. By modifying the criteria for a positive test to be a fall in urine free cortisol of more than 90 percent, the test had 100 percent diagnostic specificity for Cushing's disease. Importantly, the interpretation of this test can be further complicated by partial suppression with dexamethasone in some patients with an ectopic ACTH syndrome (i.e., bronchial carcinoid tumor). Poor compliance is also a serious problem if the test is done on an outpatient basis, which many third-party carriers now require. In addition, some patients with severe depression and a few with alcoholism have plasma hormone levels and responses to dexamethasone that are indistinguishable from Cushing's disease.

Because the high-dose dexamethasone suppression test may not reliably separate Cushing's disease from an ectopic ACTH syndrome, a cor-

ticotropin-releasing hormone (CRH) stimulation test is occasionally required. With this test, patients with an ectopic ACTH syndrome typically
have no increase in plasma cortisol or ACTH, whereas patients with pituitary ACTH-dependent Cushing's disease have an increase in both hormones. According to a study by Kay and Crapo, the CRH stimulation
test has 91 percent sensitivity and 95 percent specificity for the diagnosis
of an ectopic ACTH syndrome compared with 89 and 100 percent specificity for the overnight high-dose dexamethasone suppression test.

Regardless, the differentiation between pituitary and ectopic causes remains uncertain in up to 15 percent of patients with Cushing's syndrome.
Patients whose high-dose dexamethasone suppression tests do not meet
strict criteria and the CRH stimulation test is equivocal require inferior
petrosal sinus sampling for ACTH. In this procedure plasma venous
ACTH is obtained simultaneously from both inferior petrosal sinuses and
a peripheral vein in the basal state and after stimulation with ovine CRH.
When the ACTH concentration in the inferior petrosal sinus was twofold or more higher than that in the peripheral blood, the test had a 95 percent diagnostic accuracy; when it was three-fold or more higher in
samples obtained a few minutes after CRH, the diagnostic accuracy was
99.5 percent. When both these criteria were met, the diagnostic specificity was 100 percent in differentiating Cushing's disease from ectopic
Cushing's syndrome. Why put a patient through such vigorous testing?
Because the stakes are high: an incorrect diagnosis may result in persistent
ectopic Cushing's syndrome on one hand and hypopituitarism after unnecessary pituitary surgery on the other hand. Also, pituitary Cushing's
disease may recur in up to 21 percent of patients with Cushing's disease
who undergo transsphenoidal pituitary adenectomy.

Biochemical testing in our patient suggested ACTH-dependent Cushing's disease and her MRI showed a 2-cm pituitary adenoma that was excised by transsphenoidal adenectomy. One year after surgery her
Cushing's syndrome has fully abated and her 24-hour urine cortisol is
normal.

 ## CLINICAL PEARLS

- Cushing's syndrome should be suspected in a patient with diabetes
  mellitus, hypertension, and obesity.
- Findings favoring Cushing's syndrome are: central obesity, supraclavicular fat pads, muscle weakness, and wasting.

- The overnight dexamethasone suppression test (1 mg po at 11 PM followed by serum cortisol at 8 AM) normally suppresses serum cortisol to <5 μg/dL (<3 is more specific) but estrogen, phenytoin, and other drugs interfere with the test.

- The most reliable screening test for Cushing's disease is a 24-hour urine for free cortisol.

- After the diagnosis of Cushing's syndrome is established, the next test to perform is a high-dose dexamethasone suppression test to identify ACTH-dependent Cushing's disease.

- Inferior petrosal sinus ACTH sampling may be necessary to differentiate pituitary-dependent Cushing's disease from ectopic Cushing's syndrome.

REFERENCES

1. Flack MR, Oldfield EH, Cutler GB, et al. Urine free cortisol in the high-dose dexamethasone suppression test for differential diagnosis of Cushing's syndrome. *Ann Intern Med* 116:211, 1992.

2. Orth DN: Differential diagnosis of Cushing's syndrome. *N Engl J Med* 325:957, 1991.

3. Oldfield EH, Doppman JL, Nieman LK, et al. Petrosal sinus sampling with and without corticotropin-releasing hormone for the differential diagnosis of Cushing's syndrome. *N Engl J Med* 325:897, 1991.

4. Loriaux DL, Nieman L. Corticotropin-releasing hormone testing in pituitary disease. *Endocrinol Metab Clin North Am* 20:363, 1991.

5. Kaye TB, Crapo L. The Cushing's syndrome: An update on diagnostic tests. *Ann Intern Med* 112:434, 1990.

57-YEAR-OLD MAN WITH CHRONIC FATIGUE AND ACUTE RESPIRATORY FAILURE

A 57-year-old man, who had worked full-time as a painter until 6 months ago, presented to the emergency department with a 6-month history of cough and fatigue, and 2 days of confusion. Shortly after arrival he required intubation for acute respiratory failure.

Three months earlier, he had been hospitalized for *Staphylococcal* pneumonia and was discharged with home oxygen and a prolonged course of oral antibiotics. However, since discharge he reported continuing difficulty with fatigue, productive cough, and intermittent fever, as well as a 10-pound weight loss. He denied orthopnea, chest pain, nausea, vomiting, or diarrhea and was taking no other medications. He had not smoked for 25 years and there was no history of recent travel or other illnesses.

PHYSICAL EXAMINATION

VITAL SIGNS: Temperature, 101.9°F (38.8°C); pulse, 80; blood pressure, 106/65 mmHg; respiration, 2

GENERAL: Chronically ill-appearing, intubated male

HEENT: Eyes: extraocular muscle movement normal; mild bilateral facial muscle weakness

NECK: No thyromegaly or lymphadenopathy

LUNGS: Scattered rhonchi

CARDIAC: No murmurs, gallops, or rubs; no JVD; peripheral pulses 2+ throughout

ABDOMEN: Soft, non-tender, no hepatosplenomegaly

EXTREMITIES: No edema

NEUROLOGIC: Strength: neck flexors, MRC grade 3; elbow flexors and
extensors, MRC grade 4; shoulder abductors, MRC grade 5

LABORATORY FINDINGS

WBC, 20.6 K/μL (2% band form neutrophils, 69% segmented neutrophils, 24% lymphocytes, 5% monocytes); Hb, 13 g/dL; electrolytes:
sodium 139 mmol/L, potassium 3.4 mmol/L, chloride 92 mmol/L, bicarbonate 41 mmol/L; blood urea nitrogen and creatinine: normal; arterial
blood gases on room air (prior to intubation): pH 7.22, P_{CO_2} 110 mmHg,
P_{O_2} 40 mmHg, HCO_3 42 mmol/L; chest x-ray and chest computed tomography (CT) shown (Figs. 9-1 and 9-2).

What is the likely diagnosis and how should the patient be treated?

This patient has myasthenia gravis with crisis.

The chest x-ray demonstrates the "sail" sign, which is the triangular
radiographic density projecting from the right side of the mediastinum
(the light arrows in Fig. 9-1 mark the "sail" with effacement of the right
heart border and the dark arrows mark the right lower lobe consolidation
and collapse). This sign results from an enlarged thymus gland that may
project from either side of the mediastinum and should prompt confirmation of a mediastinal mass by CT. (The asterisk in Fig. 9-2 marks the
mass.) The thymus is more commonly seen on chest x-ray in the superior mediastinum of children and adolescents, in whom it may be a normal finding. In adults, however, the thymus becomes progressively
smaller with age and can be identified by chest CT in only 17 percent of
those over age 50 years.

An estimated 25,000 people in the United States have myasthenia
gravis. It is about twice as common in women as men, and may occur at
any age, but its peak incidence is in the sixth and seventh decades in men,
and the second and third decades in women.

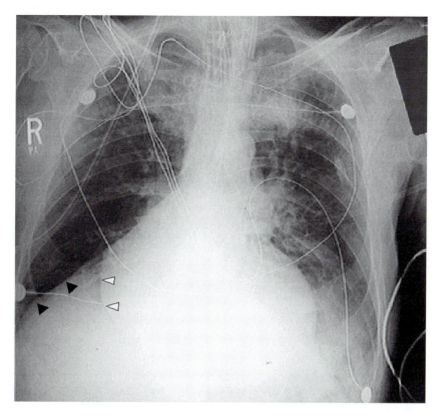

Figure 9-1.
PA chest x-ray.

The fundamental defect in this disorder is failure of neuromuscular transmission. This occurs as a consequence of specific anti-acetylcholine receptor antibodies that block active binding sites, damage the postsynaptic membrane, and accelerate receptor degradation. In addition, the neuromuscular junctions have simplified postsynaptic folding and a widened synaptic interface that further impairs transmission (see Fig. 9-3). As repeated muscle contractions reduce the levels of presynaptic acetylcholine, muscle weakness develops. The origin of the autoimmune component of this disease is not clear, but the thymus appears to be involved: about 75 percent of the patients have thymic abnormalities, either hyperplasia (85%) or thymoma (15%), and thymectomy may substantially improve the weakness.

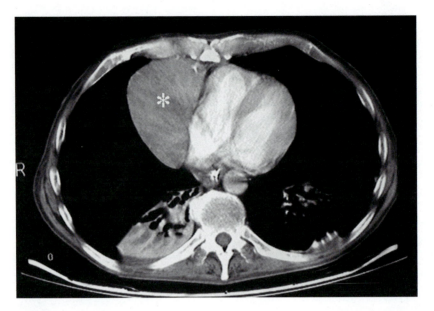

Figure 9-2.
Chest CT scan.

The cardinal features of myasthenia are weakness and fatigue. The weakness is typically progressive, particularly in muscles that are used repetitively, and partially improves after rest. The illness often begins with transient attacks of weakness that are manifest over several weeks or months. However, a generalized, more rapidly evolving course is not uncommon, particularly in those with a thymoma. Infections or other systemic disorders often exacerbate the weakness.

The muscles innervated by cranial nerves are commonly the first involved, causing ptosis and diplopia. Affected facial muscles produce a flattened smile, and difficulty with chewing; bulbar involvement causes nasal speech, difficulty swallowing, and tracheal aspiration of liquids and food. Neck flexor weakness often correlates with the degree of bulbar involvement and as such, is a useful marker for those at risk for respiratory failure. *Myasthenic crisis* is present when the patient requires intubation and mechanical ventilation. Although 15 percent of patients have disease limited to the extraocular and eyelid muscles, most patients will eventually develop generalized weakness. In a few patients, severe generalized weakness will be their initial manifestation.

The history and physical examination often provide the first clues to the diagnosis. Weakness after sustained or repetitive muscle contraction strongly suggests the diagnosis. Ptosis after sustained elevation of the eyelids, dysphonia after prolonged speaking, and weak head flexion after a period of resistance are clues. Confirmation of the diagnosis should be obtained before treatment is initiated, because other conditions mimic myasthenia and treatment is not without complications (Table 9-1).

Confirmatory tests include the anticholinesterase test, repetitive nerve stimulation, and an assay for anti-acetylcholine-receptor antibody. Edrophonium (Tensilon), a rapidly acting anticholinesterase drug, has its onset of action within 30 seconds and its effect dissipates within 5 minutes. A test is considered positive if there is unequivocal improvement in the strength of a previously weak muscle. The diagnosis also may be established by electrophysiologic testing, in which a series of repetitive shocks produce a progressive decrement in the compound muscle action potential amplitude by 15 percent or more (Fig. 9-4). This test has a sensitivity of about 80 percent. Anti-acetylcholine receptor antibodies are detected in 85 percent of all myasthenic patients; however, the sensitivity drops to 50 percent in those with weakness limited to the ocular muscles.

A serum thyroid-stimulating hormone (TSH) should be obtained because there is an increased incidence of Graves' disease in patients with myasthenia gravis—3 to 8 percent of whom are thyrotoxic, which may exacerbate the muscle weakness. Because other autoimmune disorders also occur with greater than expected frequency, a rheumatoid factor and antinuclear antibody should also be obtained.

Currently there are four methods of therapy: anticholinesterase medications, thymectomy, long-term immunosuppression, and short-term immunotherapy. Most patients initially respond to pyridostigmine (Mestinon),

TABLE 9–1   Differential Diagnosis of Myasthenia Gravis

Congenital myasthenic syndromes
Graves' disease
Intracranial mass lesions
Botulism
Drug-induced myasthenia
Lambert-Eaton syndrome
Hyperthyroidism
Progressive external ophthalmoplegia

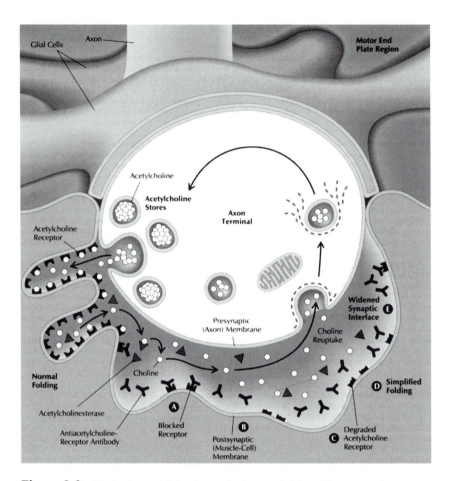

Figure 9-3. The fundamental defect in myasthenia gravis is failure of neuromuscular transmission. The failure is the consequence of specific antiacetylcholine-receptor antibodies that block active binding sites (A), damage the postsynaptic membrane (B), and accelerate receptor degradation (C). In addition, the neuromuscular junctions have simplified postsynaptic folding (D) and a widened synaptic interface (E), both of which further impair transmission. As repeated muscle contractions reduce the levels of presynaptic acetylcholine, muscle weakness develops.

but improvement often wanes over several months, and most require additional therapy. Thymectomy, which has a near zero operative mortality, is controversial in the absence of thymoma. Some centers recommend it for patients with generalized disease under the age of 50, citing a remission in about one-third and improvement in half of the patients. When weakness is not adequately controlled by these measures, immunosuppressants should be considered, including corticosteroids, azathioprine (Imuran), and cy-

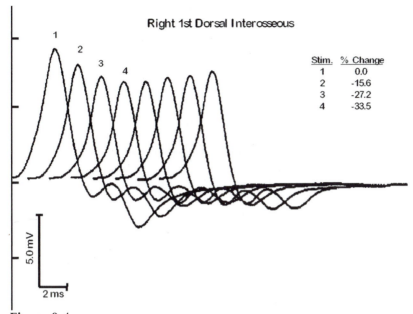

Figure 9-4.
Patient's electromyogram (EMG).

closporine (Sandimmune). A myasthenic crisis or severe exacerbation is often treated with plasmapheresis or intravenous immune globulin.

This patient had detectable anti-acetylcholine receptor antibodies and was treated with pyridostigmine, corticosteroids, and plasmapheresis. After a period of stabilization, a thymectomy was performed that revealed a benign thymoma. He was discharged after a prolonged hospital course and has continued to do well on pyridostigmine and a tapering dose of corticosteroids.

 CLINICAL PEARLS

- Myasthenia gravis is an autoimmune disorder that is about twice as common in women as men.
- Seventy-five percent of individuals with myasthenia have an abnormal thymus, usually owing to hyperplasia.
- Weakness and fatigue of facial muscles (e.g., ptosis) are frequently the first symptoms.
- The eyes alone are involved in about 15 percent of patients (typically males) with myasthenia.

- Diagnosis may be confirmed by a positive Tensilon or EMG test, or antibody serology.
- Therapy typically includes: anticholinesterase drugs, thymectomy, and immunosuppressants.

REFERENCES

1. Drachman DB. Myasthenia gravis. *N Engl J Med* 330:1797–1810, 1994.
2. Seybold ME. Myasthenia gravis: A clinical and basic science review. *JAMA* 250:2516, 1983.
3. Morgenthaler TI, Brown LR, Colby TV, et al. Thymoma. *Mayo Clin Proc* 68:1110–1123, 1993.
4. Chapman S. The sail sign. *Br J Hosp Med* 46:399–400, 1991.

54-YEAR-OLD WOMAN WITH BACK PAIN

A 54-year-old woman presented with a 3-week history of severe low back pain. She had chronic back pain, type 2 diabetes mellitus complicated by retinopathy and neuropathy, and cryptogenic cirrhosis with esophageal varices previously treated with a transjugular intrahepatic portosystemic shunt (TIPS). She had been hospitalized elsewhere with fever, chills, and back pain. She was treated with nonsteroidal anti-inflammatory drugs (NSAIDs) and a 3-day course of oral cefixime after blood cultures grew *Streptococcus agalactiae* (Group B streptococcus), although a source of the infection had not been identified. At discharge, she was afebrile and had some improvement in her pain. The following day, she presented to our emergency room with hematemesis and was admitted to the intensive care unit. Her medications were NPH and regular insulin, naproxen, and amitriptyline. She was allergic to penicillin. She had a 30 pack-year tobacco history, but did not drink alcohol.

PHYSICAL EXAMINATION

VITAL SIGNS: Temperature, 100.4°F (37.9°C); pulse, 100; respiration, 20; blood pressure, 138/70 mmHg
GENERAL: Chronically ill
HEENT: Poor dentition
NECK: No lymphadenopathy or thyromegaly
LUNGS: Clear
CARDIAC: Normal
ABDOMEN: Mildly distended, normoactive bowel sounds; no hepatosplenomegaly; no ascites

EXTREMITIES: No cyanosis or edema
BACK: Tenderness over lumbar paraspinal muscles
NEUROLOGIC: Nonfocal
RECTAL: Guaiac positive, no masses

LABORATORY FINDINGS

WBC, 8.3 K/μL (81% neutrophils, 15% lymphocytes); Hb 11.1 g/dL (MCV 89 fl), platelets 288 K/μL; prothrombin time, partial thrombo-plastin time, electrolytes, and urinanalysis, all normal; serum glucose, 306 mg/dL; Westergren erythrocyte sedimentation rate (ESR), 123 mm/hr; chest x-ray was normal.

HOSPITAL COURSE

An emergent esophagogastroduodenoscopy revealed 2+ distal esophageal varices and a large clot in the body of the stomach without active bleed-ing. A portal venogram showed stenosis of the TIPS that was successfully opened with angioplasty. On the second hospital day, she spiked a tem-perature to 102.7°F (approx 38.9°C) and her back pain seemed worse. Blood cultures grew *Streptococcus agalactiae*. Her lumbosacral MRI is shown (Fig. 10-1).

What is the likely diagnosis and how should the patient be treated?

This patient has acute osteomyelitis (OM). The MRI reveals diskitis at the L5-S1 level with adjacent osteomyelitis of the vertebral bodies of L4 and L5 and the posterior elements of L4 through S1. Cellulitis of the overlying paraspinous muscles is also present. The term *acute osteomyelitis*, used clinically to signify a newly recognized bone infection, classically presents with fever, chills, bone pain, and local swelling. Bone tenderness is consistently present. *Chronic osteomyelitis* refers to a relapse of a previ-ously treated or untreated infection dominated by prolonged low-grade

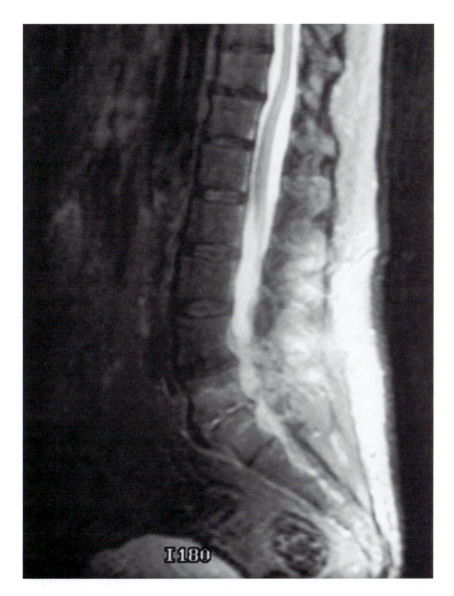

Figure 10-1.
MRI of lumbosacral spine.

inflammation. Clinical signs persisting for more than about 14 days roughly correlate with chronicity that may result in a draining sinus tract or fistula.

Bone becomes infected from the blood stream, a contiguous infection, or vascular insufficiency. The principal histologic features of acute OM are microorganisms, neutrophils, and thrombosed vessels. The hallmark of chronic OM is ischemic necrosis of bone, with separation of the bony devascularized fragments, called sequestra.

Hematogenous OM most commonly develops under age 15 and over age 50. The most frequently affected bones are the tibia, femur, and humerus in children, and the vertebrae, sacroiliac, and sternoclavicular joints in adults. Other factors predispose to hematogenous development of OM (Table 10-1). In children, bacteria have a predilection for the metaphysis of long bones, an area of reduced blood flow and scarce neutrophils that provides a sanctuary for pathogen proliferation. In adults, bacteria reach the vertebrae via spinal arteries and spread to the endplate, disk space, and adjacent vertebrae. The most common sites of involvement are the lumbar spine for bacterial infections, the thoracic spine for mycobacterial infections (Pott's disease), and the cervical spine for infections caused by intravenous drug use. Bacteremia occurs in more than half the patients but is frequently absent in vertebral body or fungal infections and in those with a Brodie's abscess (a circumscribed lytic lesion in the metaphysis). A single bacterial species, typically *Staphylococcus aureus*, is usually responsible for hematogenous OM, regardless of the patient's age. However, gram-negative organisms, especially *Escherichia coli*, account for about one-fourth of vertebral infections (Table 10-2). Patients with chronic illnesses such as cirrhosis and diabetes mellitus (our patient) are at especially high risk of developing invasive Group B streptococcal infection.

TABLE 10–1   Risk Factors for Hematogenous Osteomyelitis*

Male gender	Dental infections
Intravascular catheters	Hemodialysis
Intravenous drug use	Hemoglobinopathies
Trauma	GI infections (e.g., salmonellosis)
Bacterial endocarditis	Chemotherapy, radiation therapy
Burns	Immunodeficiency states
Skin/soft tissue infections	Genitourinary infections

*Adapted from O'Hanley P, Swartz MN. *The Scientific American Medicine CD-ROM.* New York, Osteomyelitis Scientific American Medicine Inc, 1997.

TABLE 10–2   **Bacterial Agents and Associated Conditions in Osteomyelitis★**

ORGANISM(S)	ASSOCIATED CONDITION
S. aureus	Most frequent in all types of osteomyelitis
Coagulase-negative Staphylococci	Foreign bodies
S. aureus, Pseudomonas aeruginosa, Serratia marcescens, Enterobacteriaceae, group G streptococci	Intravenous drug use, nosocomial infection, immunodeficient states
Streptococci, Salmonella species, S. aureus	Hemoglobinopathy, sickle cell disease
Group B streptococci	Cirrhosis, diabetes mellitus, neurogenic bladder

★Adapted from Lew DP, Waldvogel FA. Current concepts: Osteomyelitis. *N Engl J Med* 1997;336:999–1007; O'Hanley P, Swartz MN. *The Scientific American Medicine CD-ROM.* New York, Osteomyelitis Scientific American Medicine Inc, 1997.

Soft tissue infections may contaminate bone by direct extension or by contamination during reconstructive orthopedic procedures, an increasingly more common event. Typically, the only signs of OM spreading from a contiguous infection are low-grade fever and pain, which may be mistakenly attributed to the soft tissue infection. The diagnosis is often not made until the infection has progressed to a chronic stage. *S. aureus* is usually isolated, but these infections typically also involve gram-negative organisms and anaerobes. Blood cultures are rarely positive and isolation of the responsible organism(s) depends on stains and cultures of aspiration or bone biopsy specimens.

OM related to vascular insufficiency occurs almost exclusively in diabetics with neuropathy involving the feet, which predisposes to frequent trauma and pressure sores. Inadequate tissue perfusion hampers the inflammatory response, leading to impaired soft tissue healing and spread of the infection to bone. If a sterile surgical probe can touch bone without causing pain, a diagnosis of osteomyelitis is clearly established. Polymicrobial infections are common but staphylococci are usually isolated. The diagnosis is dependent on isolation of the organism(s) from the blood or

CASE 11

17-YEAR-OLD MAN WITH SHORTNESS OF BREATH

A previously healthy 17-year-old man presented to the emergency room after developing acute chest pain and shortness of breath while taking a shower. He described the chest pain as sharp, pleuritic, and substernal in location, without radiation. He denied any other symptoms (recent fever or chills), but did note a persistent non-productive cough, which began approximately 1 week prior, that he attributed to a viral illness. His family history was notable only for congestive heart failure in his maternal grandmother. He denied HIV risk factors, illicit drug use, or recent trauma, and was taking no medications. He had smoked up to 2 packs of cigarettes per day for the past 4 years and drank alcohol regularly on the weekends.

PHYSICAL EXAMINATION

VITAL SIGNS: Temperature, 97.9°F (36.6°C); pulse, 82; respiration, 24; blood pressure, 136/70; height, 6' 1"; weight, 70 kg

GENERAL: Age-appropriate man in mild respiratory distress

HEENT: Unremarkable

NECK: No lymph node enlargement

LUNGS: Diminished breath sounds bilaterally; hyperresonance to percussion bilaterally

CARDIAC: Soft S_1 and S_2, otherwise normal

ABDOMEN: Unremarkable

EXTREMITIES: No edema

NEUROLOGIC: Unremarkable

LABORATORY FINDINGS

WBC 7.8 K/μL (9% band form neutrophils, 64% segmented neutrophils, 21% lymphocytes, 3% monocytes, 2% eosinophils); Hb, 9.5 g/dL; electrolytes, normal; chest x-ray shown. (Fig. 11-1).

What is the likely diagnosis and how should this patient be treated?

This patient has pulmonary eosinophilic granuloma (PEG) (pulmonary Langerhans' cell granulomatosis, Histiocytosis X). The chest x-ray reveals large bilateral pneumothoraces and diffuse, symmetric reticulonodular infiltrates.

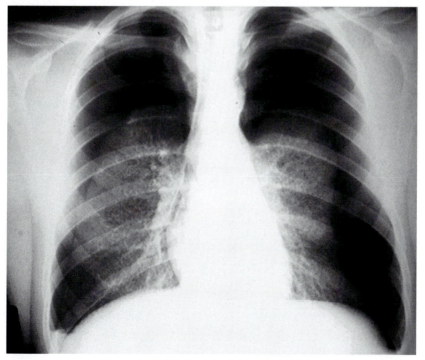

Figure 11-1.
PA chest x-ray.

A distinct disease entity, pulmonary eosinophilic granuloma is one of a spectrum of disorders known as Langerhans' cell granulomatosis (histiocytosis) or more commonly, Histiocytosis X.

This group of disorders is characterized histopathologically by destructive granulomatous lesions that contain Langerhans' cells. These cells have characteristic pentalaminar plate-like cytoplasmic organelles known as Birbeck granules, which are detectable only by electron microscopy (Fig. 11-2, arrows). The etiology of this disease is uncertain, but recent evidence suggests it is a clonal proliferative disease. Other disorders in this spectrum include *Hand-Schuller-Christian disease*, characterized by bony defects, gingival hyperplasia, exophthalmos, and diabetes insipidus; and *Letterer-Siwe disease*, a multi-system disorder with rapid progression and poor outcome. Infants and young children appear to be predominantly affected, but these disorders have been described in all ages. Adult patients are more likely to have single organ involvement (e.g., PEG).

With PEG, young men are more commonly and severely affected. Moreover, more than 90 percent of patients are current smokers and 97 percent have been regular smokers at some time. Heavy smoking appears to be more important than total tobacco consumption.

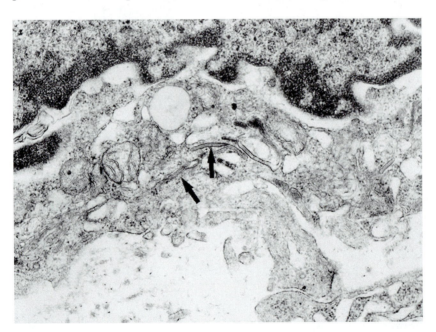

Figure 11-2.
Birbeck granules.

Up to 25 percent of patients are asymptomatic when the disease is found on routine chest x-ray. When the disease becomes symptomatic, cough and exertional dyspnea are common complaints. The presenting complaint may be chest pain, which if acute and pleuritic, is likely the consequence of a spontaneous pneumothorax, a complication that occurs in up to 14 percent of patients. Of considerable diagnostic importance, this is one of only a few disorders associated with simultaneous bilateral spontaneous pneumothoraces. Chest pain may also be a manifestation of cystic bone lesions (eosinophilic granulomas), which occur commonly in the ribs, skull, and pelvis. Central diabetes insipidus may occasionally be seen with PEG as a result of pituitary infiltration by histiocytes.

In contrast to other interstitial lung diseases in which auscultation is characterized by dry, end-inspiratory ("Velcro"-like) crackles, the breath sounds in PEG are typically normal or diminished, particularly with advanced disease. Advanced PEG may manifest signs and symptoms of pulmonary hypertension.

As opposed to acute eosinophilic pneumonia, peripheral blood eosinophilia is not present in PEG and laboratory studies are typically not helpful. The chest x-ray in PEG is classically described as showing diffuse, symmetric, reticular, or reticulonodular opacities with cysts or honeycombing. Initially, the nodules appear stellate but gradually evolve into irregular parenchymal markings, nodular enlargement with cavitation, and eventually honeycombing and bullous formation. Compared with other interstitial lung diseases, two radiographic features are unique to PEG: preservation of lung volumes despite progressive disease, and central honeycombing in the upper and mid-lung zones with costophrenic angle sparing. High-resolution chest CT (HRCT) is more sensitive and specific than chest radiography in the evaluation of interstitial lung diseases, and in PEG demonstrates nodules and thin-walled cysts that are virtually diagnostic (Fig. 11-3).

Histologic tissue confirmation, sometimes obtained by transbronchial biopsy or more often by open lung biopsy, is the most definitive test. Once obtained, light microscopy together with immunocytochemical techniques and, if needed, electron microscopy establish the diagnosis.

As a result of the great variability in the natural history of this disorder, few therapeutic guidelines exist. Asymptomatic patients are best left untreated because the disorder often resolves without therapy. Patients should be strongly encouraged to quit smoking. Those with low diffusing capacities, recurrent pneumothoraces, or multiple organ system involvement (particularly skin) often have a poor prognosis. Unfortunately,

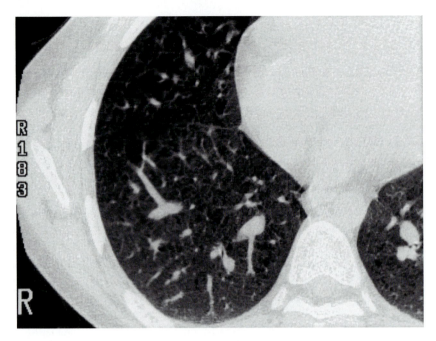

Figure 11-3.
High-resolution chest CT.

treatment with a variety of cytotoxic agents has not had a clear impact on this disease.

Following a workup for malignancy, this patient was found only to have PEG. However, he developed recurrent left-sided pneumothoraces over a 3-month period following discharge. He was subsequently treated with cyclophosphamide, methotrexate, vinblastine, prednisone, and left-sided chemical pleurodesis. At last follow-up, he reported persistent mild exertional dyspnea and was weaning from corticosteroid therapy.

 CLINICAL PEARLS

- PEG, Hand-Schuller-Christian, and Letterer-Siwe diseases are collectively termed Histiocytosis X.
- Granulomatous lesions that contain Langerhans' cells are diagnostic of PEG.
- Cigarette smoking has a strong association with PEG.

- Classic chest x-ray findings of PEG are symmetric, reticular, reticulonodular densities with cysts.
- The definitive diagnosis requires histopathologic confirmation.
- The natural history is extremely variable and the best treatment is uncertain.

REFERENCES

1. Travis W, Borok Z, Roum JH, et al. Pulmonary Langerhans cell granulomatosis (histiocytosis X): A clinicopathologic study of 48 cases. *Am J Surg Pathol* 17(10):971–986, 1993.
2. Soler P, Kambouchner M, Valeyre D, et al. Pulmonary Langerhans' cell granulomatosis (histiocytosis X). *Annu Rev Med* 43:105–115, 1992.
3. Graf-Deul E, Knoblauch A. Simultaneous bilateral spontaneous pneumothorax. *Chest* 105:1142–1146, 1994.
4. Kulwiec EL, Lynch DA, Aguayo SM, et al. Imaging of pulmonary histiocytosis X. *Radiographics* 12(3):515–526, 1992.
5. Willman CL, Busque L, Griffith BB, et al. Langerhans'-cell histiocytosis (histiocytosis x): A clonal proliferative disease. *N Engl J Med* 331:154–160, 1994.

45-YEAR-OLD WOMAN WITH ANEMIA AND RENAL FAILURE

A 45-year-old married homemaker who had previously been in good health presented with a 5-day history of nausea, vomiting, diarrhea, and myalgias. She reported 10 to 12 watery bowel movements per day. Presuming she had the flu, she treated herself with fluids and acetaminophen. Three days prior to admission, she noted a dark color and a decrease in output of urine. In addition, she developed bilateral flank pain, abdominal fullness, bloody stools, and fever. She denied chest pain, shortness of breath, arthralgias, odynophagia, dysuria, or skin rash. She took no medications regularly. Her family and friends were healthy and without recent illnesses. She did not recall eating undercooked meat or unusual foods recently. She did not drink alcohol or smoke tobacco. She had no recent travel history, although she had participated in clean-up efforts following a local flood 1 week prior to the time her symptoms began.

PHYSICAL EXAMINATION

VITAL SIGNS: Temperature, 101°F (38°C); pulse, 92; respiration, 19; blood pressure, 142/90 mmHg.
GENERAL: Pale
HEENT: Eyes: no scleral icterus. Oropharynx: few soft palate petechiae
NECK: No thyromegaly
LUNGS: Clear

CARDIAC: Hyperdynamic precordium; regular rate and rhythm; grade II/VI systolic murmur over left upper sternal border; no rub; normal jugular venous pulse

ABDOMEN: Normoactive bowel sounds, soft, diffusely tender; no hepatosplenomegaly

EXTREMITIES: No edema

NEUROLOGIC: Alert and oriented; normal strength and sensation throughout

SKIN: No lesions, normal turgor

LABORATORY FINDINGS

WBC, 13.9 K/μL (3% band neutrophils, 82% segmented neutrophils, 9% lymphocytes); Hb, 9.7 g/dL (MCV 91 fl); reticulocyte count (corrected) 0.8% (normal, 0.3–2.0); platelets, 30 K/μL; peripheral blood smear (Fig. 12-1); electrolytes: sodium, 128 mmol/L, potassium, 5.1 mmol/L,

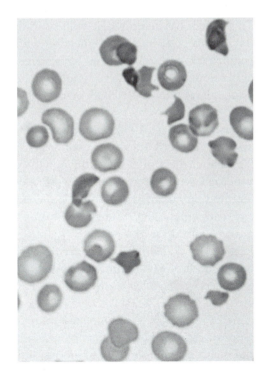

Figure 12-1.
Peripheral blood smear. (See Plate 6.)

chloride, 93 mmol/L, bicarbonate 18 mmol/L; blood urea nitrogen, 101 mg/dL, creatinine 10.6 mg/dL; calcium, 3.4 meq/L (normal, 4.3–5.2); phosphorus, 4.6 (normal, 2.5–4.5); lactate dehydrogenase, 4726 U/L (normal, 0–625); total bilirubin, 0.9 mg/dL (normal, 0–1.5); prothrombin time, 10.5 seconds (normal, 10.0–13.0); partial thromboplastin time, 28 seconds (normal, 24–34); fibrin degradation products titer, 1:2 (normal, negative); protamine sulfate gelation, negative; erythrocyte sedimentation rate (Westergren), 19 mm/hr (normal, 0–20); urinalysis, patient unable to produce urine.

What is the likely diagnosis and how should this patient be treated?

This patient has hemorrhagic colitis and the hemolytic-uremic syndrome (HUS) as a consequence of infection with *Escherichia coli* O157:H7. The peripheral blood smear shows schistocytes ("helmet cells") and a paucity of platelets, typical of microangiopathic hemolytic anemia and thrombocytopenia as seen with HUS or thrombotic thrombocytopenic purpura (TTP).

First isolated in 1982, *E. coli* serotype O157:H7 has become recognized as an important cause of both epidemic and sporadic disease throughout the world. Since the initial reports of a gastrointestinal illness associated with the consumption of undercooked ground beef from a fast-food restaurant chain, much has been learned about the epidemiology, pathophysiology, and clinical manifestations of this disease.

Recognized by its somatic (O) and flagellar (H) antigen designation, *E. coli* O157:H7 is believed to cause disease by its ability to produce either or both of two toxins, referred to as Shiga-like (similar to the toxin produced by *Shigella dysenteriae*) toxins I and II. Although other serotypes of *E. coli* (e.g., O26:H11, O103:H2) can produce similar toxins and illnesses, *E. coli* O157:H7 is the most common. It is responsible for the majority of cases of HUS, a major cause of acute renal failure in children, and is also a common cause of bloody and non-bloody diarrhea. Overall, an estimated 21,000 infections per year are believed to occur in the United States alone.

The majority of outbreaks have occurred from transmission of the organism in undercooked ground beef. It is estimated that approximately 1 percent of healthy cattle harbor the bacteria in their intestines, and that during slaughter a large amount of meat can become contaminated. Other major sources of transmission are fresh-pressed apple cider, raw milk, unchlorinated water, fecally contaminated lakes, and person-to-person contamination. For unclear reasons, infections with this organism occur predominantly during the warmer months of the year, with a peak incidence from June through September. It most commonly afflicts young children and elderly persons, although the highest morbidity and mortality occur in the elderly.

The ascending and transverse colon, which are most often affected, show edema and submucosal hemorrhage that may be manifest as "thumbprinting" on barium-enema and plain-film radiologic examinations. The mucosa appears edematous and hyperemic on endoscopic examination, showing patchy superficial ulcerations and in some cases, pseudomembranes. As seen in the toxin-mediated *Clostridium-difficile*–associated colitis, the histologic appearance is often one of a combination of infectious and ischemic patterns of injury.

E. coli O157:H7 attaches to the mucosal surface of the gut producing one or both of the Shiga-like toxins, which may act locally and systemically. Toxins and associated inflammatory mediators cause vascular injury, allowing their access into the systemic circulation. There is strong evidence that toxemia is the primary pathogenic mechanism responsible for the spectrum of systemic clinical manifestations, which are more likely to develop in patients presenting with bloody diarrhea than nonbloody diarrhea. The toxins are believed to produce vascular endothelial injury that ameliorates the anticoagulant properties of the endothelium, thus causing intravascular thrombosis.

There is a broad range of clinical manifestations in infected individuals. It may manifest simply as an asymptomatic infection, or in severe cases, cause painful abdominal cramping and bloody diarrhea (hemmorhagic colitis), complicated by the hemolytic-uremic syndrome, thrombotic thrombocytopenic purpura, and in some cases, death. The illness typically begins with abdominal cramps and nonbloody diarrhea, which becomes bloody within a day or two, prompting patients to seek medical attention. Although bloody stools are common in this infection, the diagnosis must not be dismissed in their absence. As many as 65 percent of patients had only nonbloody diarrhea in some of the reported outbreaks in the United States. Patients with nonbloody diarrhea tend to have a less severe course and are less likely to develop complications, such as HUS, TTP, or even death. Half the affected patients also have nausea and vomiting. However, unlike other bacterial diarrheas, *E. coli* O157:H7 is often accompanied by little or no fever, which may sway the clinician to consider only non–infectious enteric diseases.

Although symptoms of *E. coli* O157:H7 infection usually subside in about 1 week, about 6 percent (mostly young children and the elderly) develop the hemolytic-uremic syndrome, a complication that occurs in up to 30 percent of patients with hemorrhagic colitis. HUS is characterized by microangiopathic hemolytic anemia, thrombocytopenia, renal failure, and central nervous system manifestations. It develops predominantly in young children and the elderly and has a mortality rate of nearly 10 percent in the former and 90 percent in the latter. Risk factors include bloody diarrhea, leukocytosis, fever, and use of antimotility agents.

Thrombotic thrombocytopenic purpura (TTP) is characterized by the classic pentad of findings: fever, renal failure, thrombocytopenia, microangiopathic hemolytic anemia, and neurologic sequelae. TTP occurs in as many as 8 percent of patients with hemorrhagic colitis from *E. coli* O157:H7 and represents a more extensive form of vascular disease than that which occurs with the hemolytic-uremic syndrome. Clinically, TTP tends to have less severe renal involvement but more profound neurologic manifestations than the HUS. The reported cases of TTP associated with *E. coli* O157:H7 have occurred in adults.

Routine stool cultures do *not* detect the presence of *E. coli* O157:H7 and most clinical laboratories do not not routinely screen for this organism. As a result, when infection is suspected, the clinicians must specifically order a culture for *E. coli* O157:H7. Since the recovery rate of the organism from stool is highest within the first 6 days of the illness, cultures should be sent early. Other more sophisticated tests are available in reference laboratories for confirmation of the diagnosis or in those clinically suspicious patients with negative cultures.

No specific treatment of this infection has proven efficacious. Therefore treatment is supportive. Patients at high risk for developing HUS should be monitored closely with blood counts, peripheral blood smears and urinalyses, and should not be treated with antimotility agents. Management of the hemolytic–uremic syndrome is also supportive and may require dialysis, plasmapheresis, and intravenous immune globulin.

Prevention by means of public education and public health initiatives are the most important measures for combating this infection and its devastating complications. Counseling patients regarding the sources of infection, particularly with respect to the risk of eating undercooked ground beef and proper handwashing in institutional settings (e.g., daycare centers, nursing homes), is important. Proposed public health measures are routine laboratory screening of all grossly bloody stool specimens, mandated reporting of all *E. coli* O157:H7 infections to state health departments, and establishment of an expanded surveillance system with appropriate follow-up.

Our patient required hemodialysis and received five plasmapheresis treatments. She was discharged home on hospital day 10 with improving renal function. She had no evidence of renal impairment 1 year later.

CLINICAL PEARLS

- *Escherichia coli* O157:H7 infections produce a spectrum of manifestations, ranging from none (asymptomatic carrier) to hemorrhagic colitis complicated by HUS or TTP.
- *E. coli* O157:H7 infection is common and should be considered in all patients with diarrhea, particularly bloody diarrhea.
- The pathogenesis of *E. coli* O157:H7 is mediated via shiga-like toxins I and II.
- Undercooked ground beef is the most common source of infection, but person-to-person transmission may also occur.
- The diagnosis may be established by timely stool culture for *E. coli* O157:H7, which must be explicitly ordered since it is not routinely included in stool cultures.
- Treatment is supportive with management of complications as necessary.
- Preventive measures, including public and physician education and implementation of public health policies to prevent this infection, are important.

REFERENCES

1. Su C, Brandt LJ. *Escherichia coli* O157:H7 infection in humans. *Ann Intern Med* 123:698–714, 1995.
2. Boyce TG, Swerdlow DL, Griffin PM. *Escherichia coli* O157:H7 and the hemolytic-uremic syndrome. *N Engl J Med* 333:364–368, 1995.

36-YEAR-OLD WOMAN
WITH FATIGUE

A 36-year-old woman with no significant past medical history presented to her local physician with a 2-month history of progressive fatigue, early satiety, left upper quadrant fullness, and a 10-pound weight loss. She denied nausea and vomiting, diarrhea, hematemesis, hematochezia, fevers, or night sweats, and was taking no medications. Her menses were regular and without excessive bleeding. The family history was notable only for adult onset diabetes in her paternal grandfather. She was married, had two healthy children, and worked full-time as a graphics designer. She did not smoke tobacco or drink alcohol and reported no recent exposures or travel.

PHYSICAL EXAMINATION

VITAL SIGNS: Temperature, 97.9°F (approx 36.5°C); pulse, 82; respiration, 16; blood pressure, 136/70

GENERAL: Age appropriate female in no acute distress

NECK: No thyromegaly

LUNGS: Clear

CARDIAC: Normal

ABDOMEN: Normal bowel sounds, soft, non-tender, no hepatomegaly; spleen palpable 9 cm below the left costal margin

LYMPH: No lymph node enlargement

EXTREMITIES: No edema

SKIN: Warm and moist

disorder of uncertain cause. Individuals with significant radiation exposure are at increased risk.

The natural course of the disease is typically biphasic, and at times triphasic. Most patients present in the chronic phase, and are either asymptomatic with only an elevated white blood cell count or have mild, nonspecific symptoms. The incidence of asymptomatic cases has increased dramatically over the last 10 years, probably as a result of routine blood testing with annual physical examinations. When present, symptoms may include progressive fatigue, left upper quadrant discomfort, early satiety, anorexia, or weight loss. Splenomegaly, at times massive, is the hallmark physical finding and is present in more than 90 percent of cases. In addition, 10 to 40 percent of patients have hepatomegaly. Lymph node enlargement is very uncommon and if detected, suggests an accelerated course or blastic transformation of CML.

The chronic phase lasts approximately 4 to 5 years before evolving into a more aggressive phase. Eventually, all patients will transition to the blastic phase, which is clinically similar to an acute leukemia. The change may be abrupt or, more commonly, progressive and is characterized by increasing resistance to therapy, and the development of organomegaly, thrombocytosis or thrombocytopenia, anemia, malaise, weight loss and fevers. This is termed the accelerated phase of CML. Extramedullary involvement of lymph nodes, bone, skin, and soft tissue also may become manifest. Although clinically not well demarcated from the accelerated phase, the blast crisis phase is diagnosed when 30 percent or more blasts (usually myeloid) are present in the bone marrow or peripheral blood. In addition, further cytogenic evolution often occurs during this phase; double Ph-chromosomes, chromosome 17 abnormalities, and trisomy 8 are the most common. Mutations of the P53 oncogene, with subsequent loss of P53 function, may account for progression in about 25 percent of CML patients. The median survival of a patient in the accelerated phase of the disease is 12 to 18 months, whereas it is 3 months once the blast crisis phase appears.

The white blood cell (WBC) count is often $> 100,000/\mu L$ at the time of presentation. The differential is left-shifted, with an orderly progression of granulocytic cells at all stages of maturation (see Fig. 13-1). Infections are rarely seen at the time of diagnosis because neutrophil function remains near-normal during the early phases. Characteristically, the leukocyte alkaline phosphatase (LAP) is low. About 50 percent of patients have platelet counts in excess of 450,000 /μL and one-third have a hemoglobin concentration < 11 g/dL. The bone marrow is typically hypercellular, with as much as a 20:1 myeloid-to-erythroid ratio (normal 2:1). The serum lactate dehydrogenase and uric acid are often high, reflecting increased cell turnover. Serum vitamin B_{12} and transcobalamin levels are often 10 times the normal values as a consequence of increased transcobalamin production by neutrophils.

The diagnosis of CML rests on finding splenomegaly, marked myelopoiesis and the Ph-chromosome. Although in the past the Ph chromosome was not detected in 5 to 10 percent of cases, it is now almost always found by polymerase chain reaction (PCR) techniques.

During the chronic phase, the goal of treatment is to decrease myelopoiesis to control symptoms. Leukapheresis is often necessary for a WBC count >200,000/μL, painful splenomegaly owing to splenic infarction or if leukostasis develops; a syndrome characterized by confusion, dyspnea, priapism, and venous thrombosis. Otherwise, disease control may be achieved with a variety of chemotherapeutic agents. Busulfan and hydroxyurea have been used successfully in more than 70 percent of patients; however, busulfan has more side effects and increases the subsequent risk of marrow transplantation and now is used less often.

Despite disease control, transformation to the blast phase occurs. Therefore, a secondary goal of treatment is to induce cytogenetic remission. Three strategies have been employed to date: intensive chemotherapy, interferons, and bone marrow transplantation (BMT). Although choosing the appropriate therapy has many considerations, only allogeneic BMT provides a potential for cure. Fifty to seventy percent of patients who present in the chronic phase and receive an HLA-matched sibling BMT achieve long-term disease-free survival. Because the prognosis worsens 1 year after the diagnosis and during the accelerated or blastic phases of the disease, early identification of donors is important.

After the first year, about 20 percent of patients each year transform from the chronic to the blastic phase and about 85 percent of all CML patients die in the blastic phase. A high-risk group with a median survival of only about 2 years is identified by the following: a high white count, splenomegaly, hepatomegaly, thrombocytosis or thrombocytopenia, circulating blasts, basophilia, additional cytogenetic abnormalities, and an older age.

This patient was initially treated with hydroxyurea and subsequently underwent a successful allogeneic BMT.

CLINICAL PEARLS

- CML is a stem cell disorder characterized by an overproduction of myeloid cells.
- CML accounts for up to 15 percent of all adult leukemias.
- CML is associated with the Philadelphia (Ph) chromosome, a balanced translocation between chromosome 9 and 22; t (9;22) (q34;q11).
- Most patients present in the chronic phase and are either asymptomatic or have fatigue, weight loss, early satiety, or left upper quadrant fullness.
- The hallmark physical finding is a large spleen that may be massive.
- Allogeneic BMT offers the only opportunity to cure CML.

REFERENCES

1. Cortes JE, Talpaz M, Kantarjian H. Chronic myelogenous leukemia: A review. *Am J Med* 1996; 100:555–570.
2. Kantarjian HM, Deisseroth A, Kurzrock R, et al. Chronic myelogenous leukemia: A concise update. *Blood* 1993; 82(3):691–703.
3. Kurzrock R, Gutterman JU, Talpaz M. The molecular genetics of philadelphia chromosome-positive leukemias. *N Engl J Med* 1988; 319:990–998.

43-YEAR-OLD MAN WITH JOINT PAIN

A previously healthy 43-year-old male construction worker presented with a 1-week history of diffuse arthralgias. He described pain in all of his joints, but particularly in his ankles, wrists, and hands. Over the prior 2 days, he noted difficulty with standing because of hip and ankle pain. He also reported a recent viral illness, associated with fatigue, cough, rhinorrhea, and fever. He was treated with antibiotics and an antitussive agent with only minimal improvement in his symptoms. He denied chills, myalgia, sore throat, nausea, vomiting, diarrhea, chest pain, or shortness of breath. Medications on admission were clarithromycin and guaifenesin syrup. His family history was remarkable for type II diabetes and coronary artery disease. He was married, had two healthy children, and did not smoke tobacco, drink alcohol, or use illicit drugs. He denied recent infectious, occupational exposures, or recent travel.

PHYSICAL EXAMINATION

VITAL SIGNS: Temperature, 101.5°F (38.5°C); pulse, 98; respiration, 18; blood pressure, 126/76 mmHg
GENERAL: Moderately obese
HEENT: Normal
NECK: No lymphadenopathy or thyromegaly
LUNGS: Clear
CARDIAC: Normal
ABDOMEN: Normoactive bowel sounds, soft, nontender; no hepatosplenomegaly
EXTREMITIES: No cyanosis or edema

NEUROLOGIC: Nonfocal

MUSCULOSKELETAL: Normal range of motion; all joints nontender to palpation and without swelling, erythema, or warmth

SKIN: Tender red nodules over the pretibial surface of both legs (Fig. 14-1)

LABORATORY FINDINGS

WBC, 6.7 K/μL (normal differential); Hb, 13.6 g/dL (MCV 83 fL); platelets, 328 K/μL; electrolytes, glucose, urea nitrogen, and creatinine, normal; calcium, 4.5 meq/L (normal 4.3–5.2); erythrocyte sedimentation rate (Westergren) 84 mm/Hr; urinalysis normal; liver function tests normal; chest x-ray shown (Fig. 14-2).

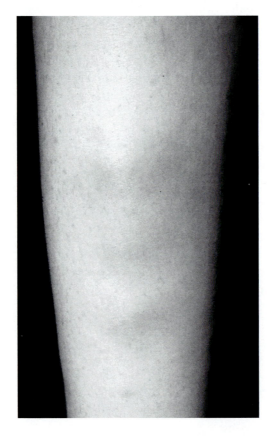

Figure 14-1.
Nodules over right lower extremity. (See Plate 8.)

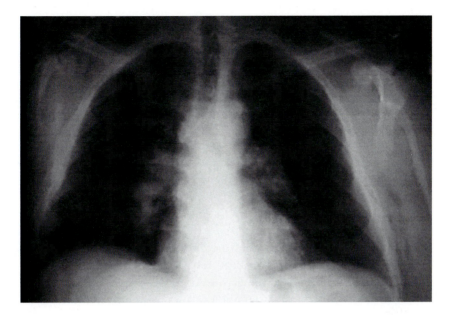

Figure 14-2.
PA Chest x-ray.

What is the diagnosis and how should this patient be treated?

This patient has sarcoidosis manifested as Loefgren's syndrome. This is an acute presentation of sarcoidosis characterized by fever, erythema nodosum (Fig. 14-1), bilateral hilar adenopathy (Fig. 14-2), and arthralgia or arthritis.

Sarcoidosis is a systemic disease of unknown etiology, characterized pathologically by the presence of noncaseating granulomas in affected organs. Clinically, the disease may present acutely or subacutely and may have a self-limited course, or it may become chronic with episodic exacerbations and remissions. Although it may affect any organ system in the body, the lung is most commonly affected. As a result, most patients present with acute or insidious respiratory complaints, or are asymptomatic but have an abnormal chest x-ray. Skin, eye, and lymph node involvement are also common.

Sarcoidosis occurs throughout the world, affecting all ethnic groups and ages, with a slight predilection for females. Most patients present between the ages of 20 and 40 years. There is tremendous diversity in its incidence and prevalence among certain ethnic and racial groups. For instance, in the United States it occurs 10 times more often among African-Americans than Caucasians, whereas in Europe the disease affects mostly Caucasians. In addition, its severity and pattern of organ involvement also differ according to race and ethnic background. In African-Americans, the disease often presents more acutely and severely than in other races; extrathoracic involvement is more common in Puerto Ricans, African-Americans, and Scandinavians.

Although much has been learned about the immunopathogenesis of this disease, its etiology remains unknown. Some of the difficulty relates to the heterogeneous expression of the disease. It also overlaps clinically with other disorders. Last, diagnostic tests to identify the disorder are nonspecific and may result in misclassification. Genetic and environmental factors are believed to play important roles. Interestingly, sarcoidosis occurs more commonly in monozygotic than dizygotic twins and familial forms of the disorder are not uncommon. Exposure to a number of organic and inorganic agents is associated with granulomatous diseases that are often clinically indistinguishable from sarcoidosis. In particular, a variety of microorganisms can induce granulomatous inflammatory changes; however, definitive proof that sarcoidosis is a result of an infectious agent remains elusive.

Sarcoidosis is believed to be a consequence of an over-exuberant cellular immune response to an antigen, mediated primarily by activated helper T lymphocytes. After stimulation by an antigen, macrophages release interleukin-1 (IL-1), which induce T-cell activation. The activated T lymphocytes then release a variety of mediators, including interleukin-2 (IL-2, T-cell growth factor), which attract and activate more T cells and other immune effector cells, including mononuclear phagocytes. The activated T cells also produce B-cell mediators, which cause polyclonal B-cell stimulation and hypergammaglobulinemia. Together, these processes result in an acute, or occasionally chronic, cascade of inflammation characterized granuloma formation. These same mediators may stimulate proliferation of fibroblasts, contributing to the development of fibrosis.

The clinical manifestations of sarcoidosis result from the granulomatous process or the impaired function that it causes. In the United States, sarcoidosis typically presents in three forms: an asymptomatic form (10–20 percent of cases), an acute or subacute form (20–40 percent of cases), and an insidious form (40–70 percent of cases). Individuals present-ing with the acute or subacute form usually develop symptoms over a pe-riod of a few weeks. These symptoms often include constitutional complaints of fever, fatigue, malaise, anorexia, or weight loss. Respiratory symptoms may include cough, dyspnea, or a retrosternal chest discomfort. In addition to Loefgren's syndrome, the Heerfordt-Waldenstrom syn-drome (uveoparotid fever) also occurs acutely and is typified by fever, parotid enlargement, anterior uveitis, and facial nerve palsy. The insidious form of sarcoidosis typically develops over months, is dominated by respi-ratory complaints alone, and commonly progresses to chronic sarcoidosis.

Respiratory tract involvement occurs in virtually all patients with sar-coidosis at some point in the course of their disease. It manifests most often as an interstitial lung disease, characterized by dry rales, restricted lung volumes, and impaired gas exchange. Typical symptoms are dyspnea, particularly with exercise, and a dry cough. Occasionally, endobronchial granulomas will cause segmental or lobar stenosis with obstruction to air-flow resulting in wheezing or atelectasis. Pleural effusions are seen in less than 5 percent of patients, and are usually unilateral lymphocytic exu-dates. Upper respiratory tract involvement may occur in up to 20 percent of patients, usually manifested by nasal congestion.

Intrathoracic and peripheral lymph node enlargement is very common in sarcoidosis. Hilar lymphadenopathy seen on chest x-ray occurs in up to 90 percent of patients. Peripheral nodes are also frequently involved, but rarely pose a clinical problem. Twenty-five percent of patients with sarcoidosis have skin involvement. The most common skin lesions are ery-thema nodosum, plaques, maculopapular eruptions, subcutaneous nodules, and lupus pernio. Erythema nodosum consists of bilateral, tender red nod-ules, typically located on the anterior surface of the legs. Although it is not specific for the diagnosis, it is very common in the acute form and por-tends an excellent prognosis. Lupus pernio is characterized by indurated violaceous lesions primarily on the nose, cheeks, lips, and ears, which are rare but can become very disfiguring with erosion into bone.

About 5 to 10 percent of patients have cardiac involvement, half of whom have electrocardiographic abnormalities (conduction abnormali-ties, arrhythmias). Other manifestations include infiltrative cardiomyopa-thy, pericarditis, and papillary muscle dysfunction. Early diagnosis is important in cardiac sarcoidosis to provide prompt, appropriate treatment and to improve overall prognosis.

The eyes are involved in about 25 percent of patients, at times causing blindness. Most often, anterior uveitis causes the rapid onset of blurred vision, photophobia, and tearing, usually that resolves spontaneously over the course of a year. A seventh cranial nerve (facial) palsy is the most common nervous system manifestation of sarcoidosis, although almost any part of the central nervous system can become involved and up to 5 percent of patients are so affected. Other central nervous system presentations may include hypothalamic (diabetes insipidus) and pituitary abnormalities, optic nerve dysfunction, chronic meningitis, and the effects of space-occupying lesions. Neurosarcoidosis should be considered in those cases in which deficits appear in both the central and peripheral nervous systems.

Bone lesions are seen in 5 percent of patients and typically involve cysts, punched-out lesions, or lattice-like radiographic changes in the hands and feet (Figs. 14-3 and 14-4). The joints are involved in up to 50 percent of cases, commonly associated with migratory or transient arthralgias in large joints. Bone marrow involvement occurs in up to 40 percent of cases, but rarely causes hematologic abnormalities.

Hepatic and splenic involvement is common but is usually not clinically apparent. Nephrocalcinosis rarely occurs as a result of hypercalcemia

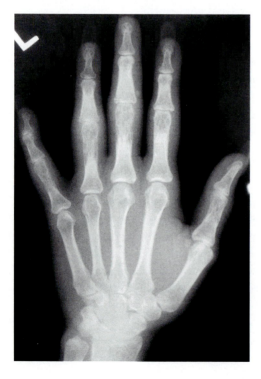

Figure 14-3.
Cystic bone lesions.

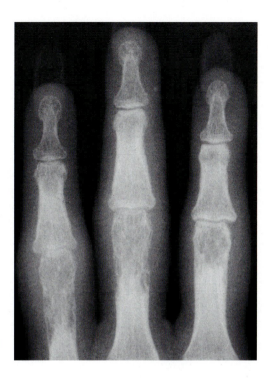

Figure 14-4.
Cystic bone lesions (magnified
image of Fig. 14-3).

from ectopic 1,25-dihydroxyvitamin D produced by the granulomas. Bilateral parotid gland enlargement is a classic feature of sarcoidosis, but is seen clinically in less than 10 percent of patients.

The diagnosis is made by a constellation of clinical, radiographic, and histologic findings. Although a variety of tests are available, including serum angiotensin-converting enzyme (SACE) level, skin anergy, bronchoalveolar lavage fluid analysis, and gallium-67 scanning, none are diagnostic and most have limited specificity. Therefore, the definitive diagnosis should only be made with a biopsy (usually skin or transbronchial lung) in the context of an appropriate clinical setting. Even with a diagnostic biopsy, a thorough history must be taken to exclude other causes of granulomatous inflammation (Table 14-1). Newman and associates have recommended a minimal baseline of tests to be performed on all newly diagnosed sarcoidosis patients.

The overall prognosis for patients with sarcoidosis is good, although the initial clinical presentation and chest x-ray are often the best measures of prognosis. Stage I disease (hilar adenopathy without parenchymal infiltrates on chest x-ray) remits in 60 to 80 percent of cases, stage II (hilar adenopathy with infiltrates) remits in 50 to 60 percent of cases, and stage

TABLE 14-1   Causes of Granulomatous Diseases

CAUSE	DISEASE
Infectious Agents	
Mycobacteria	Tuberculosis
	Atypical mycobacterial infections
Fungi	Histoplasmosis
	Coccidioidomycosis
Bacteria	Brucellosis
	Chylamydial infection
	Tularemia
Spirochetes	Treponemal infections (e.g., syphilis)
Parasites	Leishmaniasis
	Toxoplasmosis
Occupational and Environmental Exposure	
Organic or inorganic agents	Hypersensitivity pneumonitis (e.g., bacteria, fungi, animal proteins, isocyanates)
	Chronic beryllium disease
	Granulomatous disease related to other metals
	Talc
	Methotrexate-induced pneumonitis
Other Conditions	
Neoplasia	Lymphoma
	Tumor-related granulomas
Autoimmune disorders	Wegener's granulomatosis
	Primary biliary cirrhosis
	Churg-Strauss syndrome
Other	Sarcoidosis

*Adapted from Crystal RG. Sarcoidosis, in *Harrison's Principles of Internal Medicine.* Isselbacher KJ, Braunwald E, Wilson JD, et al (eds). New York, McGraw-Hill, 1994, pp 1679–1684.

III (infiltrates without adenopathy) remits in 30 percent of cases. The best prognosis is with Loefgren's syndrome. In about 15 to 20 percent of patients, the disease remains active or recurs intermittently. Unfortunately, no tests can reliably predict the overall clinical course of the disease. Instead, periodic clinical evaluations focused on affected organs are necessary. In addition, close monitoring of cardiac and pulmonary involvement, the leading causes of morbidity and mortality, is important.

Corticosteroids are the treatment of choice, despite the lack of well-controlled trials documenting improvement in long-term outcome. A variety of other agents have been used (methotrexate, chloroquine, cyclosporine) with limited efficacy. The most important decision is when to begin treatment, knowing that approximately half of the patients will remit spontaneously. Although clear guidelines are lacking, most clinicians initiate treatment for symptomatic pulmonary involvement, or for objective evidence (serial pulmonary function studies) of progressive pulmonary impairment, or in patients with significant systemic symptoms, malignant hypercalcemia, and extrapulmonary involvement that leads to functional impairment.

Our patient had pulmonary function studies (minimal obstructive and restrictive ventilatory defect with a normal diffusing capacity), fungal serologies (negative), PPD (negative), SACE level 61 U/L (normal, 8–52), and bronchoscopy performed. Bronchoalveolar lavage revealed a T helper-to-supressor ratio of 28:1; transbronchial biopsy demonstrated noncaseating granulomas and fibrosis. An opthalmology evaluation found no eye pathology. Because of the patient's significant systemic symptoms (fevers, arthralgias) he was treated with prednisone 40 mg daily for 12 weeks, followed by a taper.

 ## CLINICAL PEARLS

- Sarcoidosis is a systemic disease of unknown etiology, characterized pathologically by noncaseating granulomas.
- It is most common between 20 and 40 years of age, with a slight predilection toward females.
- There is tremendous diversity in incidence and prevalence for certain ethnic and racial groups.
- It typically presents in three forms: an asymptomatic form (10–20 percent of cases), an acute or subacute form (20–40 percent of cases), and an insidious form (40–70 percent of cases).

- Pulmonary involvement occurs in virtually all patients at some point in their disease.
- The diagnosis is made by a constellation of clinical, radiographic, and histologic findings.
- Loefgren's syndrome is an acute form of sarcoidosis characterized by fever, erythema nodosum, bilateral hilar adenopathy, and arthralgia or arthritis.

REFERENCES

1. Newman LS, Rose CS, Maier LA. Sarcoidosis. *N Engl J Med* 1997; 336:1224–1234.
2. Crystal RG. Sarcoidosis, in *Harrison's Principles of Internal Medicine*. Isselbacher KJ, Braunwald E, Wilson JD, et al (eds). New York, McGraw-Hill, 1994, pp 1679–1684.

54-YEAR-OLD WOMAN WITH BACK PAIN

A 54-year-old postmenopausal woman with a history of hypothyroidism following a partial thyroidectomy for a benign colloid adenoma in 1973, and a history of lumbar disc disease presented with complaints of chronic low back pain and fatigue. She had a 10-year history of chronic back pain. One year ago an MRI revealed a bulging L5-S1 disc without nerve root impingement. She controlled her pain successfully with exercises and taking analgesics only occasionally. Her fatigue, although progressive, was believed to be related to personal problems. She was recently hospitalized for chest pain and palpitations, and was noted to have mild hypercalcemia. Her regular medications included Synthroid, estrogen, and metoprolol. She denied weight loss, nausea or vomiting, dyspnea, or constipation. She took no over-the-counter medications or supplements, except for an occasional acetaminophen. Married with two healthy children, she worked full-time as a dental hygienist. There was no family history of cancer or thyroid disease. She had never smoked and used alcohol only rarely.

PHYSICAL EXAMINATION

VITAL SIGNS: Temperature, 99.0°F (37°C); pulse, 80; respiration, 20; blood pressure, 112/72 mmHg
GENERAL: Appeared younger than stated age
HEENT: Normal
NECK: Thyroidectomy scar, no lymph node enlargement
LUNGS: Clear
CARDIAC: Normal

ABDOMEN: Normal bowel sounds, soft, non-tender; no hepatosplen-
omegaly
EXTREMITIES: No edema
NEUROLOGIC: No motor or sensory deficits; normal strength; negative
straight leg raise
SKIN: No lesions

LABORATORY FINDINGS

WBC, 6.3 K/μL (normal differential); Hb, 14.1 g/dL; platelets, 330 K/μL;
electrolytes, urea nitrogen, and creatinine, normal; calcium, 5.4 meq/L
(normal 4.3–5.2); phosphorous 3.5 mg/dL (normal 2.5–4.5); intact PTH
96.2 (normal 11.0–54.0); thyroxine, thyroid stimulating hormone normal; urinalysis normal; lumbosacral spine films (Fig. 15-1).

What is the likely cause of this patient's symptoms and why does she have back pain?

This patient has primary hyperparathyroidism. Her back x-rays show osteopenia, which is probably causing her back pain and is likely due to a
loss of mineral density caused by osteoporosis, hyperparathyroidism, or
more likely, both disorders.

Primary hyperparathyroidism (PHP) is a common endocrine disorder
of calcium hemostasis. It is caused by an abnormally increased secretion
of parathyroid hormone (PTH), leading to high circulating PTH levels,
which eventually cause hypercalcemia and hypophosphatemia. Although
extensive bone disease and nephrolithiasis were the most common presenting features of PHP in the past, the diagnosis is now usually established in an asymptomatic patient who has had a multi-channel chemistry
panel done for an unrelated reason. The estimated prevalence of PHP in
the population is at least 1 percent, making it one of the most common
endocrine disorders, trailing only diabetes mellitus and hypothyroidism in
frequency. It can occur at any age, but is most common in the fifth and
sixth decades, affecting women two to three times more often than men,
a difference that increases with age.

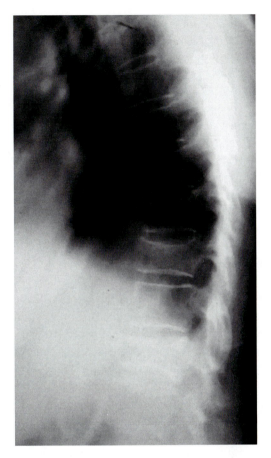

Figure 15-1.
Lumbosacral spine x-ray.

A single hyperfunctioning parathyroid adenoma is the cause of hyperparathyroidism in over 80 percent of the cases. It usually involves one of the inferior parathyroid glands, but in about 10 percent of the cases the adenoma is located in the thymus, thyroid, mediastinum, pericardium, or behind the esophagus. Diffuse parathyroid gland hyperplasia accounts for another 15 to 20 percent of the cases, about half of which are from kindreds affected with one of the multiple endocrine neoplasia (MEN) syndromes, which are transmitted as autosomal dominant traits. MEN I typically affects the pituitary, pancreas, and parathyroids, whereas MEN IIA comprises medullary thyroid carcinoma, hyperparathyroidism, and pheochromocytoma. Multiple adenomas and parathyroid cysts are very uncommon, and parathyroid carcinoma is very rare.

The majority of parathyroid adenomas originate from a single cell line (monoclonal) that has likely undergone genetic changes. One of these changes, identified in a small subset of adenomas, involves a chromosomal rearrangement whereby the 5' regulatory region of the PTH gene, located on the short arm of chromosome 11, is juxtaposed to the *PRAD1* oncogene on the long arm of the same chromosome. Over-expression of *PRAD1* can lead to an acceleration of mitosis and increase the proliferation of parathyroid cells. Other proposed mechanisms include inactivation of tumor-suppression genes and various mutations involving calcium-sensing and vitamin D receptors. Parathyroid hyperplasia may also result from a proliferation of monoclonal cells, which is controversial but has been identified in the parathyroid hyperplasia of MEN I.

Although patients are often asymptomatic at the time of diagnosis, vague constitutional symptoms such as depression, subjective weakness, and poor concentration, are common. These symptoms are believed to be part of poorly characterized neuropsychiatric syndrome associated with PHP. Patients with more advanced disease may present with symptoms primarily involving the kidneys and skeleton. Although much less common than in the past, up to 20 percent of patients with PHP have nephrolithiasis (usually composed of either calcium oxalate or calcium phosphate). Conversely, about 5 percent of patients who present with nephrolithiasis have PHP. It is therefore reasonable to screen all patients with kidney stones, especially women, with a serum calcium measurement. Renal function may be impaired by nephrocalcinosis and also by extreme hypercalcemia itself.

The classic skeletal disease of PHP, *osteitis fibrosa cystica*, is rarely seen today. The most sensitive x-ray sign of this is subperiosteal bone resorption at the radial aspects of the middle phalanges. Other rarely seen x-ray findings are resorption of the distal phalanges and clavicle, a "salt and pepper" appearance of the skull, and bone cysts caused by brown tumors that result from intense osteocyte stimulation by PTH. Overt bone disease is now very uncommon because the disease typically is discovered much earlier than it had been in the past. Bone mineral densitometry (BMD) provides a more accurate and sensitive method for detecting hyperparathyroid bone disease. PTH has an effect on both cortical and cancellous bone. It has a catabolic effect on cortical bone (appendicular skeleton), which is best demonstrated by a reduced BMD of the distal one-third of the radius, and it has an anabolic effect on cancellous bone (axial skeleton), which can be demonstrated with reduced BMD of the lumbar vertebrae. Paradoxically, hyperparathyroidism appears to provide some protection against the loss of cancellous bone that typically occurs with menopause.

Other presentations may include neuromuscular, gastrointestinal, and rheumatologic manifestations. Proximal muscle weakness, fatigability, and muscle atrophy may be so profound as to suggest a primary neuromuscular disorder. Vague abdominal complaints, constipation, and peptic ulcer disease or pancreatitis may also occur. Pseudogout rarely may be the initial presenting feature.

A detailed history to elicit the typical symptoms and a physical examination that looks for musculoskeletal abnormalities is important in the initial evaluation. The patient should be questioned about a personal or family history of endocrinopathies, medications (specifically diuretics, lithium, and calcium-containing antacids), and a history of exposure to therapeutic neck irradiation during childhood. Diuretics and oral antacids may cause hypercalcemia or may unmask hyperparathyroidism, whereas lithium and therapeutic irradiation causes PHP. The physical examination may provide clues for an alternative explanation for hypercalcemia such as malignancy or MEN syndromes.

Hypercalcemia is the laboratory hallmark of PHP. More than 90 percent of the cases of hypercalcemia are caused by PHP and malignancies. Patients with malignancy usually have serum calcium levels above 12 mg/dL and are symptomatic, whereas those with PHP typically have a lower serum calcium ($<$12 mg/dL) or intermittent hypercalcemia. A patient with PHP will rarely present with severe, life-threatening hypercalcemia, referred to as a hypercalcemic crisis. The free serum calcium should be estimated from the serum albumin level and the ionized calcium level measured directly. Other findings are hypophosphatemia, hypercalciuria, hyperchloremic metabolic acidosis (caused by a renal tubular bicarbonate leak induced by PTH), and increased 1,25-dihydroxyvitamin D.

A diagnosis of PHP is established with the highly sensitive and specific immunometric assay for intact PTH. An assay is also available for PTH-related protein (PTH-r), the humoral mediator of malignancy-associated hypercalcemia. The two clearly distinguish between PHP and hypercalcemia of malignancy: in PHP the intact PTH is high and PTH-r is low or undetectable, whereas in most patients with hypercalcemia or malignancy, PTH-r is high and intact PTH is normal or low. Most nonparathyroid causes of hypercalcemia are also associated with a low serum PTH due to negative feedback inhibition of parathyroid secretion by hypercalcemia. One of the exceptions to this is chronic lithium therapy causing hypercalcemia with an elevated PTH. Withdrawal of the drug is usually required to confirm the diagnosis. Biochemical markers of bone metabolism (osteocalcin, N-telopeptide) may indicate that the patient is undergoing mild bone loss, but their measurement is usually unnecessary. In contrast, BMD measurement with DEXA provides a very accurate noninvasive assessment of bone involvement with hyperparathyroidism, giving information that may be important in reaching a decision about surgery. A reduction in cortical bone density of more than two standard deviations below that for age-matched controls (Z-score) is an indication for surgery.

The large number of asymptomatic hypercalcemic patients being diagnosed with PHP has provoked serious questions about its management, since no long-term data are available to support parathyroidectomy—the only current definitive treatment—in this situation. To establish surgical guidelines, a Consensus Development Conference on the Management of Asymptomatic Primary Hyperparathyroidism was convened by the National Institutes of Health in 1991 (Table 15-1). According to these guidelines, only about half of the patients with PHP meet the criteria for surgery at the time of diagnosis.

When surgery is performed by an experienced parathyroid surgeon, it is curative in over 90 percent of the cases. Although no existing imaging procedure is more effective than an experienced surgeon for locating abnormal parathyroid glands in patients who have not undergone previous neck surgery, preoperative parathyroid localization is considered essential for patients undergoing a second operation. The need for parathyroid imaging in patients undergoing an initial exploration, however, remains controversial. Scintigraphy with ^{99m}Tc-sestamibi has largely replaced

TABLE 15-1   **Indications for Surgery**

Serum calcium >2.99 mmol/L (12 mg/dL)
Marked hypercalciuria (>9.98 mmol/day)
Any overt manifestation of PHP
   Nephrolithiasis
   Osteitis fibrosa cystica
   Classic neuromuscular disease
Markedly reduced cortical bone density
Reduced creatinine clearance in the absence of other cause
Age <50 years

^{99m}Tc-pertechnetate, and ^{201}Tl chloride subtraction scintigraphy for parathyroid imaging because of its superior sensitivity (~95% before the first operation and ~70% before reoperation) and negligible false-positive rate. Positron emission tomography, another technique recently applied to parathyroid imaging, is of uncertain value at present. After successful surgery, serial BMD measurement usually demonstrates increased bone density at multiple skeletal sites, but particularly in those with predominantly cancellous bone such as the vertebral spine and femoral neck.

In patients who do not meet the criteria, are unfit for surgery, or are unwilling to have it, it is prudent to measure serial calcium every 6 months, urinary calcium and creatinine every 12 months, and bone mineral density every 1 to 3 years. There often is little progression of disease as assessed by these parameters, suggesting a benign course in such patients. Medical management of PHP, although limited in efficacy, includes good hydration, avoidance of thiazide diuretics, a moderate calcium intake, and avoiding immobility. Estrogen therapy has been advocated for postmenopausal women with PHP. Oral phosphate therapy is not recommended because it raises PTH secretion and increases the long-term risk of metastatic calcification. New therapies with calcimimetic agents that are now under development offer new and effective medical management.

There are reports of increased mortality from cardiovascular disease and malignancy in patients with primary hyperparathyroidism. One recent large study of 435 patients with primary hyperparathyroidism found that the level of serum calcium was an independent predictor of mortality.

Our patient had bone mineral densitometry performed that revealed a significant reduction in cortical bone density at the distal radius. A parathyroid sestamibi scan demonstrated increased focal activity inferior to the right lobe of the thyroid gland. At surgery, a 1-cm adenoma was identified in the right inferior parathyroid gland, which was successfully resected. She has noted some improvement in her symptoms of depression. Her PTH has normalized and she continues on calcium supplementation for her osteopenia; she is scheduled for bone mineral densitometry in 1 year.

 ## CLINICAL PEARLS

⟡ PHP is a common disorder of calcium hemostasis caused by an increased secretion of parathyroid hormone.

- The majority of patients are asymptomatic at the time of diagnosis.
- It is most common in the fifth and sixth decades and has a higher predilection in women.
- Hypercalcemia and an elevated serum intact PTH level is the laboratory hallmark of PHP.
- Over 80 percent of cases are the result of a single hyperfunctioning parathyroid adenoma.
- Bone mineral densitometry provides an accurate and sensitive method for the detection of hyperparathyroid bone disease.
- Surgery is curative in over 90 percent of cases.

REFERENCES

1   Zahrani AA, Levine MA. Primary hyperparathyroidism. *Lancet* 1997; 349:1233–1238.
2.   Silverberg SJ, Bilezikian JP. Evaluation and management of primary hyperparathyroidism. *J Clin Endocrinol* 1996; 81:2036–2040.
3.   Consensus development conference panel. Diagnosis and management of asymptomatic primary hyperparathyroidism: Consensus development conference statement. *Ann Intern Med* 1991; 114:593–597.
4.   Turton, DB, Miller, DL. Recent advances in parathyroid imaging. *Trends Endocrinol Metab* 1996; 7:163–168.
5.   Collins MT, Skarulis MC, Bilezikian JP, et al. Treatment of hypercalcemia secondary to parathyroid carcinoma with a novel calcimimetic agent. *J Clin Endocrinol Metab* 1998; 83:1083–1088.
6.   Nemeth EF, Steffey ME, Hammerland LG, et al. Calcimimetics with potent and selective activity on the parathyroid calcium receptor. *Proc Natl Acad Sci USA* 1998; 95:4040–4045.
7.   Wermers RA, Khosla S, Atkinson EJ, et al. Survival after the diagnosis of hyperparathyroidism: A population-based study. *Am J Med* 1998; 104:115–122.

77-YEAR-OLD MAN WITH SHOULDER PAIN AFTER A MYOCARDIAL INFARCTION

A 77-year-old man with a history of arthritis and an abdominal aortic aneurysm repair presented to the emergency room with a 2-hour history of chest pain associated with nausea and diaphoresis. He had no history of prior myocardial infarction or hypertension and was taking no medications. His admission ECG was consistent with an acute inferior-posterior myocardial infarction, but despite prompt thrombolytic therapy, his pain and ECG changes persisted. Cardiac catheterization revealed an inferior-posterior wall motion abnormality and a totally occluded proximal right coronary artery that was opened with angioplasty; however, he developed bradycardia and hypotension, requiring a pacemaker and balloon pump. Peak creatinine kinase was 4500 U/L (MB 850 ng/ml). Over the ensuing 48 hours, he was weaned from the balloon pump and the pacemaker was removed. In spite of this, he developed persistent shoulder and back pain, intermittent nausea, and emesis.

PHYSICAL EXAMINATION

VITAL SIGNS: Temperature, 100.9°F (38°C); pulse, 82; blood pressure, 110/70 mmHg (left) 112/74 mmHg (right); respiration, 18
GENERAL: Agitated, confused, complaining of bilateral shoulder pain
LUNGS: Bilateral basilar rales
CARDIAC: No murmurs, gallops or rubs; 2 cm of JVD, pulses 2+ throughout

ABDOMEN: Unremarkable

EXTREMITIES: No edema

LABORATORY FINDINGS

Electrolytes normal; WBC, 22.3 K/mL (1% bands, 85% PMNs, 6% lymphocytes, 8% monocytes); Hb, 13.2 g/dL; chest x-ray revealed mild congestive heart failure and bilateral atelectasis; ECG is shown (Fig. 16-1).

What is the likely diagnosis and how should this patient be treated?

This patient ruptured the posterior wall of his left ventricle after sustaining an acute transmural, inferoposterior myocardial infarction. The electrocardiogram demonstrates persistent ST segment elevation 48 hours after successful angioplasty.

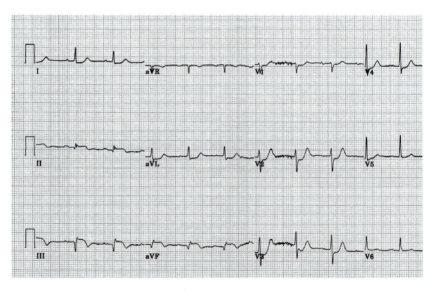

Figure 16-1.
Electrocardiogram.

Most deaths that occur during hospitalization for acute myocardial infarction are due to severe left ventricular dysfunction or a mechanical complication of the infarction, such as severe mitral regurgitation from papillary muscle rupture, right ventricular infarction, or rupture of the intraventricular septum or the left ventricular free wall.

About 10 percent of fatal myocardial infarctions are due to rupture of the free wall of the left ventricle from a large transmural infarction caused by occlusion of a single large vessel with poor collaterals. Rupture of the lateral wall is most common. This usually occurs in the setting of an acute occlusion of the left circumflex artery causing an inferoposterolateral infarction. Myocardial rupture typically occurs within 5 days, but may occur as late as 3 weeks after the infarct. It happens more frequently in women, hypertensives, and elderly patients having their first myocardial infarction. Other possible risk factors include the late administration of thrombolytic therapy and use of corticosteroid or NSAIDs.

Myocardial rupture appears to be a stuttering process of thrombus propagation and hemorrhage within the myocardium. The resulting pericardial inflammation may wall off the rupture, producing a pseudoaneurysm of the left ventricle.

The clinical presentation varies. There may be an acute myocardial tear causing hemopericardium with cardiac tamponade and electrical-mechanical dissociation. Or the course may be more subacute, manifested by pericarditis-type chest pain, vomiting, agitation, and transient bradycardia with hypotension; however, the presence of two or more of these symptoms in a patient with an acute myocardial infarction is highly predictive of a rupturing myocardium.

The diagnosis is also suggested by persistent ST segment elevation or failure to develop the typical T-wave inversion of myocardial infarction. Both findings are consistent with localized pericarditis and are very different from the usual pattern of an acute transmural infarction. Typically, the acute 1 to 5-mm ST segment elevation seen with an uncomplicated infarction recedes, without intervention, to ≤3 mm within 1 to 2 days, and the T waves become inverted within 1 to 3 days. The most negatively inverted T waves usually occur in the leads that at first show the most ST segment elevation.

Patients with symptoms or ECG changes that suggest myocardial rupture, especially during the first week after an acute myocardial infarction, should be urgently evaluated for this complication.

In an urgent situation, immediate pericardiocentesis will provide temporary relief of pericardial tamponade and confirm the diagnosis prior to emergency surgical repair. In a less acute situation, the diagnosis is easily established with echocardiography, with or without guided pericardio-centesis. Reports from large medical centers experienced in the management of this complication indicate that a long-term survival rate of 50 percent can be achieved with surgical repair of a subacute rupture. The results are much less favorable with an acute rupture.

This patient became acutely unstable and developed electrical mechani-cal dissociation. He was unresponsive to an ACLS protocol, including peri-cardiocentesis. Postmortem examination confirmed a large inferoposterior myocardial infarction with posterior wall rupture and hemopericardium. There was no evidence of an old myocardial infarction. The shoulder pain was likely referred pain as a consequence of diaphragmatic irritation, not uncommonly seen with an inferoposterior myocardial infarction.

 CLINICAL PEARLS

- Myocardial rupture accounts for 10 percent of the deaths from acute myocardial infarction.
- This usually occurs within 5 days of an acute myocardial infarction. Chest pain, emesis, agitation, hypotension, and bradycardia suggest the diagnosis.
- Persistent ST segment elevation and failure of the T-waves to invert after an acute MI suggest rupture.
- Long-term survival can be achieved by emergency surgery in pa-tients with subacute rupture.

REFERENCES

1. Oliva PB, Hammill SC, Edwards WD. Cardiac rupture, a clinically predictable complication of acute myocardial infarction: Report of 70 cases with clinicopathologic correlations. *J Am Coll Cardiol* 1993; 22:720–726.
2. Reeder GS. Identification and treatment of complications of myo-cardial infarction. *Mayo Clin Proc* 1995; 70:880–884.
3. Lopez-Sendon J, Gonzalez A, Lopez de Sa E, et al. Diagnosis of subacute ventricular wall rupture after acute myocardial infarction: Sensitivity and specificity of clinical, hemodynamic and echocardio-graphic criteria. *J Am Coll Cardiol* 1992; 19:1145–1153.

74-YEAR-OLD WOMAN WITH A RASH AND SHORTNESS OF BREATH

A 74-year-old woman with a history of hypertension presented with a chronic rash, low-grade fevers, and shortness of breath. She reported a 5-week history of an urticarial rash that began on her trunk and spread to her extremities and head. Following a failed course of topical anti-fungal therapy and prednisone, she was admitted to her local hospital and treated with a 14-day course of IV methylprednisolone. Her hospital course was complicated by hyperglycemia, hypertension, progressive weakness, and fatigue. Medical records revealed blood eosinophilia and a punch biopsy consistent with urticaria. After gradual improvement in her symptoms and rash, she was discharged to home. Two days later, she presented to The Ohio State University Health Sciences Center with worsening fatigue, shortness of breath, and persistent low-grade fevers.

Medications on admission included prednisone 20 mg po bid, diltiazem, glyburide, xanax, and hydroxyzine. She had a non-productive cough, but denied nausea, vomiting, diarrhea, chest pain, or syncope. She did not drink alcohol or smoke tobacco. She denied recent travel, pet or insect exposures, and the use of new medications, soaps, or personal hygiene products. However, she did recall cleaning her basement 3 months earlier, after area flooding caused her septic tank to overflow.

PHYSICAL EXAMINATION

VITAL SIGNS: Temperature, 100.1°F (37.7°C); pulse, 88; respiration, 20; blood pressure, 120/78 mmHg
GENERAL: Mildly obese
HEENT: Normal
NECK: No lymphadenopathy or thyromegaly
LUNGS: Clear
CARDIAC: Normal
ABDOMEN: Mildly distended, normoactive bowel sounds; no hepatosplenomegaly
EXTREMITIES: No cyanosis or edema
NEUROLOGIC: Nonfocal
SKIN: Confluent erythematous macular rash over the trunk, buttocks, and groin; scattered papular erythematous lesions on the extremities with evidence of excoriation

LABORATORY FINDINGS

WBC 4.9 K/μL (normal differential); Hb, 12.8 g/dL (MCV 84 fl), platelets, 242 K/μL; electrolytes: sodium 129 mmol/L, potassium 4.6 mmol/L, chloride 95 mmol/L, bicarbonate 22 mmol/L; urea nitrogen, 30 mg/dL; creatinine, 0.8 mg/dL; arterial blood gas, pH 7.44, P_{CO_2} 37 mmHg, P_{O_2} 100 mmHg, H_{CO_3} 25 mmol/L, O_2 sat. 98%; chest x-ray, normal

HOSPITAL COURSE

Shortly after admission the patient began to complain of diffuse abdominal pain. Abdominal films and ultrasound were unremarkable. Stool, urine, and blood cultures were negative. On hospital day 5, the patient became confused and was noted to be hypoxic. A repeat chest x-ray revealed a five-lobe infiltrate. Cerebrospinal fluid and blood cultures grew *Klebsiella* pneumoniae. A Gram stain of the bronchoalveolar lavage (BAL) specimen is shown (Fig. 17-1).

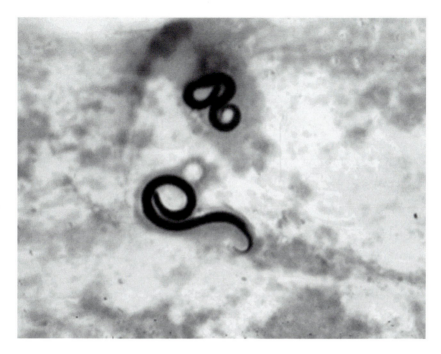

Figure 17-1.
Gram stain of BAL specimen. (See Plate 9.)

What is the likely diagnosis and how should this patient be treated?

This patient has the hyperinfection syndrome of *Strongyloides stercoralis* infection. The BAL specimen demonstrates the characteristic filariform larvae of this helminthic parasite.

Intestinal parasitic nematode infections are one of the most common infections worldwide. The fecally transmitted forms are endemic in tropical and subtropical regions, and in certain temperate climates, including the southeastern United States. Transmission of these organisms may occur whenever there is human fecal contamination or exposure. Although the severity of most intestinal nematode infections is dependent upon the acquired worm burden, in Strongyloidiasis, the disease may progress months to years after exposure as a consequence of internal auto-infection.

Strongyloides stercoralis is the organism responsible for Strongyloidiasis. Infection begins after filariform larvae from a fecally contaminated source penetrate the skin or a mucous membrane and enter the venous circulation. They follow venous blood flow to the lungs, cross into the airways, ascend the tracheobronchial tree, and are then swallowed (Fig. 17-2). The tiny (2-mm-long) adult female worms embed in the small bowel mucosal wall where they reproduce by parthenogenesis. They are rarely found in stool specimens because they inhabit the bowel tissue and not the lumen. Their eggs hatch almost immediately to form rhabditiform larvae that are evacuated in the feces.

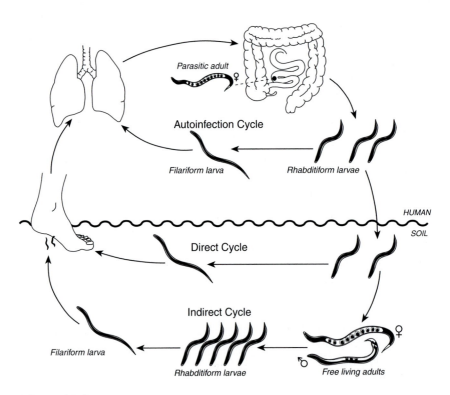

Figure 17-2
Life cycle of Strongyloides stercoralis.

The rhabditiform larvae can then develop into a free-living organism (indirect cycle) or into infective filariform larvae (direct cycle) depending on local conditions (Fig. 17-1). Importantly, the seriousness of this infection has to do with the ability of the rhabditiform larvae to develop into filariform larvae while in the bowel. These invasive larvae can then cross the mucosal surface (via intestinal mucosa or perianal skin) and enter the venous circulation to establish an "autoinfection" cycle. As a result, the infection may progress after a single, possibly remote, exogenous exposure.

The clinical features of this disease reflect the degree of gastrointestinal, pulmonary, and skin involvement by the organism. Most infected individuals have low worm burdens and are asymptomatic; however, when symptoms do occur they are often short-lived and appear at irregular intervals. The most common gastrointestinal symptoms are postprandial abdominal pain, nausea, vomiting, or diarrhea. Pulmonary involvement is manifested by cough, wheezing, and dyspnea. Larva currens is the pathognomonic skin lesion seen in chronic strongyloidiasis. It is a rapid evolving (up to 5–10 cm/h) serpiginous rash that is a consequence of the filariform larva migrating in the skin. A chronic urticarial rash may also occur, with fixed urticarial wheals involving the trunk and extremities.

The hyperinfection syndrome develops when there is a rapid acceleration of the autoinfection cycle with subsequent increase in the worm burden. Corticosteroids and other immunosuppressant agents are responsible for the majority of cases in the United States. It typically presents insidiously with nonspecific gastrointestinal symptoms as a result of the worms disrupting the integrity of the bowel mucosa. Further progression may lead to diffuse pulmonary infiltrates with respiratory failure, gram-negative (owing to enteric flora from damaged bowel) sepsis, and meningitis. Disseminated strongyloidiasis occurs when filariform larvae spread to organs outside the gastrointestinal and respiratory tracts.

Unfortunately, strongyloidiasis is a very difficult diagnosis to establish. The parasite load in most infected individuals is very low and the larval output is irregular. The definitive diagnosis requires direct visualization of the organism and no test is 100 percent sensitive. In fact, a single stool examination will detect only about 30 percent of uncomplicated infections. The sensitivity increases to 50 percent with three samples and nearly 100 percent with seven samples. Alternative diagnostic tests include concentrated stool examination, duodenal sampling, and serologic assays. Blood eosinophilia may be present early, but is often mild and nonspecific.

Thiabendazole remains the treatment of choice for strongyloidiasis. The standard dose in the United States is 25 mg/kg in three divided daily doses for two consecutive days. In the hyperinfection syndrome, treatment should be administered for 7 to 10 days or more, until parasites can no longer be detected. Because of its numerous side effects, most experts argue against empiric therapy in patients only suspected of having strongyloidiasis, and suggest aggressive measures to establish the diagnosis. Ivermectin, a novel agent with similar efficacy to thiabendazole and fewer side effects, has recently received FDA approval.

Fulminant strongyloidiasis has a very poor prognosis, but some patients have been cured. Our patient developed multi-organ system failure and died on hospital day 21. Her exposure likely occurred while cleaning after the septic tank overflowed. Importantly, because corticosteroids can activate strongyloidiasis, it may not be advisable to treat patients from an endemic area or following a suspicious exposure with immunosuppressants until infection has been ruled out.

CLINICAL PEARLS

- Intestinal nematode infections are among the most common infections worldwide.
- *Stronglyloides stercoralis* is the organism responsible for strongyloidiasis.
- This organism's virulence is in it's ability to establish an "autoinfection" cycle after a single and sometimes remote exposure.
- The symptoms reflect the organ systems involved in its life cycle (skin, gastrointestinal, and pulmonary); larva currens is the pathognomonic skin lesion.
- Strongyloidiasis is the most difficult parasitic infection to diagnose.
- A rapid increase in worm burden, usually caused by immunosuppresants (e.g., corticosteroids) leads to the *hyperinfection syndrome*, typically manifest by pulmonary infiltrates, gram-negative sepsis, and meningitis.

REFERENCES

1. Heyworth MF. Parasitic diseases in immunocompromised hosts: Cryptosporidiosis, isosporiasis, and strongyloidiasis. *Gastro Clin North Am* 1996; 25:691–707.

2. Liu LX, Weller PF. Strongyloidiasis and other intestinal nematode infections. *Infect Dis Clin North Am* 1993; 7:655–682.
3. Liu LX, Weller PF. Drug therapy: Antiparasitic drugs. *N Engl J Med* 1996; 334:1178–1184.

34-YEAR-OLD WOMAN WITH DIABETES MELLITUS

A 34-year-old African-American woman with type 1 diabetes mellitus presented to establish herself as a new patient shortly after moving into town. She had no complaints and was feeling well. She felt that her diabetes, diagnosed when she was 13 years old, had been under fairly good control. She had experienced only a few episodes of diabetic ketoacidosis as a youngster and had not been hospitalized for over 20 years. She seemed to have a good understanding of the management of her disease and had experienced no significant episodes of hypoglycemia. She was taking Lente insulin 20 units and regular insulin 5 units before breakfast, and Lente insulin 10 units before bedtime. Her recorded fasting blood glucose concentrations, which she brought to the office, ranged from 130 to 140 mg/dL but she did not check her blood glucose levels later in the day. Her last glycated hemoglobin three months ago was 8.9 percent (normal, 4.8–7.8%). She performed aerobic exercises occasionally, did not use tobacco or alcohol, and took no other drugs. She saw an ophthalmologist and gynecologist annually.

PHYSICAL EXAMINATION

VITAL SIGNS: Temperature, 98.4°F (approx 36.8°C); pulse, 98; respiration, 24; bp 148/92 mmHg; weight, 108 pounds; height, 64 inches
GENERAL: Thin, otherwise normal woman
HEENT: Eyes: fundus (Fig. 18-1)
NECK: No thyromegaly
LUNGS: Clear

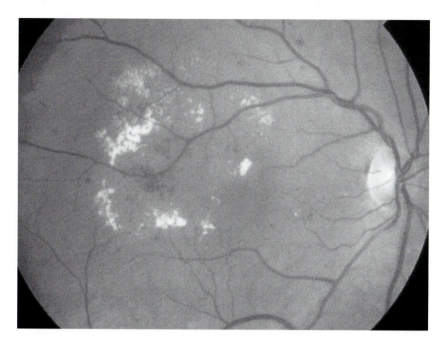

Figure 18-1.
Fundoscopic exam of right eye. (See Plate 10.)

CARDIAC: Normal

ABDOMEN: Normal

EXTREMITIES: Feet: no excoriations or other skin lesions; normal dorsalis pedis and posterior tibialis pulses

NEUROLOGIC: Light touch perception decreased on both legs to the knees; vibratory sensation diminished in legs and feet; muscle strength normal

SKIN: No lesions

LABORATORY FINDINGS

WBC, 4.3 K/μL (normal differential); Hb, 13.4 g/dL; platelets, 196 K/μL; electrolytes, normal; urea nitrogen, 22 mg/dL; creatinine, 1.1 mg/dL; serum glucose, 241 mg/dL; serum glycosylated hemoglobin, 8.5%; urinalysis, normal; no protein; urine microalbumin, 330 mg/24 hours.

What is the likely diagnosis and how should this patient be treated?

This patient's diabetes is not being well controlled and she has evidence of early microangiopathy causing diabetic nephropathy, retinopathy, and neuropathy. Her fundus reveals changes consistent with non-proliferative diabetic retinopathy (formerly known as background diabetic retinopathy), which include intraretinal hemorrhages, yellow hard exudates, and cotton wool spots.

The earliest clinical evidence of diabetic nephropathy is the appearance of low but abnormal levels (>30 mg/day) of albumin in the urine (Table 18-1). Referred to as microalbuminuria, this is the earliest indication of incipient nephropathy. Without specific intervention, most patients with this finding (80 percent) increase their urinary albumin excretion rate

TABLE 18–1   Clinical Evidence of Diabetic Nephropathy

| | | NEPHROPATHY | |
TEST FOR MICROALBUMIN*	NORMAL	INCIPIENT MICRO-ALBUMINURIA	CLINICALLY OVERT ALBUMINURIA
24-hour urine collection	<30 mg/ 24 hour	30–300 mg/ 24 hour	>300 mg/ 24 hour
Timed collection	<20 μg/ minute	20–200 μg/ minute	>200 μg/ minute
Spot collection	<30 μg/mg creatinine	30–300 μg/mg creatinine	>300 μg/mg creatinine

*Because of variability in urinary albumin excretion, two of three specimens collected within 3 to 6 months should be abnormal before considering a patient to have progressed to the next diagnostic category. Urinary albumin excretion may be increased over baseline by exercise within 24 hours, infection, fever, heart failure, marked hyperglycemia, and hypertension. Modified from American Diabetic Association Guidelines on the Management of Diabetic Nephropathy.

about 10 to 20 percent per year, developing overt nephropathy with clinical albuminuria (>300 mg/24 hours) over 10 to 15 years. Once this occurs, the glomerular filtration rate (GFR) falls at a highly variable rate, ranging from 2 to 20 mL/minute each year, leading to end-stage renal disease (ESRD) in about half of the patients within 10 years.

About 20 to 30 percent of patients with type 1 or 2 diabetes develop nephropathy, but a considerably smaller fraction progress to ESRD. Nevertheless, diabetes is the most common cause of ESRD in the United States. Although a much smaller fraction of patients with type 2 diabetes progress to ESRD, they constitute over half the patients starting on dialysis, because of their much greater prevalence than type 1 diabetics. Among patients with type 2 diabetes mellitus, there is substantial racial and ethnic variability in the development of ESRD, with African Americans, Native Americans, and Hispanics (especially Mexican-Americans) having much higher risks of developing ESRD than Caucasians. If nephropathy has not occurred after 25 to 30 years of diabetes, the risk of developing it begins to decrease. The duration of diabetes, diabetes control and, perhaps, family history of hypertension are all risk factors for nephropathy.

Recent studies have demonstrated that the onset and course of diabetic nephropathy can be ameliorated to a significant degree by several interventions. However, most of them have their greatest impact only when instituted very early in the development of this complication. Routine urinalysis should be performed yearly in adults with diabetes. If there is no proteinuria and the patient has had type 1 diabetes for over 5 years, a test for the presence of microalbumin should be done (see Table 18-1). Screening prepubertal children is unnecessary since microalbuminuria rarely occurs before puberty. Since there is marked day-to-day variability in albumin excretion, at least two or three collections done over about 6 months should show elevated levels before the diagnosis of diabetic nephropathy is made.

The Diabetes Control and Complications Trial (DCCT) and other studies have shown that intensive diabetes therapy can significantly reduce the risk of developing microalbuminuria and overt nephropathy. Strict glycemic control usually is achieved with three or more insulin injections daily or treatment with an insulin pump. In the DCCT, this resulted in about a 40 percent reduction in the occurrence of microalbuminuria. In one study, the risk of microalbuminuria in patients with type 1 diabetes was found to increase abruptly above a glycated hemoglobin value of 8.1 percent, suggesting that efforts to reduce the frequency of diabetic nephropathy should be focused on reducing glycated hemoglobin values that are above this threshold. There is a close relationship between the level of blood glucose control and the risk of complications. Patients should accordingly aim for the best level of control that can be achieved without placing themselves at undo risk of serious hypoglycemia or other hazards associated with strict blood glucose control. Some believe the goal of intensive glucose control is to reach the mean plasma glucose and glycated hemoglobin levels achieved in the intensive treatment group in the DCCT: mean blood glucose of 155 mg/dL and a glycosylated hemoglobin of about 7.2 percent. However, this degree of glycemic control is unattainable without very careful monitoring and good support for the patient. The patient under discussion should be treated more aggressively to improve her blood glucose levels. There is evidence that the cumulative incidence of diabetic nephropathy, as manifested by persistent albuminuria, among patients who have had diabetes for 25 years, has decreased substantially in the past decade, probably due to improved glycemic control.

Hypertension in patients with type 1 diabetes, which is usually caused by underlying diabetic nephropathy, typically becomes manifest when a patient develops microalbuminuria. Both systolic and diastolic hypertension seriously accelerates the progression of diabetic nephropathy. Conversely, aggressive management of hypertension substantially decreases the rate of fall of the GFR. It reduces the mortality from about 95 to 45 percent and lessens the need for dialysis and renal transplantation from over 70 percent to about 30 percent 15 years after a patient develops overt nephropathy. Hypertension is generally associated with an expanded plasma volume that decreases plasma renin activity. The goal of therapy for nonpregnant diabetic patients 18 years of age and older is to decrease blood pressure to maintain it at 130 mmHg systolic and 85 mmHg diastolic. Indeed, some suggest even lower target goals, but there is insufficient data on this issue.

Treatment with ACE inhibitors is indicated as a part of the initial therapy for patients with diabetic nephropathy. Many studies have shown that ACE inhibitors reduce the level of albuminuria and the rate of progression of renal disease in hypertensive diabetics more than that achieved by other antihypertensive agents that lower blood pressure an equal amount. ACE inhibitors have few adverse effects and may even have modest beneficial effects on lipid metabolism and insulin sensitivity. However, these drugs may exacerbate hyperkalemia in diabetic patients with renal insufficiency or hyporeninemic hypoaldosteronism. Moreover, renal function may decline in patients with advanced renal failure who are treated with this group of drugs. Cough may occur and rarely a patient develops angioedema from an ACE inhibitor. The salutary effect of ACE inhibitors is a class effect, making the choice of a specific agent a decision that depends on cost and compliance issues. This class of drugs is contraindicated in pregnant women. The new angiotensin II receptor blockers may have renal protective effects, but have not been completely studied in this regard. Thus, because of their benefits in retarding the progression of diabetic nephropathy, and their efficacy as antihypertensive agents, ACE inhibitors are the drugs of choice in the treatment of all hypertensive diabetic patients with microalbuminuria or overt nephropathy. Patients who do not tolerate ACE inhibitors should be treated with the benzothiazepine (diltiazem) or phenylalkylamine classes of calcium-channel blockers.

In addition to control of blood glucose and hypertension, dietary protein restriction may benefit patients with diabetic nephropathy. Although the effects of protein restriction are controversial, the American Diabetes Association recommends a dietary protein intake of no more than 0.8 g/kg daily (about 10 percent of calories) in a patient with overt nephropathy. It is suggested that once the GFR begins to fall, further restriction to 0.6 g/kg daily may prove useful in slowing the decline of GFR in some patients. This must be done with careful supervision since nutritional deficiency can occur that may be associated with muscle weakness and wasting.

Aside from being the earliest marker for diabetic nephropathy, albuminuria is also a marker of increased risk for cardiovascular morbidity and mortality in patients with type 1 or 2 diabetes. Accordingly, finding microalbuminuria is an indication for screening a patient for possible vascular disease and for aggressively intervening to reduce all cardiovascular risk factors—LDL cholesterol lowering, smoking cessation, treating hypertension, and instituting an exercise program.

Our patient was instructed on aggressive glycemia control and her glycosylated hemoglobin fell to 7.4 percent in 3 months. She was started on an ACE inhibitor and her microalbuminuria has remained stable for several years. Her LDL cholesterol was elevated (243 mg/dL) and a statin drug was started. Recently, she has begun to participate in an aerobic exercise program. Her funduscopic exam has remained stable.

CLINICAL PEARLS

- The earliest clinical evidence of diabetic nephropathy is an abnormal level (>30 mg/day) of albumin in the urine.
- African Americans, Native Americans, and Hispanics (especially Mexican-Americans) with type 2 diabetes have a higher than usual risk of developing end-stage renal disease from diabetes.
- Diabetic nephropathy can be ameliorated to a significant degree by several interventions: aggressive glycemia and blood pressure control, use of ACE inhibitors, and modest protein restriction.
- Hypertension in patients with type 1 diabetes is caused by the underlying diabetic nephropathy and typically becomes manifest when a patient develops microalbuminuria.
- Blood pressure in diabetic patients 18 years of age and older with nephropathy should be decreased to 130 mmHg systolic and 85 mmHg diastolic.
- Albuminuria is also a marker of cardiovascular risk.

REFERENCES

1. Krolewski AS, Laffel LMB, Krolewski M, et al. Glycosylated hemoglobin and the risk of microalbuminuria in patients with insulin-dependent diabetes mellitus. *N Engl J Med* 1995; 332:1251–1255.
2. Bojestig M, Arnqvist HJ, Hermansson G, Karlberg BE, et al. Declining incidence of nephropathy in insulin-dependent diabetes mellitus. *N Engl J Med* 1994; 330:15–18.
3. Lewis EJ, Hunsicker LG, Bain RP, et al. The effect of angiotensin-converting-enzyme inhibition on diabetic nephropathy. *N Engl J Med* 1993; 329:1456–1462.

TWO PREGNANT WOMEN WITH PERNICIOUS VOMITING

PATIENT 1

A 20-year-old African-American woman who was 8 weeks pregnant presented to the emergency department because of a 2-week history of refractory nausea and vomiting, which on four occasions contained small amounts of bright red blood. During this time she had lost about 5 pounds. She had a 1-week history of light-headedness upon standing, which on the day of admission was associated with syncope without seizure activity. She had noted swelling of her anterior neck over the past several years but had no other symptoms and was taking no medication. She had two first-trimester spontaneous abortions in the past, but 13 months earlier had a healthy girl by uncomplicated vaginal delivery.

PHYSICAL EXAMINATION

VITAL SIGNS: Temperature, 98°F (36.6°C); pulse, 117; respiration, 20; blood pressure, 138/68 mmHg (no orthostatic change)
GENERAL: Thin, ill-appearing woman in no acute distress
HEENT: Eyes: no proptosis or lid lag
NECK: Thyroid about twice the normal size without nodules or bruits (Fig. 19-1).
CARDIAC: Hyperdynamic precordium; grade II/VI aortic outflow tract murmur
ABDOMEN: Unremarkable
RECTAL: Guaiac positive stool
SKIN: Warm, moist, and smooth
NEUROLOGIC: Deep tendon reflexes normal

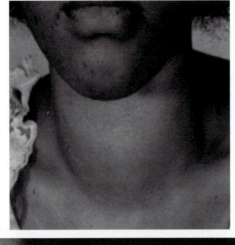

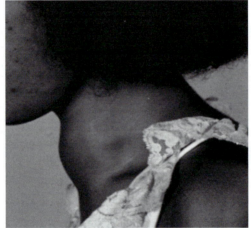

Figure 19-1.
(A) Anterior and (B) Lateral views of neck.

LABORATORY FINDINGS

Electrolytes, normal; WBC, 9200/μL, normal differential; platelet count, 224 K/μL; INR 1.1, PTT 25 sec; hemoglobin 13.0 g/dL; ESR 13 mm/hr; total thyroxine (T_4) 18.8 μg/dL (normal 5.0–11.0), *free* thyroxine index (FTI) 28.0 (normal 4.0–11.0); thyroid-stimulating hormone (TSH), <0.04 μU/mL (normal 0.2–5.0); thyroid-stimulating immunoglobulin (TSI) titer, 370 (0–130%); antimicrosomal antibody absent; quantitative β-human chorionic gonadotropin (β-hCG) 76,386 mIU/mL; fetal ultrasound, normal 8-week intrauterine pregnancy; gastroduodenoscopy, small

Mallory-Weiss tear at the esophagogastric junction without active bleeding.

PATIENT 2

A 25-year-old primigravid Caucasian woman in her ninth week of pregnancy was admitted to the obstetric service because of nausea and vomiting of 3 weeks' duration. Despite the use of promethazine, she was unable to take even liquids without vomiting and had lost about 5 pounds. She had a sore throat, but denied abdominal pain or diarrhea. She had no tremor, and had experienced no changes in vision, tachycardia, or palpitations. Ulcerative proctitis had been diagnosed during the past year.

PHYSICAL EXAMINATION

VITAL SIGNS: Temperature, 97.8°F (36.5°C); pulse, 88; respiration, 20; blood pressure, 110/90 mmHg (no orthostatic change)
GENERAL: A thin young woman
HEENT: Eyes: no proptosis or lid lag
NECK: No goiter or thyroid nodules
CARDIAC: Regular rate and rhythm; no murmurs, gallops, or rubs
ABDOMEN: Unremarkable
NEUROLOGIC: Deep tendon reflexes normal, no tremor

LABORATORY FINDINGS

Electrolytes: sodium, 136 mmol/L, potassium, 3.3 mmol/L, chloride 102 mmol/L, bicarbonate 22 mmol/L, ionized calcium 2.42 mEq/L (2.0–2.4 mEq/L); blood urea nitrogen, 5 mg/dL; creatinine, 0.6 mg/dL; serum glucose, 192 mg/dL; serum triglyceride, 93 mg/dL; hemoglobin, 12.4 g/dL; thyroid-stimulating hormone (TSH), <0.04 μIU/mL; *free* total serum thyroxine (T_4), 2.61 ng/dL (0.71–1.85 ng/dL); total triiodothyronine (T_3), 284 ng/dL (80–160 ng/dL); *free* T_3, 430 pg/dL (230–420 pg/dL); microsomal antibody absent; upper abdominal ultrasonography, no gallstones or pancreatic mass; fetal ultrasonography, normal 9-week intrauterine pregnancy.

What are the likely diagnoses and how should these patients be treated?

The first patient has thyrotoxicosis owing to Graves' disease. The second has the syndrome of hyperemesis gravidarum with mild, self-limiting thyrotoxicosis.

During a normal pregnancy, the basal metabolic rate increases about 20 percent and estrogens stimulate the hepatic production of thyroid-binding globulin (TBG). As a result, the total serum thyroxine (T_4) and triiodothyronine (T_3) concentrations rise well above normal early in pregnancy; however, serum *free* thyroid hormone concentrations remain within normal limits. Serum TSH levels fall slightly but also remain within normal limits. Despite this slight increase in thyroid activity during pregnancy, goiter usually does not develop. Therefore, the presence of a goiter during pregnancy should be regarded with suspicion.

β-human chorionic gonadotropin (β-hCG) can stimulate the thyroid; β-hCG at a concentration of 50,000 U/L is estimated to be equivalent to a TSH level of 35 μU/mL. This probably accounts for the abnormal thyroid stimulation that occurs in some pregnancies and with some trophoblastic tumors.

Thyrotoxicosis occurs in about 0.2 percent of pregnant women in the United States. Heat intolerance and fatigue of a normal pregnancy may mimic thyrotoxicosis, but most thyrotoxic patients also report weight loss, anxiety, tremor, and dyspnea. Some also may develop pernicious vomiting. These symptoms, together with the presence of a goiter and resting tachycardia, are strongly suggestive of the diagnosis. Severe thyrotoxicosis may cause preeclampsia, premature labor, heart failure, or thyroid storm, and the fetus may be small, premature, or stillborn. The diagnosis can be verified by high serum *free* T_3 and T_4 concentrations and an undetectable serum TSH concentration. Importantly, although the majority of patients presenting with thyrotoxicosis during pregnancy have Graves' disease, hyperemesis gravidarum may manifest with similar abnormalities.

The first patient has Graves' disease. It affects 1 percent of American women and has a peak incidence in the reproductive years. Antibodies such as thyroid-stimulating immunoglobulin (TSI) stimulate the TSH receptor and cause a diffuse goiter with or without infiltrative eye signs. Although thyrotoxicosis tends to remit during pregnancy, it recurs after delivery in about half the women. Antithyroid drugs, either propylthiouracil (PTU) or methimazole (MMI), are the treatment of choice. However, they must be given in the lowest possible dose because they cross the placenta and can cause fetal goiter and hypothyroidism. PTU is preferred because less of it crosses the placenta. Neither drug affects thyroid function of the breast-feeding infant. *Aplasia cutis congenita*—a rare congenital absence of skin that usually involves the scalp—is associated with MMI but not PTU therapy during pregnancy. This patient was treated with PTU.

The second patient had hyperemesis gravidarum with altered thyroid function that produced mild thyrotoxicosis. Persistent nausea and vomiting occur in up to 30 percent of pregnant women, but hyperemesis gravidarum—pernicious vomiting with weight loss over 5 percent in the first 16 weeks of gestation—occurs in only about two of every 1000 pregnancies. Thyroid function tests often become abnormal, which is believed to be related to thyroid stimulation by β-hCG. Patients with this syndrome may demonstrate a spectrum of thyroid dysfunction. Some simply have an elevation of serum thyroxine with or without suppressed TSH concentrations and experience no symptoms of thyrotoxicosis. Others have all of the symptoms seen with Graves' thyrotoxicosis and have elevated *free* T_4 and T_3 concentrations with a suppressed serum TSH concentration, but do not have a palpable goiter or antithyroid antibodies; thyrotoxicosis typically remits spontaneously in the second trimester. Therefore, most women with hyperemesis gravidarum and abnormal thyroid function tests do not require antithyroid drug therapy. This patient was not treated with anti-thyroid drugs because her symptoms abated spontaneously after a few days of hydration in the hospital.

 ## CLINICAL PEARLS

- β-hCG stimulates the thyroid gland but does not cause goiter in normal pregnant women.
- Thyrotoxic pregnant women with Graves' disease lose weight, have a goiter, and require PTU therapy.

LABORATORY FINDINGS

WBC, 8.3 K/µL (normal differential); Hb, 11.5 g/dL (MCV 90 fl); platelets, 243 K/µL; serum electrolytes, urea nitrogen, and creatinine, normal; erythrocyte sedimentation rate (Westergren), 33 mm/Hr; C3, 32 mg/dL (normal, 80–178); C4, 7 mg/dL (normal, 12–42); liver function studies, activated partial thromboplastin time, and prothrombin time, normal; anti-phospholipid antibody, negative; ANA, positive (>1:320); dsDNA, negative; cerebrospinal fluid: glucose, 99 mg/dL; protein, 50 mg/dL; WBC, 2/µL (0 polys, 70 lymphs, 19 monos, 11 macros); RBC, 9/µL; VDRL, negative; HSV PCR, negative; head MRI, see Figure 20-1.

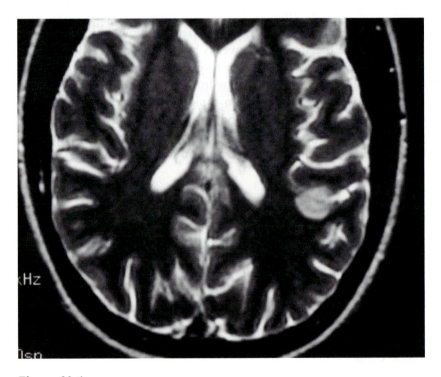

Figure 20-1
MRI of head.

What is the likely diagnosis?

This patient has neuropsychiatric lupus erythematosus (NPLE) or lupus cerebritis. The MRI demonstrates a small region of high signal intensity in the left temporo-parietal region consistent with cerebritis or infarction.

NPLE, which occurs in up to two-thirds of patients with SLE, may present with a variety of neurologic and psychiatric manifestations. Symptoms may appear at any time during the course of SLE, but typically occur within the first 2 years. They result directly from immune-mediated injury to the central nervous system (CNS) (primary events), or as the result of SLE involving other organs, complications of therapy, or both (Table 20-1). Primary events typically occur in a setting of clinically or serologically active SLE and rarely occur as an isolated event.

TABLE 20–1   **Neurologic and Psychiatric Manifestations of NPLE**

Primary Events
Vascular occlusion from immune-complex-mediated or antibody-mediated injury.
Cerebral dysfunction from antibodies to brain tissue (antineuronal, antiribosomal P protein) or cytokines
Secondary Events
Infection
Cerebrovascular accidents
Hypertensive encephalopathy
Metabolic encephalopathy
Hypercoagulable states
Drugs

*Adapted from Boumpas DT, Austin HA, III, Fessler BJ, et al. Systemic lupus erythematosus: Emerging concepts. I: Renal, neuropsychiatric, cardiovascular, pulmonary, and hematologic disease. *Ann Intern Med* 1995; 122:940–950.

The pathogenesis of NPLE is uncertain. There is a paucity of histologic findings despite severe clinical manifestations; the most frequent is multiple cerebral cortical microinfarctions. However, vasculitis and thrombosis are rare. The presenting manifestations may be focal symptoms involving the brain, spinal cord, and peripheral nervous system, but the most common are organic brain syndrome, psychiatric disturbances, and seizures (Table 20-2).

The organic brain syndrome (OBS) is characterized by various degrees of impaired cognition and memory, apathy, and disorientation, in the absence of a secondary cause (i.e., infection or drugs). OBS is estimated to affect about 20 percent of patients with SLE. However, some degree of cognitive impairment has been demonstrated by formal psychologic testing in up to 70 percent of patients with SLE and may occur without other symptoms. Severe cases may progress rapidly to delirium, stupor, or coma, whereas others may develop a slowly progressive dementia. Because cognitive deficits are often difficult to detect, a baseline evaluation should be done in all SLE patients.

Psychiatric disturbances have long been recognized as a manifestation of SLE. About 15 percent of patients with SLE develop an overt psy-

TABLE 20-2   Presenting Manifestations of NPLE

Diffuse cerebral dysfunction
   Organic brain syndrome (20%)
   Psychosis (10%)
   Major affective disorder (<1%)
Focal cerebral dysfunction
   Seizures, all types (15%)
   Cerebrovascular accidents (5%)
   Transverse myelitis (1%)
Movement disorders
Peripheral neuropathy
Autonomic neuropathy
Miscellaneous

*Adapted from Boumpas DT, Austin HA, III, Fessler BJ, et al. Systemic lupus erythematosus: Emerging concepts. I: Renal, neuropsychiatric, cardiovascular, pulmonary, and hematologic disease. *Ann Intern Med* 1995;122:940–950.

chosis. Although attributed to corticosteroid therapy in the past, the psychosis is now recognized to typically worsen after stopping steroid therapy, confirming its direct relationship to SLE in many cases. There is an association between lupus psychosis and anti-ribosomal P protein antibodies, which may help to distinguish it from drug-induced causes. Major depression, which commonly occurs in SLE, is also more typically a manifestation of SLE than a reactive process. Other less common psychiatric manifestations of SLE are anxiety, personality disorders, phobias, and manias.

Grand mal seizures, which are the most common type to occur in NPLE, are usually self-limited, although status epilepticus is not uncommon. They may occur in isolation or in association with other neurologic events such as strokes, intracranial hemorrhage, or vasculitis.

Primary NPLE is a clinical diagnosis that depends on excluding other causes of CNS symptoms, the most important of which are infection and side effects of medication. Although cerebrospinal fluid (CSF) is typically normal in NPLE, pleocytosis may be indicative of lupus cerebritis instead of infection. Electroencephalography is frequently abnormal but is nonspecific. MRI is the preferred imaging technique, because up to 80 percent of NLPE patients with a normal CT scan have an abnormal MRI. Unfortunately, the MRI manifestations are variable and none is specific for lupus cerebritis. For example, patients with OBS, psychosis, or depression often have a normal MRI, whereas patients with generalized seizures frequently have evidence of multiple, small microinfarcts, as seen in our patient. Serum antineuronal antibodies are commonly found in those patients with OBS or cognitive dysfunction, whereas antiribosomal-P antibody is seen in 45 to 90 percent of SLE patients presenting with psychosis or major depression, but none is diagnostic of the syndromes.

Treatment differs according to the clinical presentation, its severity, and underlying etiology. Patients presenting with mild diffuse manifestions may require only symptomatic treatment, whereas those with more severe or progressive diffuse presentations may benefit from immunosuppressant drugs. Corticosteroids are the agent of choice, although there have been no controlled trials proving their utility or that of other cytotoxic medications in the treatment of NLPE.

Although the majority of NPLE patients with diffuse symptoms appear to recover, studies suggest there often is residual cognitive dysfunction. Status epilepticus, strokes, and coma are poor prognostic signs. Our patient developed two additional seizures on the day of admission and was treated with phenytoin, corticosteroids, and cyclophosphamide. At the time of discharge, she had no evidence of residual deficits.

 # CLINICAL PEARLS

- NPLE occurs in up to two-thirds of SLE patients.
- The most common manifestations are organic brain syndrome, psychiatric disturbances, and seizures.
- NPLE symptoms typically occur within the first 2 years after SLE is diagnosed.
- NPLE is diagnosed in SLE by excluding other causes of neurologic and psychiatric symptoms.

REFERENCES

1. West SG. Neuropsychiatric lupus. *Rheum Dis Clin North Am* 1994; 20:129–158.
2. Boumpas DT, Austin HA, III, Fessler BJ, et al. Systemic lupus erythematosus: Emerging concepts. I: Renal, neuropsychiatric, cardiovascular, pulmonary, and hematologic disease. *Ann Intern Med* 1995; 122:940–950.
3. Ginsburg KS, Wright EA, et al. A controlled study of the prevalence of cognitive dysfunction in randomly selected patients with systemic lupus erythematosus. *Arthritis Rheumatol* 1992; 35:776–782.

54-YEAR-OLD MAN WITH OLIGURIA AND RIB PAIN

A 54-year-old man with a history of β-thalassemia, hepatitis A, and benign prostatic hypertrophy (BPH) presented to his physician with a 1-month history of decreased urine output and rib pain. He had a long standing history of BPH that had been well controlled with medication. Prostate specific antigen (PSA) was last checked 1 year ago. He denied any recent trauma to the ribs or cough. He did report progressive fatigue and generalized aching over the past 2 weeks, which he attributed to the flu. In addition, he had lost about 7 pounds over this time period. He denied hematuria, nausea/vomiting, fevers/chills, night sweats, or shortness of breath.

Medications on admission included doxazosin and aspirin. The family history was notable for thalassemia minor in his mother. He was married with two healthy children and worked as an administrator for a research foundation. He did not drink alcohol or smoke tobacco.

PHYSICAL EXAMINATION

VITAL SIGNS: Temperature, 97.4°F (36.3°C); pulse, 84; respiration, 16; blood pressure, 135/78 mmHg
GENERAL: Age-appropriate
HEENT: Normal
NECK: No lymph node enlargement or thyromegaly
CHEST: Point tenderness over the posterior 7th and 8th ribs bilaterally
LUNGS: Clear
CARDIAC: Normal
ABDOMEN: Normoactive bowel sounds, soft, nontender; no hepatosplenomegaly

EXTREMITIES: No cyanosis or edema

NEUROLOGIC: Nonfocal

RECTAL: Guaiac negative, normal sphincter tone; symmetrically enlarged and smooth prostate

LABORATORY FINDINGS

WBC, 4.9 K/μL (normal differential); Hb, 4.9 g/dL (MCV 70 fL); platelets, 205 K/μL; reticulocyte count (corrected), 0.1% (normal, 0.3–2.0%); electrolytes and glucose, normal; blood urea nitrogen, 39 mg/dL; creatinine, 4.0 mg/dL; calcium, 5.9 meq/L (normal, 4.3–5.2); LDH, alkaline phosphatase normal; prothrobin and partial thromboplastin time, normal; total protein, 10.7 g/dL (normal, 6.1–8.2); prostate specific antigen, 1.0 ng/ml (normal, 0.5–4.3); urinanalysis, normal; sulfosalicylic acid, positive; renal ultrasound: no hydronephrosis; chest x-ray: plate-like atelectatic changes of the right base; serum protein electrophoresis shown (Fig. 21-1).

What is the diagnosis?

This patient has multiple myeloma. The serum protein electrophoresis demonstrates a monoclonal spike in the gamma region, suspicious for an

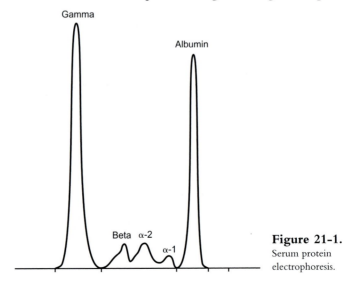

Figure 21-1.
Serum protein electrophoresis.

overproduction of IgG, which was confirmed by measurement of quantitative immunoglobulins (IgG 5341 mg/dL; normal, 576–1152).

Multiple myeloma (MM) is a malignant disorder of plasma cells. The clinical manifestations are a result of the uncontrolled proliferation and dissemination of a single clone of these cells with marrow replacement and overproduction of monoclonal protein. The cause of this disorder remains unknown; however, the transforming event likely occurs at the hematopoietic stem cell level.

MM accounts for about 10 percent of hematologic cancers and is responsible for 1 percent of cancer-related deaths. The yearly incidence is two to four per 100,000 population worldwide. The incidence increases with age and peaks during the seventh decade; the mean age at diagnosis is 62 years. It occurs more often in males than females, and in African Americans twice as often as Caucasians.

The most common complications from MM include bone destruction, infections, renal failure, anemia, and neurologic symptoms. Bone pain affects up to 70 percent of patients. The pain typically involves those sites where red marrow normally exists: the ribs, spine, sternum, clavicles, skull, and extremities (at the shoulder or pelvic girdles). Initially the pain may be intermittent and commonly involves the back and ribs. The bone lesions are caused by the proliferation of tumor cells and cytokines released by tumor cells, which stimulate osteoblasts to release interleukin-6, a potent growth factor for osteoclasts. The characteristic radiographic appearance of these lytic lesions are rounded, punched-out areas (Fig. 21-2). Because of their lytic character, radioisotopic bone scanning is usually not helpful (usually normal) and the serum alkaline phosphatase level is either normal or only slightly elevated. In addition, as a result of the bony lysis, large quantities of calcium may be mobilized, resulting in complications from severe hypercalcemia.

Bacterial infections are the next most common complication of MM. It has been estimated that over 75 percent of patients will develop a serious infection at some time in their disease course. They typically develop recurrent bouts of pneumonia, pyelonephritis, or sepsis. The most common pathogens include *Streptococcus pneumoniae*, *Klebsiella pneumoniae*, *Staphylococcus aureus*, and *Escherichia coli*; however, *S. aureus* predominates in the late stages of the disease and is responsible for the most deaths. A number of factors have been identified to account for this increased susceptibility to pyogenic infections; the majority are a consequence of quantitative and qualitative abnormalities in B and T lymphocytes. Hy-

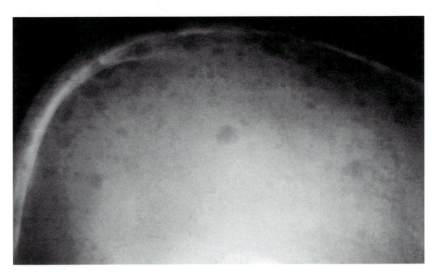

Figure 21-2.
Skull x-ray.

pogammaglobulinemia is commonly seen and is a result of decreased production and increased destruction of normal antibodies.

Hypercalcemia is the most common cause of renal failure in MM.
However, light chain (Bence Jones [BJ] protein) deposition in the
tubules, plasma cell infiltration, amyloidosis, glomerulo-sclerosis, hyperuricemia, NSAID use, hyperviscosity, and pyelonephritis all may contribute to the renal impairment. Albuminuria is rarely present early,
allowing for the easy identification of BJ proteinuria with sulfosalicylic
acid titration. The adult Fanconi syndrome (type 2 proximal renal tubular acidosis) may be an early manifestation of the tubular injury from light
chain depostion. Over time, the tubular cells become overloaded with
these proteins and large obstructing casts form, leading to distention and
destruction of the nephron (myeloma kidney). Some contrast agents may
cause light chains to precipitate within the kidney; therefore, patients
should be well hydrated prior to such procedures. Patients with MM
often have a negative anion gap, because the monoclonal protein provides additional cationic charge with subsequent retention of chloride. In
addition, pseudohyponatremia may occur in this setting from the volume
generated by the increased protein.

A severe normochromic, normocytic anemia occurs in the majority of
patients with MM. This is often multifactorial, caused by marrow re-

placement, renal insufficiency, and impaired red cell production. Blood smears can be difficult to interpret because of red cell clumping or rouleaux formation, which results from the increased globulin in the plasma causing cells to stick together (Fig. 21-3). A rapid sedimentation rate can also be seen in the setting of rouleaux formation. Clotting abnormalities may also occur due to the effect of monoclonal proteins on platelet function and clotting factors I, II, V, VII, and VIII. Although more frequently seen in primary macroglobulinemia (IgM), the hyperviscosity syndrome may occur in patients with MM with IgA or IgG proteins. The increased viscosity often interferes with circulation to the brain, eyes, lungs, kidneys, or digits. Undue sensitivity to cold by some monoclonal proteins, called cryoglobulinemia, may cause precipitation of protein at low temperatures and manifest as Raynaud's phenomenon.

Neurologic symptoms occur in a minority of patients and have a variety of causes. In approximately 10 percent of patients, plasma cell tumors cause vertebral body destruction and collapse, leading to spinal cord or

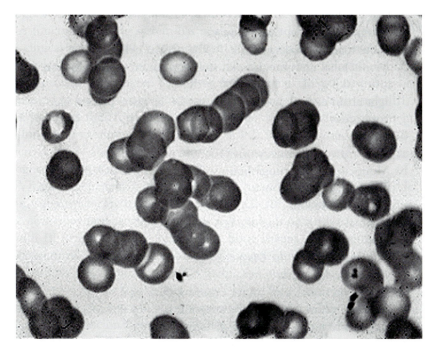

Figure 21-3
Rouleaux formation of red blood cells on peripheral blood smear. (See Plate 11.)

logeneic bone marrow transplantation has been demonstrated to cure up to 40 percent of selected patients (<55 years with an HLA-matched sibling donor). More recently, autologous transplantation has been utilized with achievement of long-term, disease-free survival.

Our patient received an autologous transplant with peripheral blood stem cells after failing standard therapy and VAD chemotherapy. He remains in remission 10 months following the transplant.

 CLINICAL PEARLS

- The incidence of MM increases with age and peaks during the seventh decade; it is more common in males and African Americans.
- The clinical manifestations are a result of a monoclonal proliferation of plasma cells.
- The classic diagnostic triad includes marrow plasmacytosis, lytic bone lesions, and serum or urine monoclonal protein.
- The most common complications include bone destruction, infections, renal failure, and anemia.
- The bone lesions are characteristically not detected by bone scanning and alkaline phosphatase is usually normal.
- Allogeneic and autologous bone marrow transplantation may provide long-term, disease-free survival in selected patients.

REFERENCES

1. Foerster J. Multiple myeloma, in *Wintrobe's Clinical Hematology*. Lee GR, Lukens J, Foerster J, et al (eds.). Athens, Malvern, PA, Lea & Febiger, 1993, pp 2219–2249.
2. Bataille R, Harousseau J. Multiple myeloma. *N Engl J Med* 1997; 336:1657–1664.
3. Alexanian R, Dimopoulos M. The treatment of multiple myeloma. *N Engl J Med* 1994; 330:484–489.
4. Schrier SL. Multiple myeloma and related serum protein disorders, in *The Scientific American Medicine CD-ROM*. New York, Scientific American Medicine, 1997.
5. Attal M, Harousseau J, Stoppa A, et al. A prospective, randomized trial of autologous bone marrow transplantation and chemotherapy in multiple myeloma. *N Engl J Med* 1996; 335:91–97.

59-YEAR-OLD WOMAN WITH A THYROID NODULE

An otherwise healthy, 59-year-old married Caucasian mother of three children was referred by her general internist for evaluation of a goiter first diagnosed when she was a teenager. At age 30, an open thyroid biopsy revealed tissue consistent with a colloid goiter and she was treated with thyroid hormone, which she stopped taking after about 1 year. Five years ago she felt the goiter was enlarging and consulted her family physician who prescribed levothyroxine 112 μg daily. Despite this therapy, the gland continued to enlarge and recently she developed hoarseness. She was advised to increase her dose of levothyroxine to 150 μg/day, but she sought another opinion. No one in the family had known thyroid disease. Mammography done 6 months ago was interpreted as normal. Her internist ordered a ^{123}I scan and referred her to our institution.

PHYSICAL EXAMINATION

VITAL SIGNS: Temperature, 98.2°F; pulse, 84; respiration, 14; bp, 146/76 mmHg

GENERAL: Normal-appearing woman with a visible goiter and a husky voice

HEENT: Normal

NECK: Thyroid: Enlarged to about twice normal size; nontender 4.0 cm firm nodule palpable in the left thyroid lobe that does not move upward with swallowing; no cervical lymph node enlargement (Fig. 22-1)

LUNGS: Clear

CARDIAC: Normal

ABDOMEN: No hepatosplenomegaly

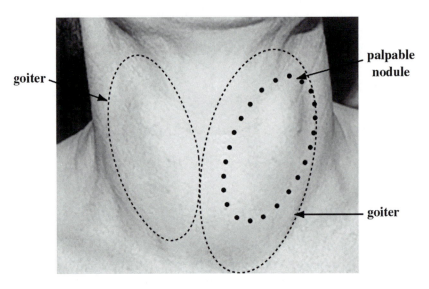

Figure 22-1
Anterior view of neck.

LABORATORY FINDINGS

TSH, 0.2 μU/mL (normal, 0.4–5.0). (The ^{123}I scan is shown in Fig. 22-2 and thyroid ultrasonography in Fig. 22-3.)

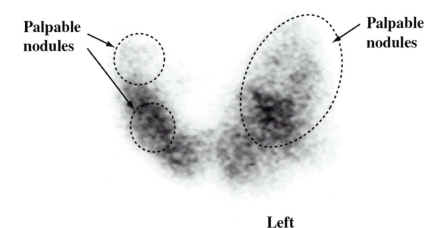

Figure 22-2
Thyroid scan.

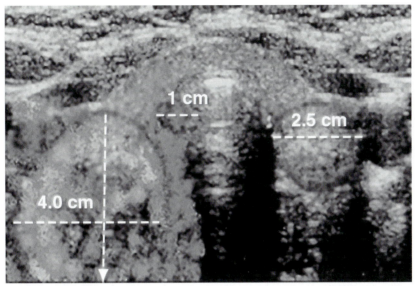

Left 6.7 cm

Figure 22-3
Thyroid ultrasound.

What is the likely diagnosis and how should this patient be treated?

This patient has an enlarging thyroid nodule in a diffuse colloid goiter associated with possible vocal cord paralysis, making a diagnosis of thyroid cancer highly likely. Although the thyroid scan and echography are both abnormal, the former showing patchy uptake of ^{123}I and the latter showing multiple nodules, neither provides adequate diagnostic information.

The frequency of palpable thyroid nodules, half of which are single on physical examination, increases throughout life, afflicting about 1 percent of an asymptomatic population around age 20 and increasing to about 5 percent in those age 50 and older. Nodules are detectable about ten times more often when the gland is examined by ultrasonography or in pathology specimens obtained at surgery or necropsy. A solitary thyroid nodule is defined as a palpably discrete swelling within an otherwise apparently normal gland, whereas a multinodular goiter is an enlarged thyroid gland with one or more palpable nodules. However, when apparently solitary thyroid nodules are studied by ultrasonography, about half the glands contain multiple nodules.

Most thyroid nodules (80%) occur in women and almost all are benign. Nonetheless, it is the concern about cancer that makes their evaluation so important. The frequency of thyroid cancer in thyroid nodules is low, around 4 percent of those subject to fine needle aspiration (FNA), and the incidence is the same whether the gland has a palpably single nodule or contains multiple nodules. This fact must be recognized by primary care physicians.

The differential diagnosis of a thyroid nodule mainly embraces the following disorders: thyroid adenoma, thyroid cancer, thyroid cyst, thyroiditis, and other inflammatory disorders. Papillary thyroid cancer is the most common thyroid malignancy. Fifteen to 25 percent of all thyroid nodules are cystic; a few are simple cysts, but the majority are hemorrhagic colloid nodules or necrotic papillary cancers.

It is important to ask about prior irradiation to the head, neck, and chest, or exposure to nuclear fallout, which remains an important clue to the diagnosis of cancer. Certain features suggest cancer in a thyroid nodule (Table 22-1). Two or more suspicious symptoms or signs, such as a rapidly growing nodule and hoarseness, suggest thyroid cancer with a high degree of probability. A nodule occurring at the extremes of age, particularly in men, is especially likely to be cancerous—the odds quadruple in men over 65. Rapid tumor growth and symptoms of local invasion also raise the probability of cancer. Growth of a thyroid nodule must be distinguished from intranodular hemorrhage that commonly occurs in benign colloid nodules, a distinction that can be made by ultrasonography. Our patient noticed growth of her nodule over several years that was not associated with intranodular hemorrhage, which should raise the suspicion of cancer. Coupled with the history of hoarseness, her clinical likelihood of cancer was very high.

A nodule larger than 1.0 cm in diameter can usually be palpated unless it lies deep within the neck. Once a nodule is palpated, the only laboratory tests usually necessary are a serum TSH level and a thyroid FNA. About 5 to 10 percent of thyroid nodules yield insufficient cytology for diagnosis. When this occurs, open biopsy often must be done to identify the pathology. When the cytology specimen is adequate to establish a diagnosis, about 4 percent are found to be malignant, about 70 percent are benign colloid nodules, and about 20 percent are highly cellular specimens showing sheets of normal or atypical follicular cells without colloid

TABLE 22–1   Relation between Clinical Findings and Malignant Thyroid Tumors

PROBABILITY OF CANCER	PATIENTS (%)	MALIGNANT (%)	CLINICAL FINDINGS
Low	44	11	No suspicious symptoms or signs
Moderate	38	14	Age <20 or >60 History of head or neck irradiation Male sex Dubious nodule fixation Nodule >4 cm in diameter and partly cystic
High	18	71	Rapid tumor growth Very firm nodule Fixation to adjacent structures Vocal-cord paralysis Enlarged regional lymph nodes

Modified from Mazzaferri EL. Management of a solitary thyroid nodule. *N Engl J Med* 1993;328:553–559. Data from Hamming JF, et al. *Arch Intern Med* 1990;150:113–116.

that are not clearly diagnostic of cancer (an indeterminate diagnosis). A thyroid scan should be done only in patients with a suppressed serum TSH level and in those with an indeterminate cytological diagnosis in an attempt to forestall surgery. A ^{123}I scan will identify the few patients with an autonomously hyperfunctioning (hot) thyroid nodule, which can be treated medically because a hot nodule is almost never caused by cancer. The others—those with malignant and indeterminate cytology—require surgery, since almost all of the former and about 20 percent of the latter have thyroid cancer found at thyroidectomy.

Thyroid hormone suppression of thyroid nodules is no longer used to diagnose thyroid cancer. This maneuver, which was widely employed before FNA became popular, has been largely abandoned because of its low diagnostic accuracy. A thyroid scan should not be done as the first diagnostic test, since most nodules are either hypofunctional (cold) or concentrate iodine with about the same avidity as the surrounding tissue (warm), findings that do not distinguish the cancerous nodule from benign thyroid nodules.

This patient had a multinodular goiter that was growing steadily over a period of 5 years. An FNA of the nodule was done immediately, yielding the cytology shown in Figure 22-4, which was interpreted as papillary thyroid cancer. Chest x-ray showed obvious pulmonary metastases (Fig. 22-5). The diagnosis of cancer was confirmed by FNA. She underwent near-total thyroidectomy, and is receiving ^{131}I therapy.

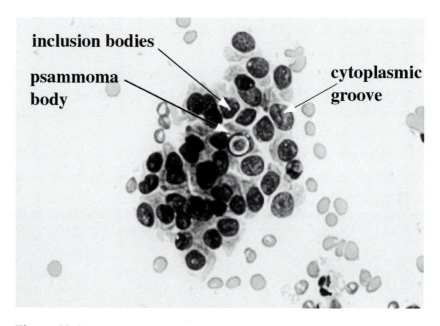

Figure 22-4
Cytology of fine needle aspiration of thyroid gland.

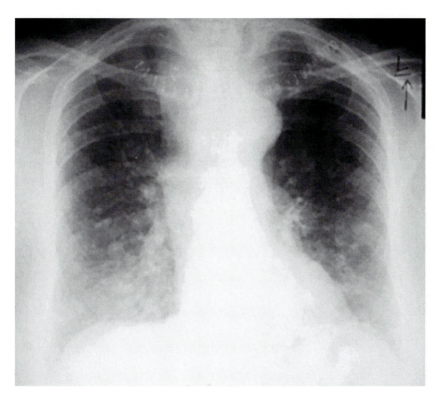

Figure 22-5
Posteroanterior chest x-ray.

 CLINICAL PEARLS

- Thyroid cancer occurs with similar frequency in an isolated thyroid nodule or a multinodular goiter.
- Most thyroid nodules are benign.
- The likelihood of thyroid cancer is high with certain historical and physical findings (see Table 22-1).
- An asymptomatic thyroid nodule may be malignant.
- The first diagnostic tests to perform on a patient with a thyroid nodule are serum TSH and FNA.
- The thyroid hormone suppression test should not be used in the diagnosis of thyroid nodules.

REFERENCES

1. Mazzaferri EL. Management of a solitary thyroid nodule. *N Engl J Med* 1993;328:553–559.
2. Hamming JF, Goslings BM, van Steenis GJ, et al. The value of fine-needle aspiration biopsy in patients with nodular thyroid disease divided into groups of suspicion of malignant neoplasms on clinical grounds *Arch Intern Med* 1990;150:113–116.
3. Belfiore LA, LaRosa GA, Guiffrida D, et al. Cancer risk in patients with cold thyroid nodules: Relevance of iodine intake, sex, age and multinodularity. *Am J Med* 1992;93:363–369.

58-YEAR-OLD FEMALE
WITH PALPITATIONS

A 58-year-old African-American woman with a history of hypertension and type II diabetes presented with a complaint of "a quivering" in her throat that awoke her from sleep. She described a similar episode earlier that day that lasted approximately 3 minutes and was associated with anxiousness, dyspnea, lightheadedness, and diaphoresis. She denied chest pain, nausea, syncope, or headache. She stated that she had experienced similar spells rarely in the past 20 years, but more commonly in the past 3 months. They never lasted more than 10 seconds and occurred now about once every 3 weeks. Each episode started abruptly and resolved spontaneously. She was not aware of a family history of tachyarrhythmias. Her medications included metformin, clonidine, hydrochlorothiazide, and estrogen. She did not drink alcohol or smoke tobacco.

PHYSICAL EXAMINATION

VITAL SIGNS: Temperature, 99.1°F (37°C); pulse, 180; respiration, 22; bp, 180/98 mm Hg
GENERAL: Anxious, mildly obese
HEENT: Eyes: Normal fundus
NECK: No thyromegaly
LUNGS: Clear
CARDIAC: Tachycardic, hyperdynamic precordium; no gallops or murmurs
ABDOMEN: Normoactive bowel sounds, no hepatosplenomegaly
EXTREMITIES: No cyanosis or edema
NEUROLOGIC: Nonfocal
SKIN: Warm and moist

LABORATORY FINDINGS

WBC, 11.7K/μL (normal differential); Hb, 14.2 g/dL; platelets, 236 K/μL, electrolytes, urea nitrogen, and creatinine, normal, serum glucose, 231 mg/dL, urinalysis, normal; electrocardiogram (Fig. 23-1).

What is the likely cause of this patient's symptoms?

This patient has supraventricular tachycardia (SVT). The electrocardiogram demonstrates inverted P waves in the ST segments (leads, II, III, and a VF, "pseudo-S") of most leads with an *RP interval* (Fig. 23-2) of less than 100 ms, all suggestive of common atrioventricular nodal reentrant tachycardia (AVNRT). Vagal maneuvers were attempted initially but failed to convert the tachycardia. She was treated with 12 mg of adenosine; this converted the rhythm to normal sinus.

SVT is any tachycardia that is initiated and maintained via atrial or atrioventricular junctional tissues. Clinically, most of the SVTs are charac-

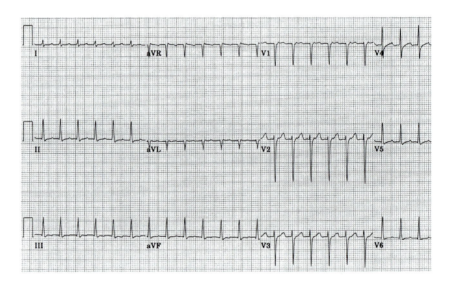

Figure 23-1
Electrocardiogram (ECG)

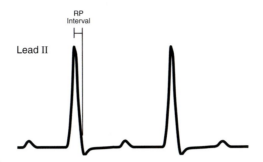

Figure 23-2
Intervals on electrocardiogram.

terized by abrupt onset and termination. In the past, this group of tach-yarrhythmias was loosely referred to as "paroxysmal atrial tachycardia." However, as a result of advances in electrophysiology, our understand-ing of the sites of origin and mechanisms of this group of arrhythmias has improved. Atrial fibrillation and atrial flutter (the most common SVTs) are also SVTs; they are somewhat unique with regard to their pathology, electrophysiology, and management and will not be further discussed.

Each of the supraventricular tachyarrhythmias (Table 23-1) arise from one of three mechanisms: reentry, enhanced automaticity, or triggered activity. Reentry is believed to be responsible for about 85 percent of SVTs and is characterized by unidirectional conduction block in a region of the myocardium or conduction tissue (Fig. 23-3). *Atrioventricular nodal reentrant tachycardia (AVNRT)* is the most common cause of paroxysmal regular SVT and accounts for about half of all patients with SVT (70% of whom are women) referred for diagnostic electrophysiologic testing.

TABLE 23-1   Types of Supraventricular
Tachycardia

Atrioventricular nodal reentrant tachycardia
Accessory pathway-mediated tachycardia
Unifocal atrial tachycardia
Multifocal atrial tachycardia
Sinus-node reentrant tachycardia
Nonparoxysmal junctional tachycardia

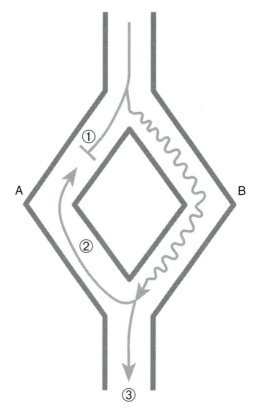

Figure 23-3 Reentry.
Rentry is responsible for 85 percent of SVTs and is characterized by unidirectional conduction block in a region of myocardium or conduction tissue (①). As a consequence of the block, the impulse propagates (slowly) over an alternative limb (B) (allowing for recovering of the original limb (A)) with retrograde (completing the reentry circuit)(②) and antegrade conduction (③).

Mechanistically, two distinct conduction pathways are demonstrable in the region of the atrioventricular (AV) node of these patients at electrophysiologic testing. One is referred to as the "fast pathway," characterized by a rapid conduction velocity and a long refractory period; the other is the "slow pathway," typified by a slow conduction velocity and a short refractory period (Figs. 23-4 and 23-5). In common AVNRT, because anterograde (atrium to ventricle) conduction continues to the ventricles almost simultaneously to retrograde (ventricle to atrium) conduction to the atrium, the QRS and P waves are recorded in close proximity. At times, the P′ waves appear negative in the inferior leads (II, III, aVF), as described for our patient.

Accessory pathways (AP) are abnormal bands of bridging myocardial tissue that form an additional connection between the atria and ventricles. AP may conduct impulses both anterograde and retrograde. During anterograde AP conduction in sinus rhythm, activation of the ventricles occurs through both the AP (ventricular preexcitation) and the normal

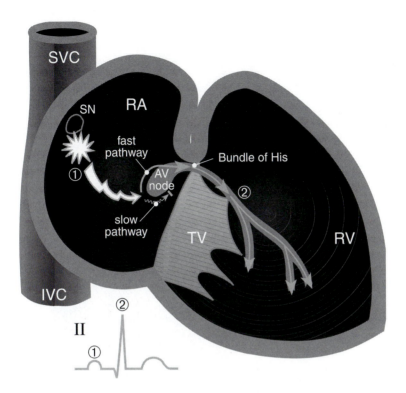

Figure 23-4 Normal sinus rhythm.
In sinus rhythm, the electrical impulse is generated in the sinus node ① and conducts rapidly through the atrial tissue to the AV node. Conduction then continues over the *fast pathway*, characterized by a rapid conduction velocity and a prolonged refractory period, over the bundle of His, bundle branches ②, Purkinje fibers, and ventricular tissue. (Abbreviations: SVC, superior vena cava; IVC, inferior vena cava; SN, sinus node; RA, right atrium; TV, tricuspid valve; RV, right ventricle)

conduction system. This is typically manifest on the electrocardiogram as a short PR interval and a delta wave, classically designated as preexcitation (Fig. 23-6). If tachycardia occurs in this setting, it is referred to as the Wolff-Parkinson-White (WPW) syndrome. However, not all APs conduct from the atria to the ventricle and cause preexcitation. Up to 25 percent of AP are capable of only retrograde conduction. This is termed *concealed AP* because of the lack of evidence by electrocardiogram when in sinus rhythm. In both instances, *atrioventricular reentrant tachycardia (AVRT)* may occur when a spontaneous atrial or ventricular premature depolarization initiates a reentrant circuit over the AP. Orthodromic AVRT (ortho-, correct, dromic-, conduction) is the second most com-

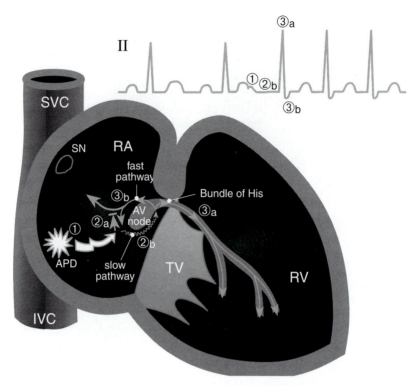

Figure 23-5 Common AV nodal reentrant tachycardia (AVNRT).
AVNRT is initiated by a premature impulse in the atrial tissue (APD) (①), which conducts quickly
to the AV node and finds the *fast pathway* of the AV node in its refractory period (unable to conduct
an impulse) and is blocked (②a). As a result, the impulse conducts slowly over the *slow pathway* because of its shorter refractory period (②b). Just before exiting the AV node, the impulse finds the *fast
pathway* recovered from its refractory state, permitting the impulse to split into two; one part con-
ducting retrograde to the atrium (③b) (completing the reentry circuit) and the other continuing normally over the bundle of His, bundle branches, Purkinje fibers, and ventricular tissue. (Abbreviations:
SVC, superior vena cava; IVC, inferior vena cava; APD, atrial premature depolarization; SN, sinus
node; RA, right atrium; TV, tricuspid valve; RV, right ventricle)

mon cause of SVT (after AVNRT) in patients without evidence of preexcitation (Fig. 23-7). In about 10 percent of patients with WPW and
AVRT, the reentrant circuit operates in the opposite fashion and is
termed antidromic AVRT. This typically occurs in patients with multiple APs and presents as a wide QRS complex tachycardia. The presence
of atrial fibrillation and atrial flutter in patients with WPW is of particular concern because of the potential for rapid anterograde conduction
over the AP. Ventricular rates of 300 bpm and faster may occur, associated with the risk of precipitating ventricular fibrillation and sudden

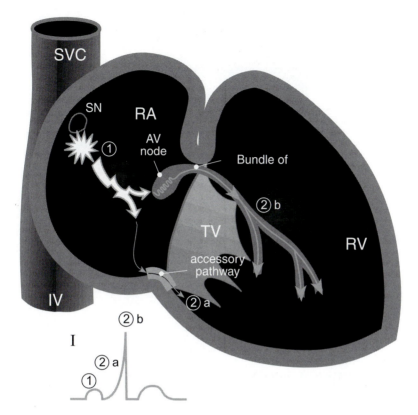

Figure 23-6 Preexcitation.

Preexcitation occurs in normal sinus rhythm when the sinus impulse (①) is conducted to both the accessory pathway (②a) and the AV node almost simultaneously, with a resultant shortened PR interval and slurring of the QRS (*delta wave*) on the electrocardiogram. (Abbreviations: SVC, superior vena cava; IVC, inferior vena cava; SN, sinus node; RA, right atrium; TV, tricuspid valve; RV, right ventricle)

death. The most important parameter in determining this risk is the refractory period of the accessory pathway(s); a refractory period greater than 250 msec has been deemed safe.

Atrial tachycardia is an SVT that arises from atrial muscle exclusive of the sinus node. Unifocal atrial tachycardia is characterized by a single P wave morphology with a rate of less than 250 bpm (atrial rates > 250 bpm are usually atrial flutter). This rhythm accounts for about 15 percent of patients with SVT and usually occurs in patients with structural heart disease. Multifocal atrial tachycardia is defined electrocardiographically as three or more different P wave morphologies with an irregular ventricu-

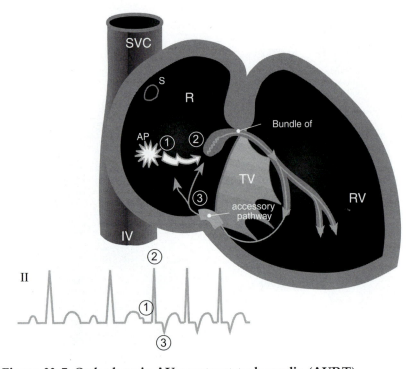

Figure 23-7 Orthodromic AV reentrant tachycardia (AVRT).
AVRT may be initiated by either a premature impulse in the atrial tissue (APD)(①) or ventricular tissue that propagates in a clockwise direction over the normal conduction system (②) and retrogradely via the accessory pathway (③) to the atrium. (Abbreviations: SVC, superior vena cava; IVC, inferior vena cava; SN, sinus node; RA, right atrium; TV, tricuspid valve; RV, right ventricle)

lar rate (usually 100–130 bpm). This rhythm occurs commonly in older patients with chronic obstructive pulmonary disease and congestive heart failure.

Nonparoxysmal junctional tachycardia is a very rare cause of SVT in adults. It is more often caused by enhanced automaticity or triggered within an injured (e.g., valve surgery, myocardial infarction, digitalis toxicity) atrioventricular junction.

The clinical presentation of patients with SVT is extremely variable. In general, patients with underlying heart disease do not tolerate rapid ventricular rates and may present with chest pain, palpitations, dyspnea, lightheadedness, or even syncope, whereas healthy individuals may experience only vague symptoms. In general, the faster the tachycardia, the more likely the patient will have symptoms. The history and physical examination are frequently helpful, particularly the pattern of onset and cessation of tachycardia and the presence or absence of heart disease, to identify the particular type. In addition, AVNRT should be considered in a patient with prominent jugular venous a-waves that match the tachycardia rate, which is a reflection of atrial contraction against a closed AV valve. Close evaluation of the electrocardiogram usually provides clues to the correct diagnosis (Table 23-2). Performing vagal maneuvers while monitoring the electrocardiogram can also improve the diagnostic accuracy.

The goal in acute treatment of SVT is to convert the tachycardia with AV nodal blocking drugs. Adenosine is the drug of choice because of its rapid onset (10–15 sec) and short duration of action (20–25 sec). About 90 percent of SVTs owing to AVRT or AVNRT are terminated with a 12-mg dose of adenosine. The calcium channel blockers verapamil and diltiazem are excellent alternatives and are preferred in patients with atrial tachycardia. However, hypotension may be caused by these drugs. Verapamil is generally not indicated in patients with congestive heart failure.

TABLE 23-2   **Electrocardiographic Clues to the Diagnosis of Common Supraventricular Tachycardias***

TACHYCARDIA	ELECTROCARDIOGRAPHIC CHARACTERISTICS
Atrioventricular nodal reentrant (AVNRT)	
Common	P waves hidden or RP < 100 ms, pseudo-S in II or III, pseudo-R in V_1
Uncommon	Inverted P waves, RP > PR
Accessory pathway-mediated	
Orthodromic atrioventricular reentrant (AVRT)	Inverted P waves, RP > PR, QRS alternans
Atrial fibrillation (Wolff-Parkinson-White)	Irregularly irregular, variable QRS
Antidromic atrioventricular reentrant (AVRT)	Inverted P waves, wide and bizarre QRS
Multifocal atrial	Variable P waves, variable rate, variable PR

*Adapted from Ganz LI, Friedman PL. Supraventricular tachycardia. *N Engl J Med* 1995;332:162–173.

23-YEAR-OLD MAN
WITH ANXIETY ATTACKS

A 23-year-old male college student with a history of asthma presented with a 2-year history of anxiety attacks associated with heavy perspiration was treated with an antidepressant and a benzodiazepine with little improvement. About 2 months prior to presenting to student health, his attacks of anxiousness, excessive perspiration, palpitations, and shortness of breath increased in severity and frequency, occurring on a daily basis and lasting 10 to 15 minutes. Between episodes he felt well and during this time was performing satisfactorily in college. On two occasions during the prior summer, while working on a factory assembly line, he felt lightheaded and was told that his blood pressure was elevated. He had lost 12 pounds over the past year.

Medications that he was taking at the time of presentation were sertraline and clonazepam, but he denied using over-the-counter or recreational drugs. He had no chest pain, syncope, headaches, diarrhea, heat intolerance, or fatigue. Family history was notable only for fibromyalgia in his mother. He did not smoke or drink alcohol.

PHYSCIAL EXAMINATION

VITAL SIGNS: Temperature, 98.2°F (36.7°C); pulse, 80; respiration, 22; bp, 118/68 mmHg
GENERAL: Thin
HEENT: Normal
NECK: No lymphadenopathy or thyromegaly
LUNGS: Clear
CARDIAC: Normal

ABDOMEN: Normal bowel sounds, soft, nontender; no hepato-splenomegaly

EXTREMITIES: No cyanosis or edema

NEUROLOGIC: Nonfocal, deep tendon reflexes 2+, fine tremor

SKIN: No lesions

LABORATORY FINDINGS

WBC, 7.3 K/L (normal differential); Hb, 14.2 g/dL; platelets, 298 K/L; electrolytes, serum glucose, urea nitrogen, and creatinine, normal; thyroid stimulating hormone (TSH), 0.88 μU/mL (normal, 0.2–5.0); urine metanephrine (total), 1180 μg/24-hours (normal, 120–700); normetanephrine, 1132 μg/24-hours (normal, 82–500); plasma dopamine, 122 pg/mL (normal, <20); plasma norepinephrine, 4863 pg/mL (normal, 217–1109); plasma epinephrine, 50 pg/mL (normal, <95); urinalysis, normal; chest x-ray, normal; abdominal CT scan shown in Fig. 24-1.

What is the likely diagnosis and how should this patient be treated?

This patient has a pheochromocytoma involving the right adrenal gland. The abdominal CT scan demonstrates a 2.8 cm right adrenal mass (arrow) (Fig. 24-1).

Pheochromocytomas are rare tumors of neuroectodermal origin that secrete catecholamines (epinephrine, norepinephrine, and rarely dopamine). They most commonly arise from the adrenal medullae, but may occur anywhere in the sympathetic nervous system (paragangliomas). Pheochromocytomas are estimated to occur in about 1 of 1000 hypertensive patients, although about half those affected have paroxysmal hypertension. Pheochromocytoma may occur at any age and is one of the most common endocrine tumors occurring in children, two-thirds of whom are males; in adults, the tumor is more common in the fourth or fifth decades of life and has a slight predilection for women. Other de-

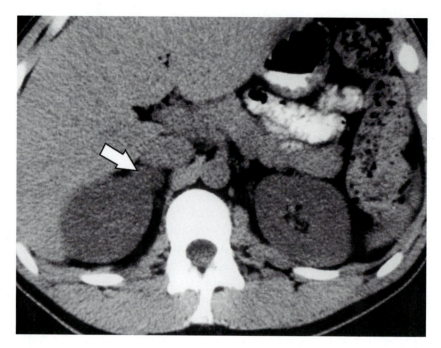

Figure 24-1
Abdominal CT scan.

mographics of this tumor have been loosely referred to as "the rule of tens" (Table 24-1).

Pheochromocytomas are encapsulated and quite vascular, averaging about 5 cm in diameter and usually weighing less than 70 g (Fig. 24-2). There is no correlation between tumor size or catecholamine concentration and the clinical or laboratory manifestations of the disease; rather, symptoms are dependent on the amount of catecholamine released into the circulation and whether the release is sustained or intermittent. Most tumors secrete both norepinephrine and epinephrine, although norepinephrine usually predominates. Rarely, the tumors may produce and secrete other substances, such as vasoactive intestinal peptide or adrenocorticotrophic hormone, which may confound the clinical diagnosis.

Most patients with pheochromocytoma present with dramatic paroxysms of hypertension accompanied by severe headache, drenching perspiration, and palpitations. The paroxysms, which may occur anywhere from once a year to several times a day, usually last 10 to 30 minutes and

TABLE 24-1   Rule of Tens

10% are bilateral
10% are extra-adrenal
10% are familial
10% are in children
10% are malignant

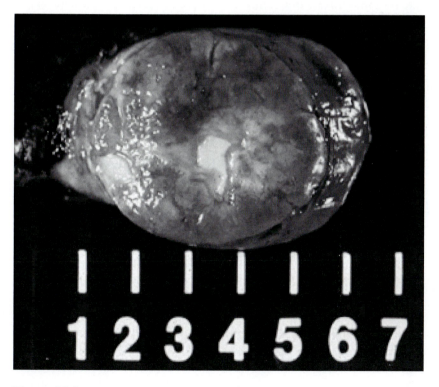

Figure 24-2
Gross pathologic specimen of pheochromocytoma.

may be precipitated by exercise, eating, assuming certain positions, taking some drugs, or undergoing surgery. Between spells, patients usually feel well and may have a normal blood pressure. Fewer than 10 percent of those with pheochromocytoma have no discernible spells. A history of paroxysmal anxiety spells followed by symptom-free intervals is helpful in distinguishing pheochromocytoma from other causes of chronic anxiety. Other less specific symptoms include tremor, pallor, weakness, nausea, and abdominal or chest pain. Weight loss is often induced by the excessive catecholamines, but obesity does not rule out the diagnosis. A family history of pheochromocytoma or other endocrine tumors is especially important.

The physical examination is usually unremarkable unless the patient is experiencing a spell, which typically produces an anxious appearance with facial pallor and inappropriate, often profuse perspiration. There may be a fine tremor of the fingers, tachycardia, and an orthostatic fall in blood pressure. Some have manifest complications of hypertension, such as retinopathy, subarachnoid hemorrhage, dissecting aneurysm, or heart failure. Abdominal pain may occur from cholelithiasis, which for uncertain reasons occurs with higher than usual frequency, particularly in patients with paroxysmal hypertension.

Pheochromocytoma, typically bilateral, occurs with greater than usual frequency in patients with neurofibromatosis and von Hippel-Lindau disease. Bilateral pheochromocytoma is also a component of familial multiple endocrine neoplasia (MEN) syndromes associated with medullary thyroid carcinoma and either hyperparathyroidism (MEN 2a) or a marfanoid habitus with mucosal neuromas (MEN 2b).

Biochemical confirmation of the clinical diagnosis is usually easy: The 24-hour urinary catecholamine and metanephrine excretion rates are high. However, reliance on this test alone may be problematic. First, it often is difficult to obtain an adequate and appropriately processed 24-hour urine collection because all medications must be stopped since many drugs interfere with the assays. Second, plasma catecholamine measurement may be a better test for small tumors because they often have rapid hormone turnover rates, releasing unmetabolized catecholamines into the circulation and causing transient but severe symptoms. Patients with large tumors often secrete more catecholamine metabolites that produce fewer symptoms and cause urine measurements to be high. Lastly, renal function may affect urine metabolites. Although not yet widely available, plasma metanephrine is the most sensitive test for pheochromocytoma.

When the clinical suspicion is high and the results of urine tests are equivocal, measurement of plasma catecholamines may be diagnostic. The usual problem, however, is the high false-positive rate (low specificity) of plasma catecholamines in hypertensive patients without pheochromocytoma who may have catecholamine levels up to 2000 pg/mL, which is in the range of pheochromocytoma. In this case, a clonidine or glucagon suppression test may be required.

Once the biochemical diagnosis has been established, anatomic localization of the tumor is necessary. CT scanning is the most widely used modality, but if intravenous contrast or radiation are contraindicated, MRI is a good alternative. Scintigraphic localization with ^{131}I-metaiodobenzylguanidine (^{131}I-MIBG), which provides anatomic and functional characterization of the tumor, is typically reserved for patients without demonstrable tumors by CT or MRI.

Surgical excision of the tumor(s) is the only definitive therapy and should be considered in all patients. Preoperative administration of an α-adrenergic blocking agent, usually for a few weeks, is essential to control the symptoms and manage hypertension. Phenoxybenzamine and prazosin are the most commonly used; however, nifedipine has recently been shown to be equally efficacious. Importantly, β-blocking agents are contraindicated in the absence of adequate α-blockade because the unopposed α_1-vasoconstrictive properties of circulating catecholamines may cause severe hypertension and cardiac ischemia, with subsequent pulmonary edema. In addition, the chronically high norepinephrine levels mimic hypovolemia that can be corrected with preoperative α-blockade and hydration, which avoids intra- and postoperative hypotension.

With appropriate surgical treatment, the 10-year survival rate of patients with benign pheochromocytoma exceeds 80 percent. Urine or plasma catecholamines or metanephrine levels should be measured 1 week after surgery and annually for about 5 years thereafter, and blood pressure should be checked monthly for the first year and then about every 6 months thereafter. Routine postoperative imaging studies are not necessary.

Our patient was treated preoperatively with phenoxybenzamine and propranolol. On the day prior to surgery, he was hydrated with 2 liters of normal saline. A laparoscopic right adrenalectomy was performed without complications or postoperative hypotension. Since surgery, he has been asymptomatic with normal blood pressure and plasma catecholamines measurements.

CLINICAL PEARLS

- Pheochromocytomas are rare tumors of neuroectodermal origin.
- Tumor size and catecholamine concentration bear no relationship to clinical manifestations or laboratory results.
- The classic presentation comprises paroxysmal hypertension, severe headache, diaphoresis, and palpitations.
- A 24-hour urine (or plasma) catecholamine and metanephrine are adequate for diagnosis in most patients.
- Bilateral pheochromocytomas occur with von Recklinghausen's neurofibromatosis, von Hippel-Lindau disease, and MEN 2a and 2b syndromes.
- Surgery is the only definitive therapy and should be considered in all patients.

REFERENCES

1. Bravo EL, Gifford RW, Manger WM. Adrenal medullary tumors: Pheochromocytoma, in *Endocrine Tumors*, Mazzaferri EL, Samaan NA (eds). Cambridge, MA, Blackwell Scientific, 1993, pp 426–447.
2. Gifford RW, Manger WM, Bravo EL. Pheochromocytoma. *Endocrinol Metab Clin North Am* 1994;23:387–404.
3. Lenders JWM., Keiser HR, Goldstein DS, et al. Plasma metanephrines in the diagnosis of pheochromocytoma. *Ann Intern Med* 1995;123:101–109.

61-YEAR-OLD WOMAN WITH HYPERCALCEMIA AND RENAL INSUFFICIENCY

A 61-year-old Caucasian woman with a history of hypothyroidism, hyperlipidemia, and symptoms of gastroesophageal reflux presented with anorexia, nausea, vomiting, headache, and weakness for the prior 2 weeks. Laboratory studies done at the referral hospital revealed acute renal failure and hypercalcemia. She had experienced two similar episodes over the past 3 years, both of which required hospitalization. During the first episode, she was treated with IV fluids and discharged without therapy because an extensive evaluation was unrevealing and her hypercalcemia had improved. During the second episode 1 year ago, hyperparathyroidism was diagnosed, a partial parathyroidectomy was performed, and her hypercalcemia improved. Records from the referring hospital revealed that a PTH assay that measured the carboxy-terminal portion of parathyroid hormone had been elevated prior to her parathyroidectomy; however, the excised parathyroid glands were normal. She had no further symptoms and denied hematemesis/hematochezia, diarrhea, weight loss, or shortness of breath. For the past 3 years there had been no change in her prescribed medications, which were levothyroxine, estrogen, amitriptyline, propranolol, gemfibrozil, and simvastatin. Family history was notable for non–insulin dependent diabetes mellitus and cerebrovascular disease. She was a married homemaker who had a healthy daughter. She did not smoke or drink alcohol and reported no recent exposures or travel.

PHYSICAL EXAMINATION

VITAL SIGNS: Temperature, 96.4°F (35.7°C); pulse, 60; respiration, 18; bp, 142/92 mmHg

GENERAL: Thin, alert, and apathetic

HEENT: Eyes: see Fig. 25-1

NECK: Well-healed scar, no thyromegaly or lymphadenopathy

LUNGS: Clear

BREAST EXAM: Normal

CARDIAC: Normal

ABDOMEN: Unremarkable

EXTREMITIES: No clubbing or edema

RECTAL: Guaiac negative, no masses

NEUROLOGIC: Nonfocal, normal strength

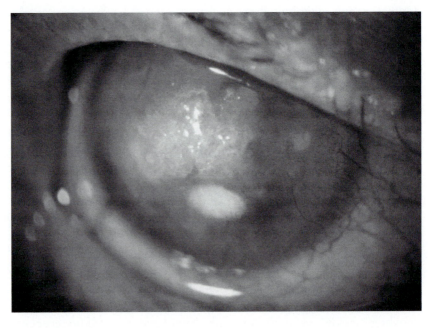

Figure 25-1
Slit-lamp examination of right eye. (See Plate 12.)

LABORATORY FINDINGS

WBC, 6.5 K/uL (normal differential); Hb, 12.2 g/dL (MCV 91 fl); serum electrolytes: sodium, 140 mmol/L; potassium, 3.3 mmol/L; chloride, 94 mmol/L; bicarbonate, 35 mmol/L; blood urea nitrogen, 44 mg/dL; creatinine, 5.3 mg/dL; serum calcium, 17.4 mg/dL (ionized, 7.92 mg/dL); phosphorus, 5.8 mg/dL; urine pH, 8.0; thyroid function, normal; liver function studies, normal; serum protein electrophoresis, normal; chest x-ray, normal; abdominal series, normal; renal ultrasound, normal

HOSPITAL COURSE

The patient was admitted and treated with IV hydration and loop diuretics. Her serum calcium and creatinine gradually improved. A neck ultrasound, parathyroid sestamibi, and abdominal CT were unremarkable. Further laboratory studies revealed: intact parathyroid hormone <2.0 pg/mL (normal, 11–54); 1,25[OH]$_2$ vitamin D 21 pg/mL (normal, 18–62); angiotensin converting enzyme 50 U/L (normal, 8–52). An esophagogastroduodenoscopy revealed a hiatal hernia and a friable-appearing pylorus.

What is the likely diagnosis and how should this patient be treated?

This patient has the milk-alkali syndrome. On direct questioning, she reported ingesting up to a bottle of calcium carbonate (TUMS®) per day, which she had recently started for relief of GERD symptoms.

The milk-alkali syndrome, as first described about 75 years ago, occurred in patients with peptic ulcer disease treated with absorbable antacids containing large quantities of alkali and calcium. At the time, it was believed to afflict 35 percent of those treated for peptic ulcer disease. In the current era of H$_2$ receptor antagonists and proton pump inhibitors, the syndrome is seen much less commonly but continues to be identified a few times per year in large hospitals. In fact, several cases have recently been reported in women who consumed calcium-containing antacids as a daily supplement for osteoporosis prevention.

The syndrome consists of a triad of hypercalcemia, metabolic alkalosis, and renal dysfunction; however, the clinical characteristics may vary depending on the duration and magnitude of calcium and alkali ingestion. Three forms have been described: acute (toxemia), intermediate (Cope syndrome), and chronic (Burnett syndrome).

The acute form typically develops within 2 to 30 days after starting calcium and alkali ingestion. Its symptoms are those of hypercalcemia and alkalosis: nausea, vomiting, anorexia, constipation, headache, vertigo, weakness, apathy or confusion, and disorientation. If the calcium ingestion continues, neurologic symptoms may progress to stupor and coma. The alkalosis and hypercalcemia are usually accompanied by hypochloremia and hypokalemia. Renal insufficiency, which develops early in the course of these metabolic abnormalities, is manifest by azotemia, elevated serum creatinine, hyperphosphatemia, proteinuria, pyuria, and granular and hyaline casts. In addition, the urine is usually alkaline.

In the intermediate form (Cope syndrome), the presenting symptoms and laboratory manifestations are similar to those of the acute form, but the history of calcium and alkali ingestion is more prolonged. Also, there may be evidence of early soft tissue calcium salt deposition in the palpebral conjunctiva manifest by conjunctivitis. Characteristically, the biochemical resolution is protracted in this form of the disorder.

In Burnett syndrome, which is the chronic form of the disorder, hypercalcemia remains a cardinal feature, but the progressive—and frequently irreversible—renal dysfunction and soft tissue calcification are the important long-term consequences. The soft tissue calcium deposits occur primarily in the conjunctiva where they cause conjunctivitis, and in the cornea where they cause band keratopathy (see Fig. 25-1), although musculoskeletal calcification and nephrocalcinosis are not uncommon.

The most important of the complex pathophysiologic events of this disorder are the effects of calcium on glomerular filtration and renal tubular bicarbonate excretion, and the effect of alkalosis on renal calcium excretion. Together, hyperphosphatemia, hypercalcemia, and alkalosis promote nephrocalcinosis and irreversible renal dysfunction.

The diagnosis is based primarily on hypercalcemia in the presence of a history of calcium and alkali ingestion. However, patients are often unaware that consuming large amounts of absorbable antacids may be harmful and often do not report them as a medication to their physician, as was the case in our patient. Although the amount of ingested calcium and alkali necessary to cause this syndrome is not well defined because of the wide individual variability in fractional calcium absorption, the majority of affected patients have ingested 5 to 10 grams of calcium per day and have had associated predisposing factors, such as renal disease or hydrochlorothiazide therapy. Importantly, the most common causes of hypercalcemia are hyperparathyroidism and malignancy, followed by other less common disorders (Table 25-1). The milk-alkali syndrome should be considered when a patient presents with hypercalcemia and renal impairment, manifestations that are invariably present in all forms of the milk-alkali disorder. Other typical biochemical features of the milk-alkali syndrome are a chloride-responsive metabolic alkalosis and urinary alkalosis. Hyperparathyroidism is usually manifest by a chloride-unresponsive metabolic acidosis and persistent hypercalcemia despite withdrawal of calcium and alkali. However, in the later stages of the milk-alkali syndrome, when the systemic pH is lowered by renal dysfunction, the response to withdrawal of calcium and alkali is delayed, which formerly made differentiating it from hyperparathyroidism difficult. The roles of parathyroid hormone (PTH) and 1,25 $(OH)_2$ vitamin D in this disorder now have been clarified. Low serum PTH and low to low-normal 1,25 $(OH)_2$ vitamin D concentrations with a history of excessive calcium ingestion are diagnostic of the milk-alkali syndrome. Serum PTH and 1,25 $(OH)_2$ vi-

TABLE 25-1   **Major Causes of Hypercalcemia**

Hyperparathyroidism
Malignancy
Sarcoidosis
Thiazide diuretics
Adrenal insufficiency
Vitamin A intoxication
Milk-alkali syndrome
Vitamin D intoxication
Aluminum intoxication

tamin D concentrations are both high in primary hyperparathyroidism. PTH assays directed to the carboxy-terminal of parathyroid hormone are difficult to interpret in patients with renal dysfunction that decreases the clearance of carboxy-terminal PTH fragments. Therefore, amino-terminal PTH or intact PTH immunoassays, which are not so altered by renal failure, should be used. Treatment of the milk-alkali syndrome is usually intravenous saline hydration, loop diuretics as needed, and withdrawal of the offending agent. Occasionally hemodialysis with a low calcium bath may be useful in patients with particularly severe hypercalcemia and renal dysfunction.

At the time of discharge from our institution, this patient's symptoms had completely resolved and her azotemia was slightly improved.

 CLINICAL PEARLS

- The milk-alkali syndrome is owing to ingestion of large amounts of absorbable calcium antacids.
- Patients with hypercalcemia should be questioned about the use of over-the-counter calcium antacids.
- The acute milk-alkali syndrome begins 2 to 30 days after ingesting calcium and alkali; symptoms range from nausea/vomiting, weakness, headache, irritability, and apathy, to stupor and coma.
- The classic triad is hypercalcemia, metabolic alkalosis, and renal insufficiency.
- Low serum PTH (intact assay) and $1,25(OH)_2$ vitamin D concentrations differentiate the milk-alkali syndrome from hyperparathyroidism.

REFERENCES

1. Abreo K, Adlakha A, Kilpatrick S, et al. The milk-alkali syndrome: A reversible form of acute renal failure. *Arch Intern Med* 1993; 153:1005–1010.
2. Muldowney WP, Mazbar SA. Rolaids-yogurt syndrome: A 1990's version of milk-alkali syndrome. *Am J Kid Dis* 1996;27:270–272.
3. Orwoll ES. The milk-alkali syndrome: Current concepts. *Ann Intern Med* 1982;97:242–248.
4. Dorsch TR. The milk-alkali syndrome, vitamin D, and parathyroid hormone. *Ann Intern Med* 1986;105:800–801.

43-YEAR-OLD MAN WITH FATIGUE AND BLURRED VISION

A 43-year-old African-American man presented with a 3-month history of fatigue and intermittent blurry vision. He reported recently getting up several times a night to urinate, but denied symptoms of hesitancy, burning, or pain on urination. Despite not feeling well, he had gained several pounds recently. Two of his four sisters and one of his brothers has diabetes mellitus. He has not had a physical examination for 10 years. He admitted smoking two packs of cigarettes per day since his teens and drank about four beers daily. He denied using recreational drugs. He worked a sedentary job as a security officer and did not participate in regular exercise.

PHYSICAL EXAMINATION

VITAL SIGNS: Temperature, 97.8°F (36.5°C); pulse, 84; respiration, 14; bp, 166/96 mmHg (right arm), 175/98 mmHg (right leg)
GENERAL: Tired-appearing, moderately obese man (weight, 245 pounds; height, 5 feet, 8 inches)
HEENT: Normal funduscopic exam
NECK: No lymphadenopathy or thyromegaly
LUNGS: Scattered rhonchi
CARDIAC: Normal
ABDOMEN: Protuberant, normoactive bowel sounds, soft, nontender; no hepatosplenomegaly or ascites
EEXTREMITIES: No cyanosis or edema
NEUROLOGIC: Deep tendon reflexes 2+; normal strength and sensation throughout
SKIN: No rashes
RECTAL: Normal prostate, guaiac negative

LABORATORY FINDINGS

WBC, 8.5 K/μL (normal differential); Hb, 15.7 g/dL; electrolytes, normal; urea nitrogen, normal; creatinine, normal; glucose (fasting), 131 mg/dL; total cholesterol, 260 mg/dL; HDL cholesterol, 27 mg/dL; LDL cholesterol, 140 mg/dL; triglycerides (fasting), 450 mg/dL; glycosylated hemoglobin, 9.5% (normal, 4.8–7.8%); urinalysis, 2+ glucose; no protein; electrocardiogram, normal; chest x-ray, normal

What is the likely diagnosis and how should this patient be treated?

This patient has type 2 diabetes mellitus, obesity, hypertension, hypercholesterolemia, and hypertriglyceridemia—syndrome X. New terminology and diagnostic criteria have been suggested for the diagnosis of diabetes mellitus by the American Diabetes Association (ADA). Previously termed non-insulin dependent diabetes mellitus (NIDDM), type 2 diabetes, or adult-onset diabetes, the term now recommended by the ADA is type 2 diabetes. It is the most prevalent form of diabetes and results from insulin resistance with an insulin secretory defect.

The new ADA diagnostic criteria for diabetes mellitus are as follows: (1) symptoms of diabetes plus casual (any time of the day without regard to the last meal) plasma glucose concentration, 200 mg/dL; (2) fasting plasma glucose (FPG), 126 mg/dL; (3) 2-hour post-glucose (using a glucose load of 75 g), 200 mg/dL.

The incidence of type 2 diabetes is significantly higher in certain ethnic populations, including African Americans, Hispanics, Pacific Islanders, and Native Americans, all of whom have a genetic predisposition to the disease. The central defect in type 2 diabetes is impaired insulin secretion, aggravated by insulin resistance. Patients with type 2 diabetes thus usually have a relative, rather than an absolute, insulin deficiency. Therefore, ketoacidosis seldom occurs spontaneously; when seen, it usually arises in association with the stress of a coexisting illness such as an infection or an acute myocardial infarction. Clinically apparent diabetes mellitus develops when insulin resistance, which is usually exacerbated by obesity, exceeds insulin secretion. Sustained hyperglycemia has a toxic effect, termed glucose toxicity, on the β-cells that further attenuates insulin secretion. In time and with increasing insulin resistance, the β-cells become completely exhausted and insulin secretion so severely impaired that the patient requires exogenous insulin.

The combination of insulin resistance, central obesity, hypertension, and hyperlipidemia is so powerful in predicting macrovascular disease in type 2 diabetes that it has been named syndrome X. This patient's lipid profile demonstrates the classic pattern seen in type 2 diabetes: hypertriglyceridemia with a low HDL. Although his LDL is only marginally elevated, his multiple risk factors place him at high risk for premature coronary atherosclerosis, and peripheral and cerebral vascular disease. He is also at risk for microvascular (eye, kidney, and nerve disease) complications of diabetes, the major determinant of which is hyperglycemia, although hypertension is also important.

Treatment for this man should begin with lifestyle interventions. He needs to be counseled on the importance of weight loss, regular moderate exercise (walking), and immediate smoking cessation. Each of these interventions will require intense management by his physician and other health care professionals, such as a diabetes nurse educator or dietician. Every attempt should be made to motivate this patient to modify his diet by reducing his daily caloric intake and the content of cholesterol and fat in his diet. The ADA recommends that a patient with type 2 diabetes eat a diet that is high in complex carbohydrates (about 50–60%) and low in fat (about 20–30%), less than 10 percent of which should be saturated. Since this patient has moderate hypertension, the sodium content of his diet should also be reduced. It is recommended that the patient attempt to lose about 1 to 2 pounds per month, which will assure a loss of body fat rather than water or muscle mass. Diet pills should generally be discouraged.

His exercise program should start with walking. More vigorous exercise such as jogging, although excellent, requires close supervision in this patient with multiple coronary risk factors and should be taken on gradually and only after a cardiac stress test.

Smoking cessation is most successful in a structured group setting and often requires a nicotine patch. The patient (and his wife if she is a smoker) should be strongly encouraged to join one of the many formal smoking cessation programs. The risk of cigarette smoking, which is independent of that of diabetes mellitus, imparts a significant increase to his already high risk of coronary artery, cerebrovascular, and peripheral vascular disease.

Before suggesting drug therapy, it is reasonable to wait about 6 months, while the patient attempts to undergo closely supervised lifestyle modifications. This entails carefully structured follow-up visits aimed at encouraging the patient and using more than one provider (nurses, dieticians, smoking cessation groups) to motivate the patient.

If the blood pressure remains elevated above 135/90 after sodium restriction, antihypertensive drug therapy is justified with a target goal of <130 mmHg systolic and <85 diastolic. A thiazide diuretic or β-blocker is not appropriate in this setting because both have adverse effects on glucose and lipid levels. An angiotensin-converting enzyme (ACE) inhibitor is a better choice, given its salutary effect on renal function and proteinuria in patients with diabetes mellitus. Calcium-channel blockers are also a reasonable choice. Long-acting β-blockers, such as terazosin or doxazosin, may have a beneficial effect on lipids.

If the patient continues to have high levels of fasting blood glucose (>120 mg/dL preprandial and >140 mg/dL bedtime glucose), or glycosylated hemoglobin (>8.5%), pharmacologic intervention is necessary. Any agent that improves glycemic control will enhance insulin sensitivity because of the overall improvement in the metabolic environment and the amelioration of hyperglycemia-induced defects in insulin action and secretion. Sulfonylurea drugs or a long-acting insulin are the main options available for initial therapy of a patient with type 2 diabetes mellitus. The sulfonylurea drugs, which are a rational choice to start with, act mainly by stimulating insulin secretion and are most effective early in the course of the disease, when the patient's β-cells maintain the capacity to secrete insulin and the patient is adhering to a diet. They may cause weight gain, which should be carefully avoided. When maximum doses of a sulfonylurea provide inadequate glycemic control, the biguanide metformin usually works, principally by improving insulin sensitivity, and can be added to the regimen providing renal function is normal. Both drugs used together are more effective than either used alone because of their different and complementary mechanisms of action. The glycated hemoglobin usually declines about 1.5 to 2.0 percent with the use of these drugs. Acarbose, a relatively new agent that can be administered in combination with either a sulfonylurea or metformin, works by delaying the absorption of glucose by blocking carbohydrate digestion. It causes a reduction in postprandial hyperglycemia and lowers glycated hemoglobin less than about 1 percent, but up to 50 percent of patients experience side effects, mainly flatulence, and many are noncompliant because it must be taken three times a day. When fasting hyperglycemia is unresponsive to intensive dietary and oral agent therapy, insulin should be started. It is best administered alone as intermediate- or long-acting insulin (NPH, Lente, or ultralente) at bedtime to reduce the fasting plasma glucose level. However, it almost invariably causes weight gain. For patients who remain in poor glycemic control (glycated Hb >8.5%) despite insulin therapy of >30 U/day given in multiple injections, troglitazone (thiazolidinedione), the new oral agent that reduces insulin resistance, should be considered. The recommended dosage range is between 200 and 600 mg/day, with the average dose estimated to be 400 mg/day. Dosing is once per day with breakfast. When diabetes is poorly controlled, despite maximum therapy, no insulin reduction is recommended, although a 10 to 20 percent reduction may be required if premeal glucose values consistently drop below 120 mg/dL. There is no increased risk of weight gain and it may improve the abnormalities associated with the insulin resistance syndrome.

This patient was only able to lose 15 pounds but stopped smoking. His hyperglycemia was controlled with a gradually increased exercise program and a timed-release sulfonylurea agent.

 CLINICAL PEARLS

- Non–insulin dependent diabetes mellitus is now termed type 2 diabetes mellitus.
- New ADA criteria for the diagnosis of diabetes are: (1) symptoms of diabetes plus a casual plasma glucose, 200 mg/dL; (2) FPG, 126 mg/dL; (3) 2-hour post-glucose (after 75 g), 200 mg/dL.
- Syndrome X is a constellation of insulin resistance, central obesity, hypertension, and hyperlipidemia that predicts macrovascular disease in type 2 diabetes.
- If the blood pressure is >135/90 after lifestyle interventions, antihypertensive drug therapy, usually with an ACE inhibitor or calcium-channel blocker, should be considered in a patient with type 2 diabetes.
- Sulfonylurea drugs increase insulin secretion and have an additive effect when combined with biguanides.
- Troglitazone (an insulin sensitizer) and acarbose (a glucose absorption inhibitor) are two new drugs for the treatment of type 2 diabetes.

REFERENCES

1. Report of the Expert Committee on the Diagnosis and Classification of Diabetes Mellitus. *Diabetes* 1997;20:1183.
2. Lewis EJ, Hunsicker L, Bain R, et al. A clinical trial of an angiotensive converting enzyme inhibitor in the neuropathy of insulin-dependent diabetes mellitus. *N Engl J Med* 1993;329:145–162.

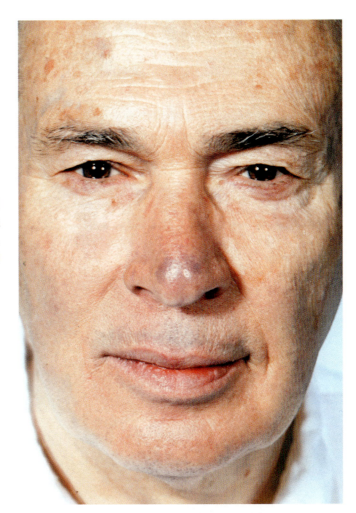

Plate 1
Blue–gray skin
pigmentation.
(See Case 2.)

Plate 2
Gingival hyperplasia.
(See Case 3.)

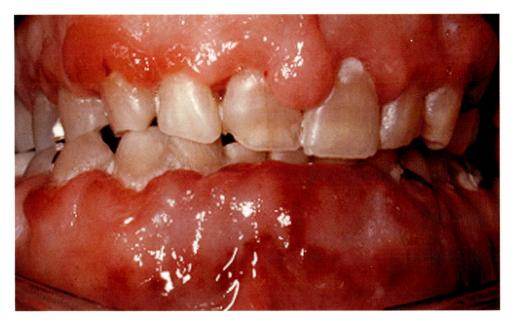

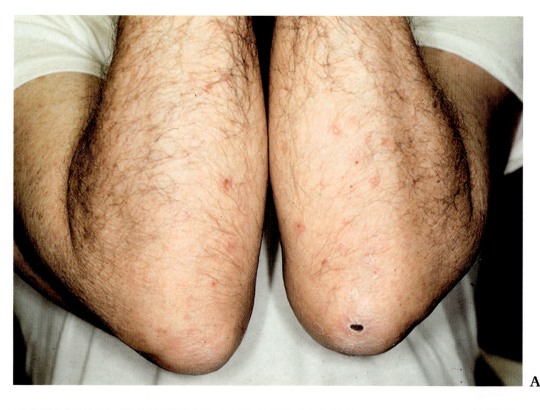

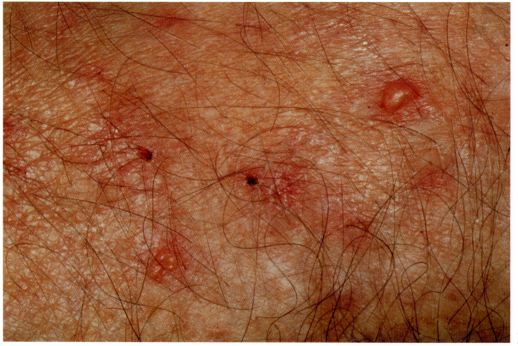

Plate 3
Dermatitis herpetiformis. (See Case 4.)

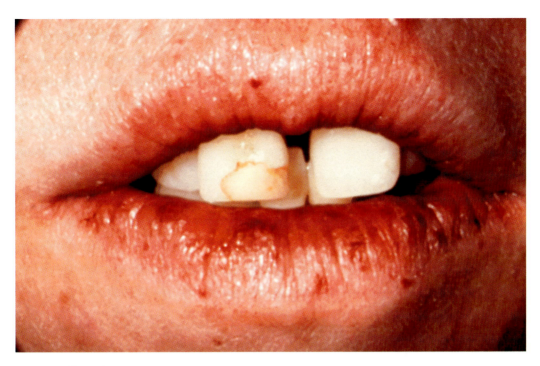

Plate 4
Punctate telangiectasias. (See Case 7.)

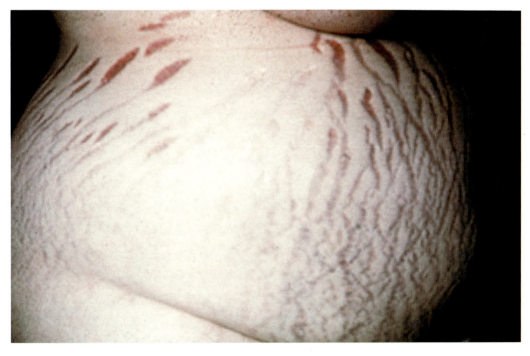

Plate 5
Skin striae. (See Case 8.)

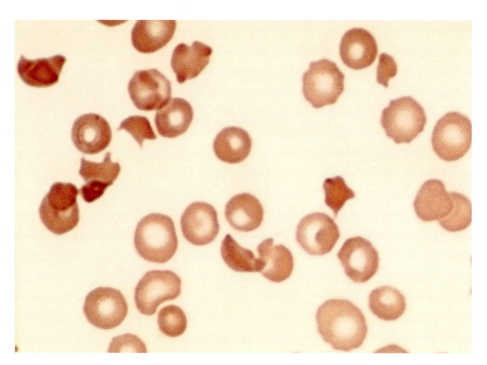

Plate 6
Peripheral blood smear. (See Case 12.)

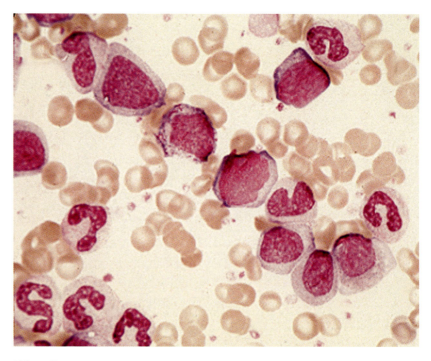

Plate 7
Peripheral blood smear. (See Case 13.)

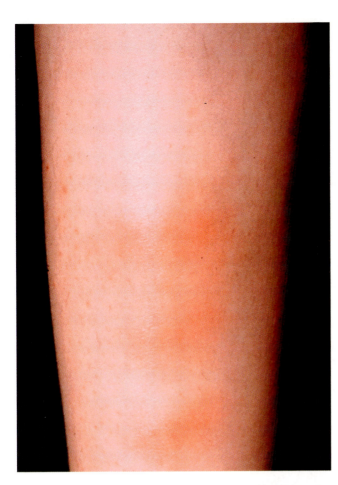

Plate 8
Nodules over right lower extremity. (See Case 14.)

Plate 9
Gram stain of BAL specimen. (See Case 17.)

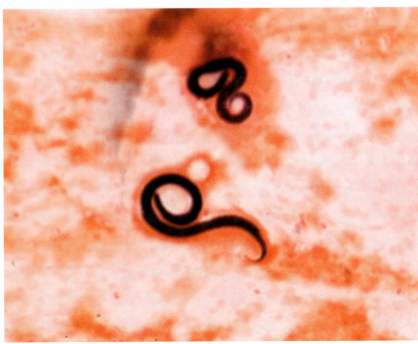

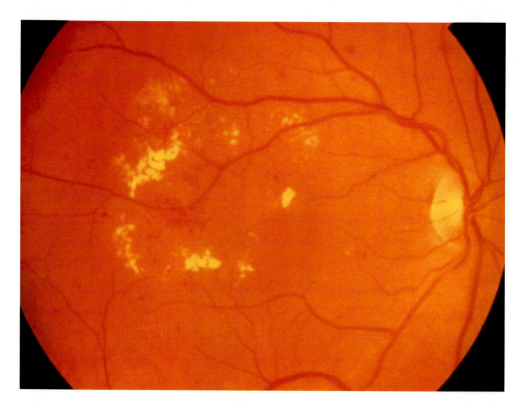

Plate 10
Fundoscopic examination of right eye. (See Case 18.)

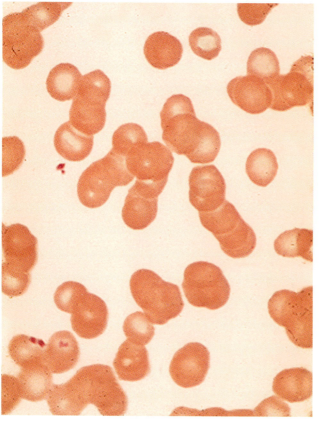

Plate 11
Rouleaux formation of red blood cells on peripheral blood smear. (See Case 21.)

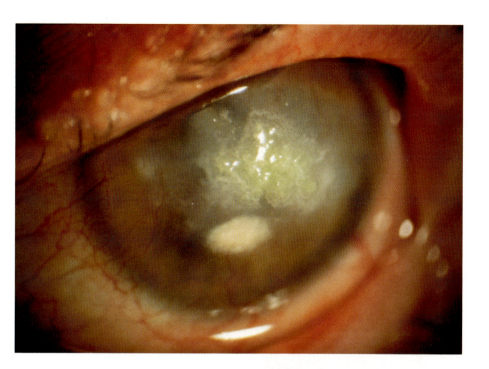

Plate 12
Slit-lamp examination of
right eye. (See Case 25.)

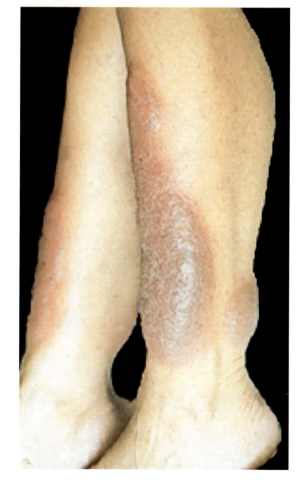

Plate 13
Skin findings on lower
extremity. (See Case 28.)

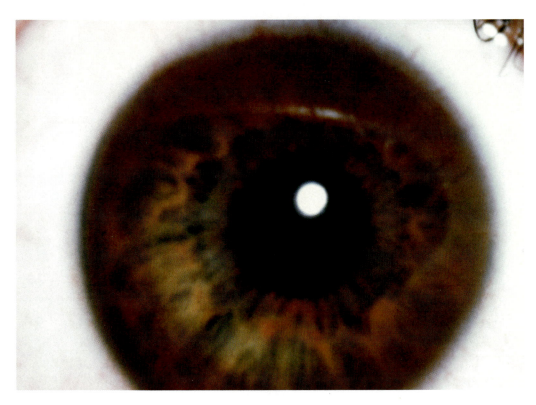

Plate 14
Kayser-Fleisher rings. (See Case 33.)

71-YEAR-OLD MAN WITH LOW BACK PAIN

A 71-year-old man with a history of hypertension, type 2 diabetes mellitus, and Parkinson's disease presented with severe low back pain that had been present for 10 years and managed with intermittent NSAID therapy. Two years previously he had been told that he had "spinal arthritis." Two months prior to this presentation he stumbled while ascending a flight of stairs, and the pain began radiating to his posterior thighs, becoming more severe and persistent. He began having difficulty ambulating and required help with his daily activities. Medications that he took regularly were glucophage, carbidopa-levodopa, indapamide, and orphenadrine. He denied fever, chills, weight loss, bowel or bladder incontinence, and chest pain. He was widowed, lived alone in a first-floor apartment, and did not drink alcohol or smoke tobacco.

PHYSICAL EXAMINATION

VITAL SIGNS: Temperature, 97.4°F (36.3°C); pulse, 84; respiration, 16; bp, 135/78 mmHg

GENERAL: Masked facies, stooped posture

HEENT: Normal

NECK: No lymphadenopathy or thyromegaly

LUNGS: Clear

CARDIAC: Grade I/VI systolic ejection murmur at left sternal border with radiation to carotids; normal carotid upstroke

ABDOMEN: Midline scar, soft, normoactive bowel sounds; no hepatosplenomegaly

EXTREMITIES: No cyanosis or edema

NEUROLOGIC: Upper extremity resting "pill-rolling" tremor and cog-wheel rigidity; deep tendon reflexes 2+; normal strength and sensation throughout

BACK: Moderate lumbosacral paraspinal tenderness; negative straight leg raise; radiation of pain and paresthesias to thighs associated with standing spinal extension

RECTAL: Normal sphincter tone

LABORATORY FINDINGS

WBC, 11.5 K/μL (normal differential); Hb, 15.7 g/dL; platelets, 354 K/μL; electrolytes, normal; urea nitrogen, normal; creatinine, normal; glucose, 181 mg/dL; urinanalysis, normal; sulfosalicylic acid, negative; lumbar spine radiographs with flexion/extension lateral projections: normal alignment, moderately severe degenerative changes with severe disk disease at all levels and limited range of motion, no lytic lesions or fractures seen; magnetic resonance imaging (MRI) of the lumbar spine (Fig. 27-1).

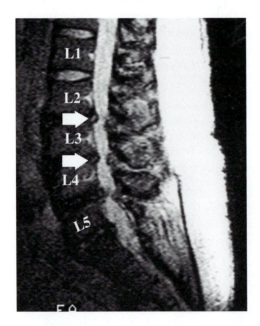

Figure 27-1
MRI of lumbar spine.

What is the likely diagnosis and how should this patient be treated?

This patient has lumbar spinal stenosis. The MRI shows loss of disk height and signal intensity at L2-3, L3-4, L4-5, and L5-S1 with disk protrusion (thick arrows) and osteophytes at each of these levels. There is also moderately severe facet arthropathy and hypertrophy of the ligamentum flavum (thin arrows). These changes caused spinal canal and lateral recess stenosis at L2-3, L3-4, L4-5, and, to a lesser extent, L5-S1.

Low back pain (LBP) is the most common musculoskeletal symptom for which people seek medical attention. Its estimated lifetime prevalence in the general population exceeds 70 percent. LBP is typically classified into acute (<12 weeks) and chronic (≥12 weeks) forms.

Acute LBP, although associated with a wide range of disorders, occasionally may be caused by serious underlying conditions such as compression fracture, malignancy, infection, or aneurysm, which the initial history and physical examination should focus on identifying. Nonetheless, most cases of acute LBP are mechanical: musculoligamentous, degenerative disk, and facet joint disease. Over 90 percent of patients with acute LBP improve within 1 month with conservative therapy, but when the pain persists, further evaluation should be considered.

Chronic LBP is caused by many mechanical and nonmechanical disorders that require a systematic approach to diagnose. In the elderly, the most common cause of chronic LBP is degeneration of osseous, articular, and ligamentous structures of the lumbosacral spine that eventually leads to osteoarthritis. Degenerative spinal stenosis occurs when osteoarthritis and compensatory soft tissue hypertrophy narrows the spinal canal and causes neural compression.

Understanding the pathophysiology of this degenerative process gives some insight into the clinical syndrome. Degeneration of the intervertebral disks occurs with aging, leading to a loss in height of the disks, which causes the vertebral bodies to move closer together. The supporting ligaments thus become lax, compromising the inherent stability of the intervertebral joints, which increases compressive and shear forces that eventually lead to osteoarthritis. Osteophytes ("spurs") begin to appear in the anterior spine at ligament attachment sites as a result of motion, whereas the facet joints and ligamentum flavum in the posterior spine hypertrophy, decreasing the space available for the nerve roots to traverse and exit the spinal canal. When the narrowing becomes critical, the vascular supply to the nerve roots is compromised, resulting in leg pain or claudication. Stenosis may involve the central canal, the lateral recess, and the intervertebral foramen, and may occur at one or more levels, but most commonly involve L3-L4 and L4-L5, as in our patient.

Lumbar stenosis usually occurs in men in their sixth or seventh decade of life. The presenting complaint is typically claudication, which denotes pain, weakness, or numbness of the leg after walking or that occurs in a certain position of spine extension, as when walking down hills or steps. Unlike claudication owing to peripheral vascular disease in which a patient must stop walking to gain relief, a patient with neurogenic claudication must sit or flex forward to increase space in the spinal canal that decreases pain and restores blood flow to the nerve roots. Several maneuvers, such as the stoop test or bicycle test, may differentiate the two forms of claudication, but their sensitivity is low. It is more important to perform a thorough vascular exam to exclude a vascular cause. It is often helpful to examine the patient sitting, standing, and immediately after walking (stress neurologic exam); however, it is not uncommon to have no localizing physical findings with spinal stenosis. Reduction in vibratory sense is the most sensitive physical finding, but its specificity for spinal stenosis is lost when there is coexisting diabetes mellitus or other peripheral nerve disorders. In contrast to lumbar disk herniation, LBP from spinal stenosis is caused by degenerative changes in the spine and not nerve root compression and rarely causes signs of nerve root tension such as a positive straight leg-raise test.

The initial evaluation should include AP and lateral spine radiographs, preferably while standing, to exclude degenerative scoliosis and spondylolisthesis. Once the diagnosis is established by history and physical examination, however, no further studies are necessary. An MRI should only be done when conservative therapy has failed to help guide further therapy. If an MRI cannot be done, a CT myelogram is a good alternative. An EMG may provide supportive evidence of abnormal physiology, but gives no information about the anatomic deformity. In patients with coexisting peripheral vascular disease, Doppler studies and a vascular consultation may be helpful.

Treatment of spinal stenosis is conservative and focused on the control of symptoms. NSAID agents, analgesics, epidural steroid injections, exercise, physical therapy, bracing, acupuncture, chiropractic treatment, and stress reduction techniques are just a few of the available treatments. Although few controlled trials have been done to document the effectiveness of any of these therapeutic modalities, multidisciplinary pain treatment programs may be helpful. A decision for surgery should be based on the anticipated quality of the patient's life after appropriate nonoperative measures have failed. Since paralysis, and bowel and bladder dysfunction rarely occur in lumbar stenosis, there are no absolute functional or anatomical criteria to warrant surgery. Decompressive laminectomy may give some relief, whereas spinal fusion may be useful for those with deformities. If no postoperative complications occur, patients are generally home within 5 days and are functionally independent within 6 weeks.

Our patient was taken to surgery for a multi-level decompressive laminectomy. He tolerated the procedure without difficulty and was sent home on the fourth postoperative day. On follow-up he reported dramatic improvement in his symptoms and was taking regular daily walks.

 ## CLINICAL PEARLS

- First exclude malignancy, infection, and aneurysm as a cause of back pain.
- Spinal stenosis occurs most commonly in males in their sixth or seventh decades.
- Claudication ameliorated by spine flexion is often the first manifestation of spinal stenosis.
- Rule out peripheral vascular disease as a cause of claudication owing to spinal stenosis.
- An MRI should be done when conservative treatment of spinal stenosis is ineffective.
- Laminectomy is for patients with disabling symptoms unresponsive to conservative measures.

REFERENCES

1. Bridwell KH. Lumbar spinal stenosis: Diagnosis, management, and treatment. *Clin Geriatric Med* 1994;10:677–701.
2. Borenstein DG. Chronic low back pain. *Rheum Dis Clin North Am* 1996;22:439–456.
3. Garfin SR. A 50-year-old woman with disabling spinal stenosis. *JAMA* 1995;274:1949–1954.

55-YEAR-OLD WOMAN WITH ANXIETY, WEIGHT LOSS, AND WEAKNESS

A 55-year-old woman presented with a complaint of a 30-pound weight loss over the past 6 months despite, according to her husband, having a voracious appetite. During this time she also noted increased anxiety, difficulty climbing stairs, palpitations, and insomnia. In addition, she reported being "hot all the time." In fact, she frequently wanted to sleep with her bedroom window open, but her husband objected because it was February and snowing outside. Her past medical history was unremarkable. She had smoked one pack of cigarettes daily for over 35 years, but denied alcohol or drug use. Her only medication was estrogen, which was started following hysterectomy for benign fibroid tumors at age 49. Her family history was notable for thyrotoxicosis in her mother. No one in the family had thyroid cancer.

PHYSICAL EXAMINATION

VITAL SIGNS: Temperature, 98.4°F (~36.9°C); pulse, 98; respiration, 14; bp, 154/76 mmHg; weight, 134 pounds; height, 64 inches
GENERAL: Thin, hyperkinetic woman with prominent eyes (Fig. 28-1)
HEENT: Eyes: normal fundus and extraocular muscle movements
NECK: Goiter with systolic bruit (Fig. 28-2)
CARDIAC: Hyperdynamic precordium; loud S_1 and S_2, grade II/VI systolic ejection murmur over the left sternal border

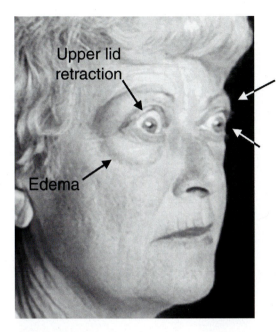

Upper lid retraction

Periorbital edema

Upper lid retraction

Proptosis

Edema

Figure 28-1
Facial features.

ABDOMEN: Normoactive bowel sounds, soft, nontender; no hepatosplenomegaly

EXTREMITIES: Hands: Figure 28-3

NEUROLOGIC: Generalized decreased muscle strength, unable to stand from a squat without assistance, difficulty standing from a seated position

SKIN: Figure 28-4

LABORATORY FINDINGS

WBC, 4.2 K/μL (normal differential); Hb, 13.6 g/dL; platelets, 181 K/μL;. electrolytes, normal; glucose, normal; urea nitrogen, normal; creatinine, normal; urinalysis, normal; serum total thyroxine, 22 μg/dL (normal, 4.5–12.0); free thyroxine, 4.6 ng/mL (normal, 0.7–1.5); thyroid ^{123}I uptake scan, diffusely enlarged goiter with homogeneous uptake of ^{123}I, 88 percent uptake at 24 hours

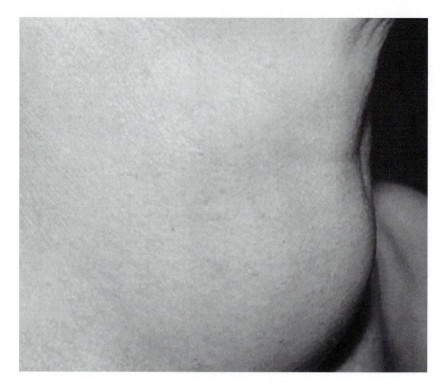

Figure 28-2
Goiter.

What is the likely diagnosis and how should this patient be treated?

This lady has thyrotoxic Graves' disease complicated by ophthalmopathy, Plummer's sign (nail pooling away from nailbed as a consequence of accelerated growth), and pre-tibial myxedema (thyroid dermopathy) (see Figs. 28-1, 28-3, and 28-4). Smoking increases the risk of Graves' disease and worsens the ophthalmopathy. She probably should be treated with antithyroid drugs. Approximately one in 300 patients has a serious adverse reaction to these drugs, which usually is agranulocytosis. Treatment with ^{131}I may temporarily worsen her ophthalmopathy. Her skin lesion

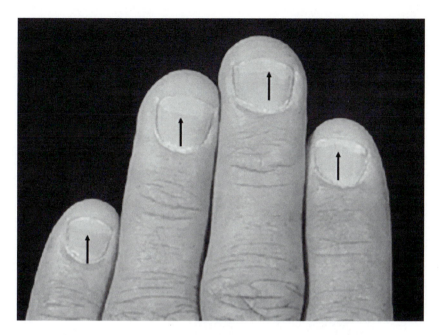

Figure 28-3
Nail beds.

will not respond to antithyroid drugs, but most likely will respond to corticosteroids.

Graves' disease is a familial autoimmune disorder in which polyclonal TSH receptor (TSHr) antibodies stimulate the synthesis and release of thyroid hormone and subsequently increase the size of the thyroid gland. Other antibodies target retro-orbital tissues, producing inflammation and exophthalmos that may result in serious morbidity. Pretibial myxedema is also an autoimmune manifestation in which antibody binds to antigens in the deep skin layers. The prevalence of Graves' disease is increased in smokers, who also have a much higher risk of developing severe ophthalmopathy. In addition, older men have a higher incidence of severe ophthalmopathy that is often unilateral.

The presence of diffuse toxic goiter with or without ophthalmopathy is sufficient to make the diagnosis of Graves' disease; however, the classic presentation, albeit less common, is the triad of diffuse toxic goiter, exophthalmos, and pretibial myxedema. Although most present with diffuse toxic goiter, some patients manifest ophthalmopathy alone and may never develop thyrotoxicosis, a condition termed euthyroid Graves' disease.

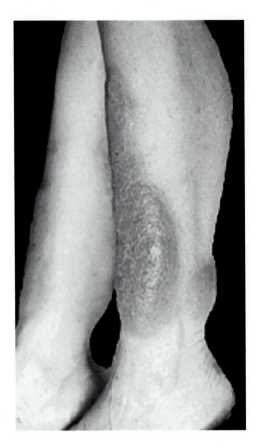

Figure 28-4
Skin findings on lower
extremities. (See Plate 13.)

This is a familial disorder without a clear pattern of inheritance, although the concordance rate in monozygotic twins is 50 percent. It typically affects middle-aged women, but can occur in both sexes at all ages. About 30 percent of patients have evidence of ophthalmopathy by examination, but most (80%) have eye muscle swelling detectable only by ultrasound or CT. Bilateral but asymmetric exophthalmos is normally seen, and because it is usually self-limiting, usually requires no therapy. Consultations with an endocrinologist and ophthalmologist are indicated for the few patients who develop severe proptosis with ophthalmoplegia and impaired vision. Pretibial myxedema is seen in about 5 percent of patients with Graves' disease, and occurs exclusively in those with ophthalmopathy. The anterior-lateral aspect of the leg is typically involved with red-brown plaques that resembles pig skin. Approximately half subside spontaneously; however, compression of blood vessels or nerves may lead to ischemia or neuropathy, and trauma (surgery) often worsens the lesions.

Symptoms of thyrotoxicosis are typically the reason patients seek evaluation. Although the diagnosis may be quite apparent by history and physical examination alone, it may be more challenging in those with subtle symptoms or coexisting diseases or conditions, such as pregnancy or old age. Overt thyrotoxicosis almost always causes high anxiety, palpitations, nervousness, restlessness, tremor, heat intolerance, and weight loss. These symptoms, however, also occur frequently with anxiety and depression, which at times may be difficult to distinguish from thyrotoxicosis. Nonetheless, certain symptoms of thyrotoxicosis are so unique that their presence makes the bedside diagnosis of thyrotoxicosis a virtual certainty. Weight loss, despite a voracious appetite and eating more than usual, is a highly specific symptom of thyrotoxicosis. This occurs with regularity only in thyrotoxicosis, diabetes mellitus, or malabsorption. Heat intolerance is another fairly specific symptom of thyrotoxicosis, especially when severe and of recent onset. Patients often relate unusual accounts of seeking cooler temperatures. On one occasion, a nervous medical student complained to us about his grades (in itself not a distinguishing feature of thyrotoxicosis); however, the diagnosis was obvious, considering the conversation occurred outside in the blistering cold while it was snowing, and the student was sweating profusely—with his jacket off and shirt sleeves rolled up! This and his goiter and tremor made the diagnosis of thyrotoxicosis obvious. Few diseases lend themselves to such instant "bedside" recognition. Muscle weakness is another important symptom. Ordinarily, patients notice difficulty climbing stairs or standing from a seated position, and may have trouble holding their arms up for an extended period, while fixing their hair, for instance.

The presence of a goiter in a symptomatic patient clinches the diagnosis of thyrotoxicosis. If exophthalmos is present, the diagnosis is Graves' disease. A CT scan of the orbit can distinguish clinically asymmetrical exophthalmos of Graves' disease from a retro-orbital tumor (Fig. 28-5). Pretibial myxedema is so unique to Graves' disease that there ordinarily is little doubt about its origin, particularly since ophthalmopathy is almost always coexistent.

Elderly patients with Graves' disease may have a much less obvious presentation. Thyrotoxicosis often is manifest only by atrial fibrillation or heart failure associated with weight loss and muscle weakness. The goiter may not be obvious and ophthalmopathy is not as common as in younger patients. Occasionally, elderly patients manifest a flat affect, giving the ap-

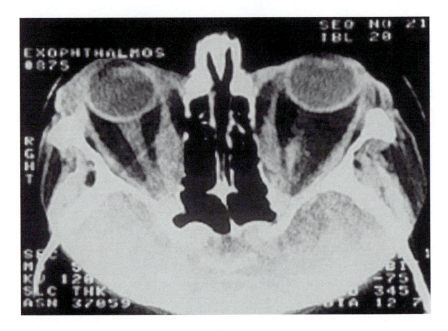

Figure 28-5
CT scan of orbits.

pearance of apathy or depression as their main manifestation of thyrotoxicosis, a syndrome termed *apathetic thyrotoxicosis*.

Once the diagnosis is identified or suspected at the bedside, it must be
confirmed by an undetectably low serum TSH and high serum free thyroxine (T4) concentration. In some patients, serum *total* triiodothyronine
(T3) alone is elevated (termed *T3 thyrotoxicosis*) and rarely only *free T3* is
elevated (a syndrome termed *free T3 thyrotoxicosis*). If the patient is clinically toxic and the free thyroid hormone levels are high, *but the serum
TSH is in the normal range or high*, the diagnosis is either a pituitary tumor
secreting TSH or pituitary resistance to thyroid hormone, two very uncommon but important diagnoses.

After a biochemical diagnosis of thyrotoxicosis is established, its cause
must be determined. It is convenient to consider the causes of thyrotoxicosis in two general categories: (1) those owing to hyperthyroidism,
which have a high thyroidal radioiodine uptake (RAIU); and (2) those
without hyperthyroidism in which the RAIU is low. The most common
causes of thyrotoxicosis with a high RAIU are Graves' disease, toxic
multinodular goiter, and an autonomously hyperfunctioning thyroid

nodule. Less common causes are abnormal thyroid stimulators, for example, β-hCG (produced by molar pregnancy or choriocarcinoma), or a TSH-secreting pituitary tumor or pituitary resistant to thyroid hormone. The most common causes of thyrotoxicosis with a low RAIU are ingestion of excess amounts of thyroid hormone, which have either an iatrogenic or factitious cause, and various forms of thyroiditis. Rarely ectopic thyroid tissue, as occurs with ovarian teratomas, can cause thyrotoxicosis with a low RAIU.

Therapy of thyroid disorders with a high RAIU is aimed primarily at curbing the secretion of thyroid hormone, whereas treatment for thyrotoxicosis with a low RAIU is generally aimed at modifying the peripheral effects of thyroid hormone, usually with β-blockers. Treatment of Graves' disease is somewhat unique because it has a natural history of spontaneous resolution over a period of years. Three choices of therapy exist: subtotal thyroidectomy, thionamides, and radioactive iodine (^{131}I). Most patients can be treated with anti-thyroid drugs or ^{131}I. The choice between the two is mainly a matter of patient and physician preference, since both are effective therapy. The thionamides—propylthiouracil (PTU) or methimazole (Tapazole)—effectively ameliorate the symptoms of thyrotoxicosis and are generally given to very thyrotoxic patients and are the preferred therapy for pregnant women and children under the age of 18. They are frequently used before surgery, and sometimes are given to very thyrotoxic patients before ^{131}I therapy. Dosage varies with the severity of thyrotoxicosis and the size of the goiter, but initial treatment is usually 50 to 100 mg of PTU given orally every 8 hours or 10 to 30 mg of methimazole once daily. Serum thyroid hormone levels fall over about 6 weeks and the dose is adjusted every 6 weeks to maintain the free serum T4 in the normal range. TSH often remains suppressed for months, which is not a reason to increase the dosage; however, it should be reduced if the TSH is high. The maintenance doses for PTU are 50 to 100 mg daily, and for methimazole 5 to 10 mg daily. Agranulocytosis occurs in about three per 1000 patients treated with antithyroid drugs and usually occurs in the first 3 months of therapy. It is less common in patients under age 40 and with less than 40 mg of methimazole daily. Clinically, it presents abruptly with fever and severe pharyngitis. Routine white cell counts may detect it before the onset of symptoms, but a low white cell count must be distinguished from the mild granulocytopenia that occurs with Graves' disease. The white cell count usually returns to normal within 1 to 2 weeks of stopping the drug. Agranulocytosis is an absolute contraindication to further thionamide therapy. The most common reaction to these drugs is an urticarial, erythematous, and pruritic skin rash. A few patients may develop cholestatic jaundice. After 1 year's treatment, permanent remission of Graves' disease after drug withdrawal is about 30 percent, but ranges from 10 to 70 percent in reported series. The remission rate doubles to around 75 percent after 2 years of therapy. The likelihood of remission is greater in those patients with a small goiter, mild thyrotoxicosis, and with a longer duration of therapy. No test can reliably predict a permanent remission.

The treatment of choice for nonpregnant thyrotoxic adults is [131]I. It is also the treatment for recurrent hyperthyroidism, but is strictly contraindicated in pregnancy. The goal is to render the patient euthyroid, although with the usual therapeutic dose (around 10 mCi) most patients develop hypothyroidism within the first year of treatment. It cures the hyperthyroidism and shrinks the goiter in practically everyone and almost no one develops recurrent thyrotoxicosis. Importantly, ophthalmopathy may be aggravated by ^{131}I therapy, although concurrent treatment with corticosteroids may prevent this complication.

Subtotal thyroidectomy is an effective and safe form of therapy that promptly renders the patient euthyroid. It is usually performed when patients cannot or will not take ^{131}I or antithyroid drugs, and for the few patients with Graves' disease who have goiters causing compressive symptoms. Surgery should also be performed if there is suspicion of thyroid cancer, which ordinarily exists in a patient with diffuse toxic goiter complicated by a hypofunctional (cold) nodule. Although some prepare patients with β-adrenergic blockers alone, most clinicians treat thyrotoxic patients scheduled to undergo surgery with antithyroid drugs until they are euthyroid to avert the risk of postoperative thyroid storm. Fewer than 1 percent of patients develop tetany owing to surgical damage to the parathyroids. Transient hypocalcemia occurs more often and is owing to an increased rate of calcium entering bones postoperatively—termed the *hungry bone syndrome*.

Some of the signs of thyrotoxicosis can be ameliorated with β-adrenergic blockers without altering the excessive thyroid function. Propranolol inhibits the peripheral deiodination of T4 to T3. It alleviates the tachycardia, arrhythmias, eyelid retraction, and tremor of thyrotoxicosis. Restlessness, myopathy, periodic paralysis, and bulbar dysfunction may also improve with propranolol.

This patient was treated with antithyroid drugs for several years and failed to respond. She was subsequently given ^{131}I and her hyperthyroidism abated. Her ophthalmopathy stabilized and required no specific therapy. Her skin lesions were treated with topical and intralesional glucocorticoid that resulted in some improvement over several years.

 CLINICAL PEARLS

- Thyrotoxicosis should be suspected in a patient with weight loss despite normal food intake, severe heat intolerance, anxiety, weakness, and tachycardia.
- Diffuse toxic goiter is almost always owing to Graves' disease, an autoimmune disorder that tends to run in families and predominantly affects young and middle-aged women.
- The diagnosis of thyrotoxicosis must be verified with high free thyroid hormone (T4 or T3) levels and a totally suppressed serum TSH level.
- Thyrotoxicosis may occur with a low thyroidal uptake of ^{123}I, which suggests thyroid hormone ingestion, thyroiditis, or ectopic thyroid hormone production.
- The three forms of therapy are subtotal thyroidectomy, antithyroid drugs, and [131]I.
- Agranulocytosis occurs in about one in 1000 patients treated with antithyroid drugs.

REFERENCES

1. Burch HB, Solomon BL, Wartofsky L, et al. Discontinuing antithyroid drug therapy before ablation with radioiodine in Graves' disease. *Ann Intern Med* 1994;121:553–559.
2. Franklyn JA. Drug therapy: The management of hyperthyroidism. *N Engl J Med* 1994;330:1731–1738.
3. Singer PA, Cooper DS, Levy EG, et al. Treatment guidelines for patients with hyperthyroidism and hypothyroidism. *JAMA* 1995; 273:808–812.

78-YEAR-OLD WOMAN WITH BLACKOUT SPELLS

A 78-year-old woman with a history of hypertension and osteoarthritis presented after experiencing three "blackout" spells. The spells occurred suddenly, without warning, and were associated with a period of un-awareness of her surroundings. Each of the episodes lasted seconds and resulted in a fall, which on one occasion caused bruising of her left shoul-der. Her husband reported "jerking movements" of her arms and legs with each spell. After the spells, she awakened quickly and was able to re-sume her activity, although she was somewhat fatigued for the remainder of the day. All of the spells occurred while seated; one happened after eat-ing in a restaurant. The owner called 911, but she refused to be taken to the emergency room. She denied chest pain, shortness of breath, nausea, diaphoresis, palpitations, weakness, or loss of bowel or bladder control during the spells. She reported excellent exercise tolerance and partici-pated in water aerobics regularly. Six months ago, a stress echocardiogram done for atypical chest pain was normal. Her regular medications were amlodipine, hydrochlorothiazide, and acetaminophen. She did not smoke and drank one glass of wine nightly.

PHYSICAL EXAMINATION

VITAL SIGNS: Temperature, 98.2°F (36.7°C); pulse, 74; respiration, 18; bp, 116/70 mmHg (lying); 120/72 mmHg (standing)
GENERAL: Thin, younger than stated age
HEENT: Normal
NECK: No thyromegaly
Lungs: Clear
CARDIAC: Regular rate and rhythm; no murmurs or gallops; normal PMI and venous pressure; no carotid bruits

ABDOMEN: Normoactive bowel sounds, soft, nontender; no hepatosplenomegaly

EXTREMITIES: Heberden's nodules; no cyanosis or edema

LABORATORY FINDINGS

WBC, 8.5 K/μL (normal differential); Hb, 13.1 g/dL; platelets, 222 K/μL; electrolytes, normal; glucose, normal; urea nitrogen, normal; creatinine, normal; urinalysis, normal; electrocardiogram, normal sinus rhythm

What is the likley diagnosis and how should this patient be treated?

Further questioning elicited that all of her syncopal spells occurred within 30 minutes after eating a meal; therefore, she likely has postprandial syncope—a commonly unrecognized cause of syncope in the hypertensive elderly patient. This form of syncope results from a significant decrease in blood pressure (>20 mmHg) within 75 minutes of ingesting a meal. The mechanism of postprandial hypotension is not fully understood but is particularly common in older hypertensive patients.

Syncope is defined as a transient loss of consciousness associated with a loss of postural tone and followed by spontaneous recovery. It is a very common abnormality, accounting for up to 6 percent of hospital admissions and 3 percent of emergency room visits, particularly among young healthy adults (up to 50%) and the elderly. Syncope can result from a variety of physiologic and pathologic changes that may lead to either a benign, self-limited course or a malignant course associated with significant morbidity.

Syncope generally occurs as a result of a transient period of inadequate perfusion to the brainstem. This may occur by three distinct mechanisms: (1) a decrease in systemic vascular resistance; (2) a decrease in cardiac output; or (3) as a result of cerebrovascular disease. The causes of syncope may be classified into four major categories based on these mechanisms (Table 29-1).

TABLE 29-1   Etiologies of Syncope

NONCARDIOVASCULAR	CARDIOVASCULAR
REFLEX-MEDIATED VASOMOTOR INSTABILITY	**DECREASED CARDIAC OUTPUT**
Vasovagal	**Obstruction to flow**
Situational	Left ventricular outflow
Micturition	obstruction
Cough	Aortic stenosis, hyper-
Swallowing	trophic CMP
Defecation	Mitral stenosis, atrial
Carotid sinus syncope	myxoma
Neuralgias	Right ventricular outflow
High altitude	obstruction
Psychiatric disorders	Pulmonic stenosis
	Pulmonary embolism,
ORTHOSTATIC HYPOTENSION NEUROLOGICAL DISORDERS	hypertension
	Atrial myxoma
	Other Heart Diseases
Migraines	Pump failure
Transient ischemic attacks	Myocardial infarction,
Seizures	coronary disease
	Tamponade, aortic
	dissection
	Arrhythmias
	Bradyarrhythmias
	Sinus node disease
	Second and third
	degree AV block
	Pacemaker malfunction
	Tachyarrhythmias
	Ventricular tachycardia
	Torsades de pointes
	Supraventricular
	tachycardia

Adapted from Kapoor WN. Syncope and hypotension, in *Heart Disease: A Textbook of Cardiovascular Medicine*, Braunwald E. (ed). Philadelphia, Saunders, 1997, pp 863–876.

Reflex-mediated vasomotor instability syndromes (neurocardiogenic, neurally mediated syncope) are a group of disorders characterized by reflex mechanisms involving afferent and efferent neural arcs, resulting in inappropriate vasodilatation or bradycardia, hypotension, and syncope. The afferent signals are received from receptors in a variety of organ systems that respond to pain, mechanical stimuli, and temperature. Vasodepressor (vasovagal, neurocardiogenic) syncope is the most common of the reflex-mediated syndromes and is the most common cause of non-cardiovascular syncope and syncope of unknown etiology. It is characterized by hypotension, with or without bradycardia, often associated with a prodrome of lightheadedness, warmth, pallor, nausea, blurred vision, or diaphoresis. Vasodepressor syncope commonly occurs in young people, often in response to fear or pain. Other predisposing factors are prolonged standing and heat exposure. Of note, elderly patients who experience vasodepressor syncope frequently do not experience prodromal symptoms and will often give a history of syncope without warning. Vasodepressor syncope usually occurs in an upright posture, with initiation of the pathophysiologic response that is the premise for the upright tilt test (Fig. 29-1). Situational syncope likely occurs with a similar reflex mechanism except that the site of afferent signal generation is different (e.g., urinary bladder, GI tract, respiratory tract).

Carotid sinus syncope occurs as a result of stimulation to the carotid sinus baroreceptors located in the internal carotid artery just above the bifurcation of the common carotid artery. It occurs predominantly in men over age 50 who have a history of coronary artery disease and hypertension. A history of syncope with sudden head turning, with shaving, or while wearing a tight collar can be elicited in up to 25 percent of affected patients. Syncope is associated with a pause (bradycardia) plus hypotension or hypotension without bradycardia. Other forms of syncope thought to be reflex-mediated include those associated with aortic stenosis, hypertrophic cardiomyopathy, atrial fibrillation, and pacemakers (pacemaker syndrome).

Orthostatic hypotension (OH) is another important and common cause of syncope, particularly in the elderly patient who may be taking cardiovascular or psychotropic drugs. Normally, assuming an upright posture is associated with peripheral venous pooling, decreased cardiac output, and a drop in blood pressure. These changes are compensated by sympathetic stimuli that induce reflex tachycardia and vasoconstriction. Thus, only a transient and small decrease in systolic blood pressure occurs while the diastolic pressure tends to increase. In patients with OH, a pro-

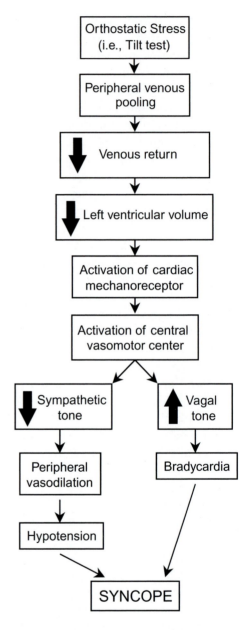

Figure 29–1
Pathophysiology of vasovagal
syncope.

found and persistent decrease in the systolic blood pressure (>20 mmHg) occurs, with or without a concomitant drop in diastolic pressure as a result of a defect in the regulation of the compensatory response. Syncope is typically brief and occurs suddenly after standing. Associated symptoms may include dizziness, blurred vision, and profound weakness, but symptoms of autonomic hyperactivity do not occur. Causes other than drugs and volume depletion are primary autonomic insufficiency (Shy-Drager, or idiopathic) and a number of secondary autonomic insufficiency syndromes (owing to diabetes mellitus, amyloidosis, and multiple CVAs).

Neurological disorders are an uncommon cause of syncope. Only 6 percent of ischemic strokes or transient ischemic attacks are associated with syncope. When they do cause syncope, concurrent neurological symptoms are almost always manifest. Seizure disorders may be associated with syncope; however, seizure-like activity that may occur with non-neurologic syncope may be difficult to differentiate from typical seizure activity. Prolonged recovery from syncope (with confusion or lethargy) is suggestive of a postictal state; this is the most reliable historical feature for identification of seizures.

Cardiac syncope occurs as a consequence of obstruction to cardiac output, myocardial ischemia with sudden pump failure, or arrhythmias. Left ventricular outflow tract obstruction caused by aortic stenosis or hypertrophic cardiomyopathy are the most common mechanical causes of cardiac syncope. Syncope in the setting of these entities typically occurs with exertion. Almost half of the patients with severe aortic stenosis experience syncope, after which the average survival without valve replacement is 2 to 3 years. Hypertrophic cardiomyopathy causes syncope in up to 30 percent of patients; these patients frequently have ventricular arrhythmias. Other important mechanical lesions include congenital heart disease, pulmonary hypertension, cardiac tamponade, and atrial myxomas. Elderly patients may present with syncope as the main manifestation of an acute myocardial infarction. Arrhythmias are also important causes of cardiac syncope. High-degree atrioventricular (AV) block may cause syncope (Stokes-Adams attack). Ventricular asystole results in an abrupt onset of unconsciousness unrelated to position. Patients with sick sinus syndrome, caused by impaired sinoatrial impulse formation or conduction, frequently present with syncope. Ventricular tachyarrhythmias generally occur in the setting of organic heart disease, but congenital syndromes (long QT interval), metabolic disturbances, and drugs may also be causative. Other tachyarrhythmias causing syncope are atrial fibrillation or flutter with rapid ventricular response, Wolff-Parkinson-White syndrome, and AV nodal re-entrant tachycardia.

A detailed history and physical examination are the most important elements in the evaluation of a patient with syncope. The history permits the clinician to discern true syncope from other entities, such as vertigo and lightheadedness. Also, the history and physical help stratify the patient's risk and provide clues for a presumptive diagnosis, which helps direct further testing, if necessary (Table 29-2). The physical examination should focus on cardiovascular and neurological abnormalities and evaluation for an orthostatic fall in blood pressure. The bedside evaluation of patients with a definable cause of syncope will identify its cause in up to 85 percent of cases. The electrocardiogram (ECG) is abnormal in about 50 percent of patients with syncope, most of whom do not have a cardiac cause. The ECG may provide clues for guiding further evaluation. Laboratory blood screening is rarely helpful.

Once the history, physical examination, and ECG are completed, directed diagnostic testing should be performed to confirm the initial clinical suspicion. The American College of Physicians has recently published clinical guidelines for guiding clinicians in the evaluation of syncope. These guidelines take into account the results of the baseline history and

TABLE 29-2   Historical Clues

HISTORY	CONSIDER
Sudden onset	Arrhythmia
Unrelated to position	
Palpitations	
No prodrome	
Onset of varying duration when upright	Reflex-mediated
Prodrome—(warm, diaphoresis, nausea	(Neurocardiogenic)
Sudden onset after standing	Orthostatic hypotension
Exertional onset	Aortic stenosis, hypertrophic CMP
	Subclavian steal (arm exercise)
	Exercise arrhythmia
Gradual onset and resolution	Metabolic, drugs
Vertebrobasilar symptoms	Cerebrovascular disease
Postictal state	Seizure disorder

Adapted from Schaal SF, Nelson SD, Boudoulas H, et al. Syncope. *Curr Prob Cardiol* 1992;17:205–264.

physical examination, likelihood of disease in a specific population, and the sensitivity and specificity of available tests. Others have suggested different approaches and algorithms. Differentiation between cardiac syncope and noncardiac causes of syncope is important because of the marked difference in prognosis. The 1-year mortality for cardiac syncope is 18 to 33 percent, compared to 0 to 12 percent for noncardiac syncope and 6 percent for syncope of unknown cause.

Treatment decisions begin with risk stratification and the identification of underlying heart disease, arrhythmias, and possibility for sudden death. Therapies for the various causes of syncope are usually quite successful if the cause is specifically defined.

Our patient reported significant improvement after stopping her diuretic, eating smaller and more frequent meals, and liberalizing her salt and fluid intake. She remains normotensive on amlodipine.

CLINICAL PEARLS

- Syncope is a very common problem among young healthy adults and the elderly.
- Syncope occurs as a result of three mechanisms: decreased systemic vascular resistance, decreased cardiac output, and cerebrovascular disease.
- Reflex-mediated syndromes (vasovagal) are a common cause of syncope in young adults.
- Orthostatic hypotension is an important cause of syncope in the elderly.
- The most important element in the evaluation of syncope is a detailed history and physical.
- The 1-year mortality for cardiac syncope (18–33%) is significantly higher than that for noncardiac syncope (0–12%).
- Postprandial syncope is an often unrecognized cause for syncope in the elderly.

REFERENCES

1. Linzer M, Yang EH, Estes III NA, et al. Diagnosing syncope. Part 1: Value of history, physical examination, and electrocardiography. *Ann Intern Med* 1997;126:989–996.

2. Linzer M, Yang EH, Estes III NA, et al. Diagnosing syncope. Part 2: Unexplained syncope. *Ann Intern Med* 1997;127:76–86.

3. Kapoor WN. Syncope and hypotension, in *Heart Disease: A Textbook of Cardiovascular Medicine*, Braunwald E. (ed). Philadelphia, Saunders, 1997, pp 863–876.

4. Manolis AS, Linzer M, Salem D, et al. Syncope: Current diagnostic evaluation and management. *Ann Intern Med* 1990;112:850–863.

5. Schaal SF, Nelson SD, Boudoulas H, et al. Syncope. *Curr Prob Cardiol* 1992;17:205–264.

6. Jansen R, Lipsitz LA. Postprandial hypotension: Epidemiology, pathophysiology, and clinical management. *Ann Intern Med* 1995;122: 286–295.

23-YEAR-OLD MAN WITH DIABETES MELLITUS AND SYNCOPE

A 23-year-old man presented for advice regarding the management of his type 1 diabetes mellitus that had been present since age 12. He had recently been having substantial difficulty controlling his blood glucose levels. Three months ago, because his morning glucose levels were around 150 mg/dL and his glycated hemoglobin was 8.3 percent (normal, 4.8–7.8%), his physician advised him to increase his insulin dosage and begin a vigorous exercise program. After several weeks, his fasting blood glucose levels dropped to between 70 and 90 mg/dL and his random blood glucose levels were never higher than 150 mg/dL. When seen in consultation, he was taking 40 units of Lente and 5 units of regular insulin before breakfast, 10 units of regular insulin 30 minutes before dinner, and 10 units of Lente insulin at bedtime. His main concern was that, for the first time ever, several weeks ago, he lost consciousness, requiring intravenous glucose administration by the emergency squad. Since then, he has experienced several other episodes of confusion and near-syncope, usually an hour or so after dinner. During the last episode he was stopped by the police for operating his motor vehicle recklessly. He reported experiencing none of the usual adrenergic hypoglycemic symptoms during these episodes. He has gained about 6 pounds recently, takes no other medications, and does not smoke, drink alcohol, or use illicit drugs. He denied impotence.

PHYSICAL EXAMINATION

VITAL SIGNS: Temperature, 97.4°F (~36.3°C); pulse, 64; respiration, 15; bp, 126/76 mmHg

207

GENERAL: Normal-appearing man (weight, 145 pounds; height, 5 feet 8 inches), good muscle mass
HEENT: Normal funduscopic exam
NECK: No lymphadenopathy or thyromegaly
LUNGS: Clear
CARDIAC: Normal
ABDOMEN: No organomegaly
EXTREMITIES: Good pulses in feet, no foot lesions
NEUROLOGIC: Deep tendon knee reflexes 3+; normal strength and sensation throughout
SKIN: No rashes or other abnormalities

LABORATORY FINDINGS

WBC, 5.5 K/μL (normal differential); Hb, 15.3 g/dL; electrolytes, normal; urea nitrogen, normal; creatinine, normal; glucose (fasting), 66 mg/dL; total cholesterol, 160 mg/dL; HDL cholesterol, 45 mg/dL; LDL cholesterol, 100 mg/dL; triglycerides (fasting), 120 mg/dL; glycosylated hemoglobin, 5.4% (normal, 4.8–7.8%); urinalysis, negative, without glucose; 24-hour urine for microalbumin, 15 mg (normal, <30); electrocardiogram, normal; serum cortisol 60 minutes after cortrosyn (250 μg im), 25 μg/dL

What is the likely diagnosis and how should this patient be treated?

This patient has type 1 diabetes mellitus (formerly termed insulin dependent diabetes mellitus or IDDM), complicated by the recent onset of *hypoglycemia unawareness*, a syndrome associated with intensified insulin therapy. This can resolve by avoiding hypoglycemia for about 1 month. His insulin regimen should be altered to raise his fasting serum glucose level to about 120 mg/dL, and his pre-dinner regular insulin may be switched to insulin lispro.

The results of the Diabetes Control and Complications Trial (DCCT) demonstrate that strict glycemic control in patients with type 1 diabetes mellitus significantly reduces the risk of complications such as retinopathy and nephropathy. Strict glycemic control usually is achieved with three or more insulin injections daily or treatment with an insulin pump. In the DCCT, this resulted in about a 70 percent reduction in the risk of diabetic retinopathy, a 40 percent decrease in the occurrence of microalbuminuria, and a 60 percent reduction in the risk of clinical peripheral neuropathy. However, patients experienced almost a threefold increase in severe hypoglycemia. Nonetheless, mean blood glucose values in the intensive therapy group remained about 40 percent above normal. Although a primary treatment goal in patients with type 1 diabetes should be a level of blood glucose control at least equal to that achieved in the intensively treated DCCT group, this may not apply to all patients and must be based on clinical judgment. Serious hypoglycemia is dangerous and more likely to occur when blood glucose control is achieved.

Severe hypoglycemia, in which blood glucose concentrations fall so low that cognitive function is impaired—or more simply, the patient requires assistance from someone else—is a dangerous complication of insulin therapy that affects up to 30 percent of patients with type 1 diabetes. In the DCCT, the incidence of severe hypoglycemia (as evidenced by seizures or hypoglycemic coma, including multiple episodes in some patients) was about three times higher in the group receiving intensive therapy than in the group receiving conventional therapy. There were 54 hospitalizations, usually brief, to treat hypoglycemia and there were three fatal motor vehicle accidents in which hypoglycemia may have had a causative role. Accordingly, this degree of rigorous control may have to be sacrificed when frequent or severe hypoglycemia cannot be avoided.

Severe hypoglycemia may result from anything that causes serum insulin and glucose concentrations to be mismatched (Table 30-1). Hypoglycemia ordinarily produces a series of symptoms beginning with those owing to epinephrine release (pallor, tachycardia, sweating, anxiety, tremor), which, if untreated, lead to symptoms of central nervous system glucose deprivation, termed neuroglycopenia, consisting of confusion, stupor, seizures (focal or generalized), coma, and death.

Some diabetic patients are particularly vulnerable to severe hypoglycemia because they do not experience these warning symptoms as blood glucose falls. Termed *hypoglycemia unawareness*, this phenomenon results from delayed and diminished neurohumoral responses to hypoglycemia. The major risk factors for this complication are a history of severe hypoglycemia, long-standing duration of diabetes, and intensified diabetes treatment. Hypoglycemia awareness can be restored by avoiding

TABLE 30-1   Common Causes of Hypoglycemia in
Patients with Type 1 Diabetes Mellitus

Insulin Therapy
Mismatch of meals and insulin injection
Erratic absorption of insulin
Abdominal injection (faster)
Deltoid or femoral region injections (slower)
Enhanced Insulin Sensitivity
Exercise (prolonged effect)
Loss of counterregulatory hormones
Hypopituitarism or adrenal insufficiency
Malabsorption
Autonomic neuropathy (25–50% have gastric or intestinal stasis
    and malabsorption)
Celiac sprue (greater than usual frequency)
Drugs
Beta-blockers
Other Concurrent Diseases
Renal failure
Hepatic failure

hypoglycemia for about 1 month. The target blood sugar level should be raised slightly during that month and the patient should be educated about this problem. One study found that the most important ways to prevent hypoglycemia were avoidance of subnormal blood glucose concentrations, reduced doses of overnight insulin after vigorous exercise, and an absolute requirement for snacks between meals and at bedtime. Understanding and dealing with *hypoglycemia unawareness* helps patients walk the fine line between excellent glycemic control and unacceptable episodes of severe hypoglycemia.

Timing of the peak action of insulin and peak blood glucose concentrations is important in avoiding hypoglycemia. This may be particularly difficult to achieve with regular insulin, which reaches a maximum action about 2 hours after injection, making it necessary to inject the insulin at least a half hour before the meal to limit the anticipated increase in serum glucose concentration. The delayed absorption of regular insulin is partly caused by its propensity to form dimers in solution, which subsequently form hexamers. Although insulin monomers and dimers diffuse rapidly from the subcutaneous space into the circulation, the size of hexamers limits their diffusion. A new analog, insulin lispro, has been formed by reversing the natural sequences of lysine and proline in the C-terminal end of the B-chain of insulin, thus preventing the formation of hexamers. Absorption of insulin lispro is faster, resulting in earlier (40 minutes) and higher peak serum insulin levels than after regular insulin. The length of time to peak activity after subcutaneous insulin lispro is independent of the dose, whereas for regular insulin the time to peak activity increases with increasing doses. As a result of its more rapid onset of action, lispro insulin must be injected just before a meal. The fasting and pre-meal glucose concentrations tend to be higher during treatment with insulin lispro than during treatment with regular insulin. Body weight increases during intensified insulin treatment, but is no more with lispro than with regular insulin. Studies of the awareness of hypoglycemia and glucose counterregulation after the administration of insulin lispro compared to regular insulin reveal similar responses for both.

Our patient's pre-dinner regular insulin was switched to lispro, and his total insulin dosage was decreased. He was educated about hypoglycemia unawareness and his target blood glucose levels were raised. The hypoglycemia episodes resolved in about 1 month.

 ## CLINICAL PEARLS

- Intensified insulin therapy reduces the risks of retinopathy (70%), neuropathy (60%), and microalbuminuria (40%), but increases the risk of severe hypoglycemia threefold.
- Severe hypoglycemia impairing cognitive function affects up to 30 percent of type 1 diabetics.
- Hypoglycemia unawareness results from abnormal neurohumoral responses to hypoglycemia.
- The major risk factors for hypoglycemia unawareness are a history of severe hypoglycemia, long-standing duration of diabetes, and intensified diabetes treatment.
- Hypoglycemia awareness can be restored by avoiding hypoglycemia for about 1 month.
- A new analog, insulin lispro, peaks faster (40 minutes) and higher after subcutaneous injection than regular insulin.

REFERENCES

1. Diabetes Control and Complications Trial Research Group. The effect of intensive treatment of diabetes on the development and progression of long-term complications in insulin-dependent diabetes mellitus. *N Engl J Med* 1993;329:977.
2. Boyle PJ, et al. Brain glucose uptake and unawareness of hypoglycemia in patients with insulin-dependent diabetes mellitus. *N Engl J Med* 1995;333:1726.
3. Cranston I, et al. Restoration of hypoglycaemia unawareness in patients with long-standing duration of insulin-dependent diabetes mellitus. *Lancet* 1994;344:283.
4. Holleman F, Hoekstra JBL. Insulin lispro. *N Engl J Med* 1997;337:176.

CASE 31

83-YEAR-OLD WOMAN WITH BACK PAIN

An 83-year-old retired female Russian physician who recently emigrated to the United States presented with a 5-month history of debilitating back pain. She described the pain as a severe "aching," localized to her mid-back. She denied bowel or bladder incontinence. Her past medical history was notable for an unspecified tachyarrhythmia and glaucoma, osteoporosis, and skeletal tuberculosis as a child, requiring right hip surgery. She reported no recent history of trauma or falls. She denied fever, chills, night sweats, fatigue, chest pain, cough, and shortness of breath, weakness, or weight loss. Her regular medications included acetaminophen, docusate sodium, and calcitonin nasal spray. There was no family history of cancer, diabetes, or coronary artery disease; her father died of tuberculosis. She did not use alcohol and was a lifetime non-smoker.

PHYSICAL EXAMINATION

VITAL SIGNS: Temperature, 98.5°F (36.9°C); pulse, 88; respiration, 18; bp, 163/100 mmHg
GENERAL: Age appropriate
HEENT: Normal
NECK: No thyromegaly
THORAX: Kyphosis
LUNGS: Clear
CARDIAC: Regular rate and rhythm; no gallops or murmurs; mild left ventricular enlargement; jugular venous pulse normal; 2+ pulses in upper and lower extremities

ABDOMEN: Normoactive bowel sounds; soft, nontender; no hepato-splenomegaly

EXTREMITIES: No cyanosis or edema; right leg was shorter than left

BACK: Palpable paraspinal fullness and tenderness over thoracic vertebrae T7–8

NEUROLOGIC: Cranial nerves II–XII intact; reflexes 2+ throughout; no sensory or motor deficits

RECTAL: Guaiac negative, normal sphincter tone

LABORATORY FINDINGS

WBC, 4.3 K/μL (65% segs, 23% lymphs, 8% monos); Hb, 16 g/dL; platelets, 288 K/μL; electrolytes, glucose, urea nitrogen, and creatinine normal; calcium, 5.3 mEq/L (normal, 4.3–5.2); phosphorus, 4.5 mg/dL (normal, 2.5–4.5); lactate dehydrogenase, 664 U/L (normal, 0–625); alkaline phosphatase, 212 U/L (normal, 0–110); blood and urine cultures negative; erythrocyte sedimentation rate 83 mm/hr (normal, 0–20); thyroxine and TSH normal; urinalysis normal; chest x-ray and thoracic spine film (Fig. 31-1); thoracic spine MRI (Fig. 31-2).

What is the likely diagnosis and how should this patient be treated?

This patient has Pott's disease, or tuberculous spondylitis. The chest x-ray reveals extensive bilateral apical calcification consistent with previous granulomatous disease. The thoracic spine film shows bony destruction of the inferior endplate of T7 and superior endplate of T8 with obliteration of the disk space and loss of height of both vertebral bodies, and an associated soft tissue paravertebral mass with areas of calcification. The thoracic spine MRI demonstrates collapse of T7 and T8 with an intervening high-signal mass within the disk space. There is paraspinal and epidural extension of the mass with cord compression. In addition, there is a high signal in the posterior elements of T7–8. A CT-guided needle biopsy of the paraspinal mass was nondiagnostic. Subsequently, an open biopsy and laminectomy procedure was performed. Microscopic examination of the

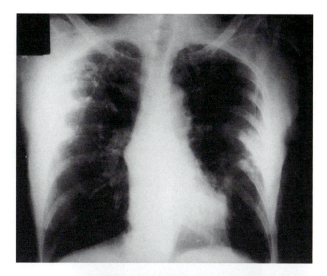

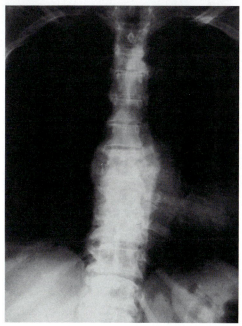

Figure 31-1
PA chest x-ray and thoracic
spine x-ray.

tissues revealed caseating granulomas and acid-fast organisms, consistent with *Mycobacterium tuberculosis*, which was confirmed by cultures.

The English surgeon Sir Percivall Pott (1714–1788) first described tuberculous spondylitis in 1779. It was one of the most common disorders seen in the early days of orthopedics. Although the worldwide incidence

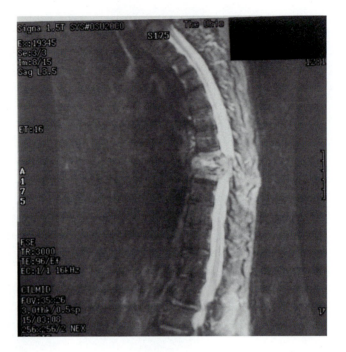

Figure 31-2
MRI of thoracic spine.

of *M. tuberculosis* (TB) is on the upswing with the advent of the AIDS crisis, skeletal involvement with the disease is relatively uncommon, occurring in only 1 to 3 percent of patients. The spine is the most common site affected, accounting for about half the cases, whereas involvement of the hip and knee account for about 15 percent each. In developing nations, skeletal TB is seen more commonly in children and teenagers, whereas in North America, it is seen predominantly in elderly patients with long-standing tuberculosis.

Development of skeletal tuberculosis is thought to occur by the hematogenous spread of organisms early in the disease course. In some, it may be the only manifestation of disease and may go unrecognized for years, similar to pulmonary involvement. In the case of spinal involvement, seeding of organisms is believed to occur through a paravertebral venous plexus (Batson's plexus), although spread through lymphatic drainage of periaortic lymph nodes has also been suggested. Infection typ-

ically involves the anterior portion of the vertebral body, eventually erod-
ing the endplates superiorly or inferiorly. Vertebral collapse and anterior
wedging of the spinal column ultimately cause instability and obvious deformities such as kyphosis or a gibbous formation. A paravertebral abscess
is typical of vertebral tuberculosis and has been demonstrated in over
50 percent of patients with the disease. The abscess usually extends an-
terolaterally, occasionally for a considerable distance, but rarely invades
the peridural space. In the upper thoracic spine, the abscess may grow
into the chest wall as a mass; in the lower spine, it may extend to the in-
guinal region or develop into a psoas abscess.

As with other causes of vertebral osteomyelitis, the usual presenting
symptom is dull, continuous back pain and the initial diagnosis is often
back strain or disk disease. Rarely, patients present with progressive paraplegia caused by vertebral compression and a complicated paraspinal abscess or mass (Pott's paraplegia). In contrast to pyogenic osteomyelitis,
spinal tuberculosis most commonly involves the thoracic vertebrae.

Radiographically, spinal TB typically appears as an osteolytic bone lesion. However, chronic infections may have calcification that increases
the bone density on spine radiograms. Importantly, vertebral fusion does
not occur in spinal tuberculosis. Involvement of any two adjacent vertebrae and the intervening disk space suggests either pyogenic osteomyelitis
or Pott's disease as opposed to malignancy, which usually does not invade
the disk space. By plain radiogram or CT scan, the presence of calcification within a soft tissue paravertebral mass is virtually pathognomonic of
a Pott's tumor. MRI is useful in evaluating the degree of spinal cord compromise as well as disk and disk space changes. Aspiration of the abscess
or open bone biopsy is often necessary to confirm the diagnosis.

Skeletal TB, including Pott's disease, is often responsive to anti-
tuberculous chemotherapy. However, in severe cases with a large abscess
or impending spinal cord compression, emergent surgical intervention
may be required for adequate drainage and spinal cord stabilization.

Following the debridement and laminectomy procedure, our patient
was placed on a four-drug regimen of INH: rifampin, pyrazinamide,
ethambutol, and pyridoxine. The organism was susceptible to all drugs
tested. The State Health Department and Epidemiology Department
were notified and PPD skin testing was performed on her family. At last
visit, 2 years after presentation, some back pain persists, but serial MRI
studies have demonstrated no change and she remains without neurologic
impairment.

CLINICAL PEARLS

- Despite worldwide resurgence in *M. tuberculosis* infections owing to the AIDS epidemic, skeletal involvement with tuberculosis remains uncommon.
- The spine is the most common site of skeletal infection with TB in adults, accounting for approximately half the cases.
- Pott's disease is thought to develop from hematogenous spread of organisms through Batson's plexus.
- A paravertebral abscess (mass) is typical of spinal tuberculosis and occurs in over half the patients.
- The most common presenting complaint is dull, aching back pain—often diagnosed as back strain or disk disease.
- CT scanning or MRI reveals the characteristic lesion and can assess neurologic compromise, but needle aspiration or open biopsy is often necessary to identify the organism.
- Pott's disease is frequently responsive to anti-tuberculous chemotherapy, but may require surgical intervention in severe cases with spinal cord compromise.

REFERENCES

1. Flamm ES. Percivall Pott: an 18th century neurosurgeon. *J Neurosurg* 1992;76:319–326.
2. Sternbach G. Percivall Pott: tuberculous spondylitis. *J Emerg Med* 1996;14:79–83.
3. Davidson PT, Horowitz I. Skeletal tuberculosis. *Am J Med* 1970; 48:72–84.
4. Rezai AR, Lee M, Cooper PR, et al. Modern management of spinal tuberculosis. *Neurosurgery* 1995;36:87–97.
5. Marcq M, Sharma O. Tuberculosis of the spine: a reminder. *Chest* 1973;63:403–408.
6. Sharif H, Morgan JL, al Shahed MS, et al. Imaging of tuberculosis and craniospinal tuberculosis: role of CT and MR imaging in the management of tuberculous spondylitis. *Radiol Clin North Am* 1995;33:787–804.

31-YEAR-OLD MAN FOUND UNCONSCIOUS AND UNRESPONSIVE

A 31-year-old man was transferred to The Ohio State University Medical Center emergency department after being abandoned in an unresponsive state at another hospital. On arrival to our emergency department, he was obtunded and unresponsive and was immediately intubated because he was unable to protect his airway. During the initial evaluation, a nearly empty bottle of amitriptyline was found in the man's pocket and he was noted to smell of alcohol. No other history was available at the time of presentation.

PHYSICAL EXAMINATION

VITAL SIGNS: Temperature, 97.6°F (36.4°C); pulse, 101; respiration, 14 (ventilator-assisted); bp, 120/75 mmHg
GENERAL: Obtunded, unresponsive
HEENT: Pupils 4 mm with no response to light
NECK: No lymphadenopathy or thyromegaly
LUNGS: Clear
CARDIAC: Slightly tachycardic, regular rate and rhythm without murmurs, rubs, or gallops
ABDOMEN: Soft, hypoactive bowel sounds; no hepatosplenomegaly

EXTREMITIES: No cyanosis, edema, or rash
NEUROLOGIC: Deep tendon reflexes 2+; unable to assess strength or sensation

LABORATORY FINDINGS

WBC, 9.8 K/μL (normal differential); Hb, 14.9 g/dL; platelets, 354 K/ μL; electrolytes: sodium, 138 mEq/L; potassium, 3.4 mEq/L; chloride, 101 mEq/L; bicarbonate, 22 mEq/L; urea nitrogen, 16 mg/dL; creatinine, 1.0 mg/dL; glucose, 197; anion gap, 15 mEq/L (normal, <12 mEq/L); measured serum osmolality, 345 mOsm/kg H_2O; arterial blood gas measurements on 100% oxygen: pH, 7.54; P_{CO_2}, 24 mm Hg; P_{O_2}, 305 mm Hg; CO_2, 15 mEq/L; ethanol level, 0.147 mg/dL; amitriptyline level, 1004 ng/mL; urinalysis: pH, 8.5; urine sediment (Fig. 32-1). ECG showed normal sinus rhythm with a normal QT interval.

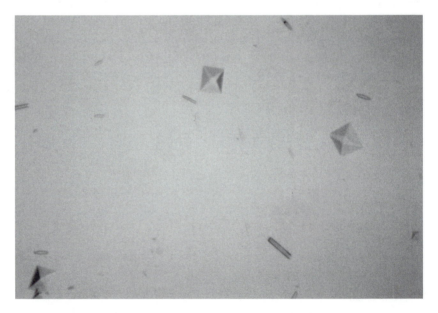

Figure 32-1
Microscopic examination of urine.

What is the patient's anion gap? What is the patient's calculated serum osmolality? What is the patient's osmolar gap? What does the urine sediment show? What is the diagnosis?

Three simple calculations must be done to recognize the diagnosis in this patient: the anion gap, the calculated serum osmolality, and the serum osmolar gap.

The anion gap is calculated from:

$$\text{Anion gap} = \text{sodium} - [\text{chloride} + \text{bicarbonate}]$$

Using this formula, his anion gap was 15 mEq/L (normal <12). The calculated serum osmolality (Osm − C) is derived from:

$$\text{Osm} - \text{C} = 2 \times \text{sodium} + [\text{glucose}/18] + [\text{BUN}/2.8]$$

His calculated serum osmolality (Osm − C) is 293 mOsm/kg H_2O (normal, 290 + 5).

The osmolar gap is calculated from the following formula:

$$\text{Osmolar gap} = [\text{measured osmolality} - \text{calculated osmolality}]$$

Using this calculation, the patient's osmolar gap is 52 mOsm/kg H_2O (normal <10).

The urine sediment shows calcium oxalate crystals (see Fig. 32-1).

This case illustrates the need for a careful diagnostic evaluation in a patient with a drug overdose, including an investigation for multiple drug ingestion. Endotracheal intubation was done to protect his airway and further evaluation was done. His serum amitriptyline level was 1004 ng/mL (therapeutic, 120–250 ng/mL) consistent with a tricyclic antidepressant overdose. This does not, however, cause an osmolar gap, which indicates the presence of another low-molecular-weight substance (e.g., ethanol) in his serum. However, ethanol does not account for his clinical picture.

The wide anion and osmolar gaps are the main clues to the correct diagnosis, which was significantly narrowed to include only diabetic ketoacidosis, alcoholic ketoacidosis, and poisoning by methanol or ethylene glycol. Calcium oxalate crystals suggested ethylene glycol intoxication. His serum ethylene glycol levels were 500 mg/L (toxicity >20 mg/dL).

TRICYCLIC ANTIDEPRESSANT TOXIC SYNDROME

Tricyclic antidepressants (TCAs) are commonly prescribed and widely used in attempted suicides, causing life-threatening problems. They account for the largest percentage of adult deaths owing to pharmaceutical agents. Through blockade of neuronal reuptake of serotonin, norepinephrine, or dopamine, TCAs exert α-adrenergic effects and a neuronal membrane-stabilizing effect. They are lipophilic and about 98 percent protein-bound (this is pH dependent) with large distribution volumes (10–50 L/kg). The half-life of amoxapine is about 8 hours, but in other TCAs ranges up to 20 hours.

Initially, TCAs produce anticholinergic effects consisting of hypotension, sinus tachycardia, mydriasis (not responding to light), dry mouth, respiratory depression, ileus, and urinary retention. The principal manifestations are in the central nervous system and heart. Generalized seizures and coma are followed by cardiovascular deaths, primarily from ventricular arrhythmias and conduction abnormalities that may occur up to 24 hours after ingestion. Myocardial depression similar to that seen with quinidine produces ECG changes that portend a poor prognosis, such as prolongation of the PR or QT intervals, widening of the QRS complex, and the appearance of bundle branch block.

Treatment begins with activated charcoal gastric lavage, which should be done within 24 hours of ingestion. Emesis should not be induced because of the risk of aspiration. Forced diuresis, hemodialysis, and hemoperfusion play no role in removal of the drug. The mainstay of treatment is sodium bicarbonate given in a dosage sufficient to raise the serum pH to about 7.48 to 7.52, which substantially increases protein binding of the drug. Inducing respiratory alkalosis by hyperventilation is not useful. Heart conduction abnormalities and hypotension often improve with sodium bicarbonate, whereas arrhythmias may correct with phenytoin (500 mg to 1 g intravenously). Lidocaine or bretylium may have a transient beneficial effect; however, quinidine, disopyramide, and procainamide are contraindicated. Cardiac monitoring for 24 hours is usually necessary after the ECG has normalized. Seizures can be treated with diazepam, phenytoin, or phenobarbital.

ETHYLENE GLYCOL POISONING

Methanol and ethylene glycol, which are two of the most toxic alcohols, have very similar properties. Both produce metabolites that cause a profound anion-gap metabolic acidosis and an osmolar gap, although methanol is worse in this regard. Ethylene glycol undergoes hepatic degradation by alcohol dehydrogenase through several metabolites that contribute to the metabolic acidosis, eventually forming oxalic acid that is precipitated in the renal tubules as calcium oxalate. This causes renal failure. The urine sediment shows needle-shaped calcium oxalate monohydrate and envelope-shaped calcium oxalate dihydrate crystals (see Fig. 32-1). The half-life of ethylene glycol in the circulation is about 3 hours, with a volume of distribution of 0.7 L/kg. Its hepatic metabolism is shorter than that of methanol, making its latent period shorter.

Ethylene glycol toxicity can be divided into three stages. *Stage 1* (30 minutes to 12 hours after ingestion) is characterized by inebriation, ataxia, and metabolic acidosis with respiratory compensation (Kussmaul's breathing), seizures, hypocalcemia, calcium oxaluria (4–8 hours after ingestion), and myoclonus. During this stage coma and death can occur from cerebral edema. *Stage 2* (12–36 hours after ingestion) is characterized by a deteriorating respiratory status manifest by tachypnea, cyanosis, pulmonary edema, and cardiomegaly. Death during this stage is usually owing to cardiovascular causes or bronchopneumonia. *Stage 3* (36–72 hours after ingestion) is dominated by renal failure from acute tubular necrosis, manifest by hematuria, proteinuria, and oliguria or anuria. Noncardiogenic pulmonary edema may occur during this stage.

Activated charcoal gastric lavage, which binds both methanol and ethylene glycol, is done promptly. Sodium bicarbonate is given intravenously at a dosage of 1 to 3 mEq/kg to normalize the arterial pH, but calcium should be monitored because this may worsen existing hypocalcemia. Ethanol, which competes with ethylene glycol (or methanol) for alcohol dehydrogenase, should be given to patients with metabolic acidosis if the ethylene glycol level is over 20 mg/dL or there are symptoms from the poisoning. It is given intravenously as a 10% ethanol solution at a loading dose of up about 10 mL/kg and a maintenance dose of about 1.4 mL/kg/hour aimed at holding the serum ethanol level between 100 mg/dL and 200 mg/dL. The maintenance rate is about doubled during hemodialysis. Ethanol treatment effectively decreases the accumulation of toxic metabolites.

Hemodialysis is the mainstay of therapy for ethylene glycol and methanol because of their low protein binding, low volume of distribution, and high water solubility. Indications for dialysis include methanol or ethylene glycol levels over 50 mg/dL, profound metabolic acidosis, renal failure, or visual symptoms developing after methanol ingestion. Maintenance of ethyl alcohol concentrations during dialysis can be achieved by adding ethyl alcohol to the dialysate bath at a concentration of 100 mg/dL or by increasing the amount of ethyl alcohol infusion. It is important to administer thiamine and pyridoxine and monitor calcium during ethylene glycol poisoning.

Our patient was treated in the medical intensive care unit with both sodium bicarbonate and ethanol infusions. Hemodialysis was not required because his ethylene glycol levels fell rapidly, acid-base status corrected promptly, and renal function remained normal. The patient had protected himself from ethylene glycol poisoning by the concurrent ingestion of ethanol. The patient's TCA and ethylene glycol levels fell without further serious sequelae and he was extubated 72 hours after admission and transferred to an inpatient psychiatric unit for further treatment.

 ## CLINICAL PEARLS

- A wide anion and osmolar gap together suggests diabetic ketoacidosis, lactic acidosis, and methanol or ethylene glycol intoxication.
- Tricyclic antidepressants cause the largest number of pharmaceutical deaths in adults.
- TCA toxicity produces cardiovascular and central nervous system effects and deaths from ventricular arrhythmias.
- TCA toxicity is treated with intravenous sodium bicarbonate to raise the pH up to 7.52.
- Ethylene glycol ingestion produces an osmolar gap and urinary calcium oxalate crystals.
- Ethanol and hemodialysis are used to treat ethylene glycol poisoning.

REFERENCES

1. Klaasen CD, Amdur MO, Doull J, et al. *Casarett and Doull's Toxicology*, 5th ed. New York: McGraw-Hill, New York, 1996.
2. Newton EH, Shih RD, Hoffman RS. Cyclic antidepressant overdose: A review of current management strategies. *Am J Emerg Med* 1994;12:376.
3. Curtin L, Kraner J, Wine H, et al. Complete recovery after massive ethylene glycol ingestion. *Arch Intern Med* 1992;152:1311.
4. Parillo JE, Bone RC. *Critical Care Medicine, Principles of Diagnosis and Management.* Chicago, Mosby-Year Book, 1995.

20-YEAR-OLD WOMAN WITH JANUNDICE

A 20-year-old woman presented to the emergency department with complaints of nausea, abdominal pain, and a yellow discoloration to her skin. Her difficulties began 3 weeks prior, when she developed nausea followed by right upper quadrant abdominal pain and jaundice over the last week. She denied fevers, chills, emesis, diarrhea, arthralgias, or myalgias. Her symptoms were unrelated to eating and she reported no history of cholelithiasis. Her past medical history was notable only for traumatic childhood lower extremity fractures. She had never received a blood transfusion and denied risk factors for hepatitis B and HIV. She was physically active and reported intentionally losing approximately 80 pounds over the last 18 months with the help of a variety of commercially available herbal preparations. Her medications included ibuprofen, azithromycin, and promethazine. There was no family history of liver disease. She did not smoke tobacco or drink alcohol.

PHYSICAL EXAMINATION

VITAL SIGNS: Temperature, 98.8°F (37°C); pulse, 88; respiration, 16; bp, 125/80 mmHg

GENERAL: Jaundice; mildly obese female

HEENT: Scleral icterus and Kayser-Fleischer rings (Fig. 33-1).

NECK: No thyromegaly

LUNGS: Clear

CARDIAC: Regular rate and rhythm; no murmurs, gallops or rubs; normal jugular venous pulse

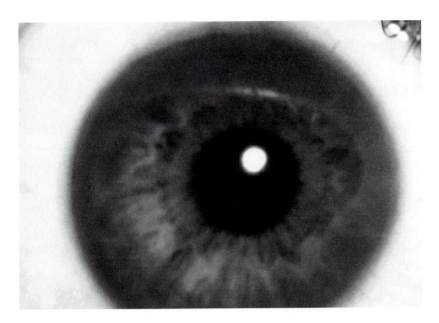

Figure 33-1
Kayser-Fleischer rings. (See Plate 14.)

ABDOMEN: Normoactive bowel sounds; soft, right upper quadrant tenderness; palpable liver tip, no splenomegaly; no ascites
EXTREMITIES: Trace lower extremity edema
RECTAL: Normal sphincter tone, guaiac negative
NEUROLOGIC: Nonfocal; normal strength and reflexes; no asterixis
SKIN: Jaundice, no telangiectasias

LABORATORY FINDINGS

WBC, 8.6 K/µL (normal differential); Hb, 13.8 g/dL; platelets, 147 K/µL; electrolytes, normal; bun, normal; creatinine, normal; international normalized ratio (INR) 2.1; PTT 85 seconds (normal, 24–34); alkaline phosphatase, 120 U/L (normal, 0–110); ALT, 80 U/L (normal, 0–60); AST, 170 U/L (normal, 0–60); LDH, 900 U/L (normal, 0–625); GGT, 290 U/L (normal, 5–85); total bilirubin, 30 mg/dL (normal, 0–1.5); and direct bilirubin, 27 mg/dL (normal, 0–0.3); albumin, 2.3 g/dL; acute abdominal series, unremarkable; right upper quadrant ultrasound revealed mild hepatomegaly and no gallstones

HOSPITAL COURSE

The patient was admitted and the following screening hepatic laboratory studies were obtained: hepatitis A, B, and C serologies were all negative, hepatitis C PCR negative; antinuclear, anti-smooth muscle, anti-liver-kidney, and anti-mitochondrial antibodies negative. Cytomegalovirus (CMV), Epstein-Barr virus (EBV), and herpes simplex virus (HSV) antibodies revealed no acute process. Serum ceruloplasmin, 19 mg/dL (normal, 20–50); alpha-1 antitrypsin, 251 (normal, 80–240)

Approximately 48 hours after admission the patient's condition deteriorated. Her WBC increased to 25 K/μL, hemoglobin dropped to 6.0 g/dL, and total bilirubin increased to 43 mg/dL. The patient remained guaiac negative. Further laboratory studies revealed: reticulocyte count (corrected), 1.6; haptoglobin, 8 mg/dL (normal, 20–230); LDH, 4800 U/L; direct Coombs' test, negative

What is the likely diagnosis and how should this patient be treated?

This patient has acute fulminant hepatic failure owing to Wilson's disease that is complicated by Coombs' negative hemolytic anemia. The diagnosis is made from close examination of the patient's eyes that reveal Kayser-Fleischer (KF) rings owing to copper sulfate deposits in Descemet's membrane of the cornea (see Fig. 33-1). They can often be seen by direct examination, but are best seen through a slit-lamp. The rings are typically 1 to 3 mm in thickness and are best seen over the outer edge of the iris in the periphery of the cornea. Although usually circumferential, they may be located only superiorly and inferiorly. However, the pigment can vary in color and the color of the patient's eyes as well as the degree and color of pigment deposition influence its visibility on direct examination. The presence of KF rings is about 90 percent sensitive and almost 100 percent specific for Wilson's disease. They were once thought to be pathognomonic of Wilson's disease but can rarely be seen in chronic familial cholestasis and primary biliary sclerosis.

Wilson's disease, or hepatolenticular degeneration, is an inherited autosomal recessive disorder of copper metabolism that has a prevalence of about 1 per 30,000 in the population. It is a disease primarily of children and young adults. About half of the patients are symptomatic by age 15 but it is rarely diagnosed after the age of 40 years. The genetic defect in Wilson's disease has recently been localized to band q14.3 on chromosome 13. This gene codes for a copper-binding transport protein, P-type ATPase, which is highly expressed in the liver and brain. A variety of gene mutations can give rise to the same phenotype and, as a consequence, most of those afflicted are compound heterozygotes with different mutations in each allele. The prevalence of heterozygous carriers in the population ranges from 1–90 to 1–180.

Normally, dietary copper is absorbed by the small intestine and processed by the liver for use as a cofactor in numerous cellular enzymatic reactions, incorporated into ceruloplasmin, or excreted in the bile. In Wilson's disease, copper uptake by the hepatocytes is preserved but excretion of copper into the bile is impaired. This leads to excessive copper in the liver and other tissues, including the brain, cornea, kidney, bone marrow, and musculoskeletal system. In addition, the incorporation of copper into ceruloplasmin is impaired. Although the physiologic role of ceruloplasmin remains poorly understood, its value is low in up to 85 percent of patients with Wilson's disease.

The clinical presentation of Wilson's disease is determined by the locations of tissue deposition. In one large clinical series, 42 percent of the patients presented with hepatic dysfunction, 34 percent with neurologic manifestations, 10 percent with hematologic abnormalities, and 10 percent with psychiatric symptoms. The majority of those who present with hepatic dysfunction are women, typically at a young age. Men more commonly present with neurologic manifestations. Hepatic dysfunction may involve a spectrum from low-grade indolent cirrhosis to acute hepatic failure. Importantly, Wilson's disease may be the most common cause of chronic liver dysfunction in children. The neurologic manifestations of Wilson's disease are widely variable and often include a number of movement disorders, including dystonia, Parkinsonism, tremor, and gait disorders. The most common neurologic manifestation is dysarthria, at times associated with abnormal facial expressions. The hematologic findings may include thrombocytopenia, neutropenia, or characteristically a Coombs' negative hemolytic anemia. The hemolysis is believed to occur as a result of direct oxidative injury by copper on the red blood cell membrane. It is rarely seen in other causes of liver disease and may precede any of the hepatic manifestations of Wilson's disease. Behavioral and psychiatric manifestations may include irritability, depression, psychosis, personality changes, and cognitive deficits. Other less common manifestations are rheumatologic disorders, renal tubular acidosis, cardiomyopathy, pancreatic insufficiency, and hypoparathyroidism.

In about 80 percent of cases the diagnosis of Wilson's disease can be established by a decrease in serum ceruloplasmin levels. Patients with Wilson's disease who have normal levels of serum ceruloplasmin are presumed to be heterozygotes. Other distinguishing laboratory studies include an increase in the 24-hour urine for copper and a high serum copper level. In the absence of conclusive clinical findings (i.e., Kayser-Fleischer rings) and laboratory studies, an increased hepatic copper content of a liver biopsy specimen is the definitive test, providing the patient does not have long-standing cholestasis. To date, genetic testing has proved difficult because of the large number of possible mutations but may be useful in studying a given family.

Treatment must be approached cautiously to avoid the development of acute encephalopathy or fulminant hepatic failure with the rapid mobilization of copper. The goal of therapy is twofold: first, lowering dietary copper and reducing its absorption; second, mobilizing tissue copper deposits. The former can be achieved with zinc or potassium salts and the latter with oral copper chelating agents, such as dimethylcysteine (penicillamine), trientine hydrochloride, dimercaprol, and zinc. Chelation therapy requires monitoring of 24-hour urine copper levels; the goal is 1 to 3 g/day. Penicillamine may be associated with significant side effects, including severe nausea, abdominal pain, leukopenia, and thrombocytopenia. In fulminant hepatic failure, chelating agents are futile but orthotopic liver transplantation is a life-saving option that is curative. Neurologic symptoms also respond poorly to therapy. Plasma exchange successfully lowers serum copper levels and may reduce the severity of hemolysis.

In addition to a slit-lamp ophthalmologic exam, our patient had a 24-hour urine copper level of 4135 μg (normal, <35) and a serum copper level of 208 μg/dL (normal, 70–155). She subsequently underwent successful orthotopic liver transplantation on day 7 of her hospitalization and has done remarkably well since then. Screening of her first-degree relatives with a history and physical examination, liver function tests, serum ceruloplasmin, and slit-lamp studies revealed no other family members with the disease.

CLINICAL PEARLS

- Wilson's disease is an inherited autosomal recessive disorder of copper metabolism that is typically diagnosed in early adulthood.
- The genetic defect has been localized to a mutation on chromosome 13 that codes for a copper-binding transport protein.
- The liver does not properly excrete copper, resulting in a buildup of copper and its deposition into a variety of tissues.
- Kayser-Fleischer rings, a low serum ceruloplasmin, or an elevated 24-hour urine copper level usually establish the diagnosis.
- Early diagnosis will prevent the irreversible deleterious effects of copper deposition on end-organ function.
- Successful treatment can be achieved with closely supervised oral chelation therapy.
- Screening first-degree family members for Wilson's disease is required.

REFERENCES

1. Brewer GJ, Yuzbasiyan-Gurkan V. Wilson disease. *Medicine* 1992; 71:139.
2. Kiss JE, Berman D, Thiel DV. Effective removal of copper by plasma exchange in fulminant Wilson's disease. *Transfusion* 1998;38:327.
3. Schilsky ML. Wilson's disease: genetic basis of copper toxicity and natural history. *Semin Liver Dis* 1996;16:83.
4. Yarze JC, Martin P, Munoz SJ, et al. Wilson's disease: current status. *Am J Med* 1992;92:643.

32-YEAR-OLD PREGNANT WOMAN WITH RESPIRATORY DISTRESS

A 32-year-old woman in her 28th week of pregnancy presented with a 2-day history of a rapidly spreading vesicular rash and progressive shortness of breath for one day. She denied hemoptysis, fever, or chills, but had diffuse pleuritic chest pain and a cough productive of scant brownish sputum. She vaguely recalled having had chickenpox as a child, and had been in good health without any significant past medical history. Her only medication was a daily prenatal vitamin. Family history was unremarkable. Her social history was positive for smoking one-half pack of cigarettes daily for many years, but she denied any alcohol or other illicit drug use. She lived at home with her husband and two children, one of whom had a similar rash.

PHYSICAL EXAMINATION

VITAL SIGNS: Temperature, 99.5°F (37.5°C); pulse, 132; respiration, 32; bp, 132/71 mmHg
GENERAL: Sitting upright on full facemask ventilation, in obvious respiratory distress
SKIN: Vesicular rash on trunk, face, and extremities, in various stages of eruption
HEENT: Oropharynx with a few raised, erythematous lesions
NECK: No lymphadenopathy or thyromegaly
LUNGS: Tachypneic, scant bibasilar crackles, otherwise clear
CARDIAC: Tachycardic and regular without murmurs, rubs, or gallops

ABDOMEN: Soft, nontender, uterine fundus palpable consistent with second-trimester pregnancy

EXTREMITIES: No cyanosis or edema, 2+ pulses throughout

NEUROLOGIC: Deep tendon reflexes 2+; normal strength and sensation throughout

LABORATORY FINDINGS

WBC, 11.1 K/μL (77% neutrophils, 13% lymphocytes, 10% monocytes); Hb 11.2 g/dL; platelets, 72 K/μL; electrolytes, glucose, urea nitrogen, creatinine, and prothrombin time, normal; arterial blood gas measurements on 100% oxygen via facemask: pH, 7.38; P_{CO_2}, 30 mmHg; P_{O_2}, 71 mmHg; CO_2, 17 mEq/L; O_2 saturation, 94%; ECG, sinus tachycardia; chest x-ray shown (Fig. 34-1); bronchoalveolar lavage fluid: 9% alveolar macrophages, 56% lymphocytes, 35% neutrophils, negative for bacteria, virus, fungus, acid-fast bacteria, or legionella.

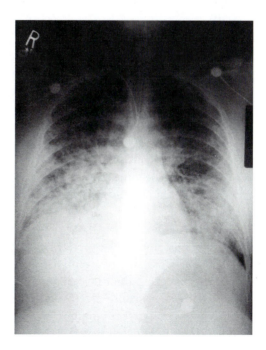

Figure 34-1
PA chest x-ray.

What is the most likely cause of this patient's respiratory distress?

This patient has varicella pneumonitis. The exposure history along with the typical skin findings should raise a strong suspicion for varicella zoster virus (VZV) infection. In seeking a definitive diagnosis in the patient with respiratory disease, a wide choice of diagnostic procedures is available. These procedures vary considerably in diagnostic reliability and specificity. Hence, an orderly sequence of test selection is mandatory, with choices based on the patient's clinical presentation and the severity and progression of the disease. This patient was initially evaluated with arterial blood gas measurements and a chest radiogram, both of which demonstrated severe respiratory compromise. The patient was admitted to an intensive care unit, where she was subsequently intubated for worsening respiratory failure. After intubation, the patient had a diagnostic bronchoscopy performed to try to help define the etiology of her respiratory failure.

The primary objectives of bronchoscopy include direct visualization of the tracheobronchial tree, including abnormalities such as tumors or granulomatous lesions, biopsy of endobronchial lesions, and lavage, brushing, or biopsy of lung regions for cultural and cytologic examinations. Both the diagnostic reach of and accessibility to bronchoscopy have been expanded by the flexible fiberoptic bronchoscope (FOB), which has made bronchoscopy more available to the physician and more acceptable to the patient. Fiberoptic bronchoscopy can be performed via transnasal or transoral routes or is easily performed through an endotracheal tube (as in this case). Fiberoptic bronchoscopy is commonly used as a diagnostic procedure on patients who are intubated and on ventilators in intensive care units. It has become particularly important in the diagnostic appraisal of patients with respiratory failure of unknown etiology or with immunosuppressed states.

Bronchoalveolar lavage (BAL) often will provide a diagnosis when induced sputa do not. This is performed by lightly wedging the bronchoscope in the distal airways, gently irrigating the air spaces beyond with saline, and analyzing the cells obtained. A normal cell differential from a BAL specimen is mainly alveolar macrophages with <1 percent neutrophils and <16 percent lymphocytes. The BAL in this case had 35 percent neutrophils, indicative of an inflammatory state, as well as 56 percent lymphocytes, raising the concern for viral infection, sarcoidosis, or hypersensitivity pneumonitis. The patient's clinical scenario was consistent with the BAL findings in the preceding, all suggestive of VZV infection.

VZV infection occurs primarily as chickenpox or herpes zoster. The VZV infection is generally considered self-limiting, with little associated morbidity and mortality. VZV pneumonitis, however, has been reported as a fatal complication and today is regarded as the most serious manifestation of disseminated VZV infection. The risk of herpes zoster is highest among patients who have received bone marrow transplants and those with Hodgkin's disease (approximately 50%), but it is considerably lower with acute leukemia or solid tumors (20 and 10%, respectively). Dissemination to the lungs is rare in immunocompromised patients with herpes zoster (5–10%).

Although varicella in adults accounts for only 2 percent of the estimated 3 to 4 million annual cases in the United States, 25 percent of the fatalities occur in this age group, reflecting a higher complication rate as compared to children. The incidence of varicella pneumonia in otherwise healthy adults has been estimated to range from 10 to 50 percent. However, several recent studies suggest that the incidence in adults may be much lower, in the range of 5 percent or less. Interestingly, some reports have indicated that 50 percent of cigarette smokers with varicella develop pneumonia, in contrast to only 3 percent or fewer of their nonsmoking counterparts. Untreated adult varicella pneumonia is fatal in about 10 percent of the cases. Although pregnant and postpartum women have an increased risk of VZV pneumonitis, the incidence rates in these subgroups are unknown. However, the mortality rate is approximately 40 percent, exceeding estimates for otherwise normal healthy adults while corresponding to rates reported for patients with cancer and bone marrow transplant recipients. Corticosteroid therapy as administered to patients with underlying renal, collagen-vascular, or other disorders has been associated with an increased risk of VZV pneumonitis. Recent reports have also indicated that conventional "low-dose" corticosteroid therapy (5–20 mg/day) may also predispose to disseminated varicella.

Fever, cough, dyspnea, tachypnea, chest pain, and hemoptysis are the hallmarks of severe VZV infection in the lungs. Early clues to pneumonia in subjects at risk are continued eruption of new skin lesions, persistent fever, and new-onset cough. The development of varicella pneumonia in the absence of fever and after the cessation of new skin lesions is exceedingly rare. In 50 to 75 percent of subjects, pneumonia is accompanied or preceded by severe and often unremitting abdominal

delivery of her baby on the ninth hospital day. The baby was delivered without incident and did well. Sadly, the patient's respiratory status continued to decline and she expired on the fourteenth hospital day. Postmortem examination revealed diffuse interstitial pneumonitis with organizing pneumonia, and cultures from the lung grew varicella-zoster.

 # CLINICAL PEARLS

- A patient's historical recollection of chickenpox is often inaccurate.
- Varicella pneumonitis is the most serious and potentially fatal complication of VZV infection in the adult.
- Smokers and pregnant women are at an increased risk for fatal VZV pneumonia.
- Clues to the development of VZV pneumonia are continual eruption of new skin lesions and persistent fever and cough, beyond the usual time course of the illness.
- Acyclovir is the treatment of choice for VZV pneumonia. Despite this treatment, patients with respiratory failure have a mortality rate of approximately 50 percent.

REFERENCES

1. Committee on Infectious Diseases of the American Academy of Pediatrics. Varicella zoster infection, in *Report of the Committee on Infectious Diseases*, 22nd ed. 1991;517–524.
2. Ventura A. Varicella vaccination: guidelines for adolescents and adults. *Am Fam Pract* 1997;55:1220–1224.
3. Feldman S. Varicella-zoster pneumonitis. *Chest* 1994;106:22S–27S.
4. Isselbacher KJ et al. *Harrison's Principles of Internal Medicine*, 13th ed. New York, McGraw-Hill, 1994.

25-YEAR-OLD WOMAN WITH EXERCISE INTOLERANCE AND ANKLE EDEMA

A 25-year-old woman was admitted to the hospital for evaluation of increasingly severe exercise intolerance and mild ankle edema that had developed 3 weeks earlier. She denied any antecedent illness, fevers, chills, orthopnea, paroxysmal nocturnal dyspnea, or other symptoms. Review of systems was positive for some joint pain and stiffness over the past 1 to 2 years as well as some recent oral aphthous ulcers. Her medical history was otherwise unremarkable. The only medicine she took regularly was an oral contraceptive.

PHYSICAL EXAMINATION

VITAL SIGNS: Temperature, 98.6°F (36.9°C); pulse, 84; respiration, 20; bp, 110/89 mmHg; paradoxical pulse, 15 mmHg

GENERAL: Thin woman who did not appear acutely ill

HEENT: Two buccal aphthous ulcers, otherwise normal

NECK: No lymphadenopathy or thyromegaly

LUNGS: Clear

CARDIAC: Mild jugular venous distention with attenuated y descents; regular rate and rhythm without murmurs, rubs, or gallops

ABDOMEN: Normoactive bowel sounds; soft, nontender with no hepatosplenomegaly

EXTREMITIES: Trace peripheral edema, tenderness over MCP joints of both hands

Integument: Normal

Neurologic: Cranial nerves intact; deep tendon reflexes 2+; normal strength and sensation throughout

LABORATORY FINDINGS

Complete blood cell count, normal; electrolytes, normal; glucose, normal; bun, normal; creatinine, normal; protein, normal; lactate dehydrogenase, normal; Westergren sedimentation rate and urinalysis, normal; blood cultures, negative; ECG, sinus tachycardia and generalized low-voltage with a rightward axis and poor R-wave progression across the precordial leads; chest x-ray showed bulging of the posterior heart border on lateral view (Fig. 35-1); transthoracic echocardiogram showed large pericardial effusion, inferior vena cava plethora, and right atrial and ventricular collapse (Fig. 35-2)

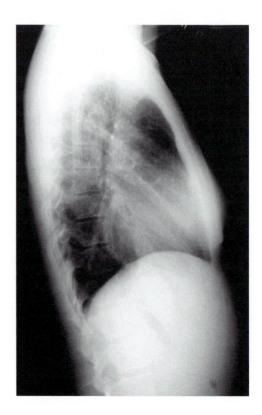

Figure 35-1
Lateral chest x-ray.

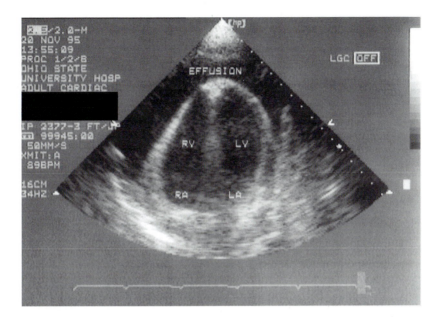

Figure 35-2
Transthoracic echocardiogram.

What is the likely diagnosis and how should this patient be treated?

The patient has pericardial tamponade. The physical exam findings of an abnormal paradoxical pulse (>10 mmHg) and attenuated y descents of the jugular venous pressure waveform, should strongly suggest pericardial tamponade. The ECG showed low voltage and the chest x-ray showed evidence of an enlarged cardiac silhouette, either secondary to chamber enlargement or pericardial effusion. Pericardial effusion with tamponade was confirmed by a transthoracic echocardiogram that showed a large pericardial effusion with echocardiographic findings consistent with tamponade physiology.

The visceral pericardium is a serous membrane that is separated by a small amount (15–50 mL) of fluid, an ultrafiltrate of plasma, from a fibrous sac, the parietal pericardium. The pericardium prevents sudden dilatation of the cardiac chambers during exercise and hypervolemia, and facilitates atrial filling during ventricular systole as a result of the development of a negative intrapericardial pressure during ejection. The pericardium also restricts the anatomic position of the heart, minimizes friction between the heart and surrounding structures, prevents displacement of the heart and kinking of the great vessels, and probably retards the spread of infections from the lungs and pleural cavities to the heart.

The accumulation of fluid in the pericardium in an amount sufficient to cause serious obstruction to the inflow of blood to the ventricles results in cardiac tamponade, a grave complication that may be fatal if not treated promptly. The three most common causes of tamponade are neoplastic disease, idiopathic pericarditis, and uremia. Tamponade also results from bleeding into the pericardial space following surgery, trauma (including cardiac perforation during procedures), tuberculosis, and hemopericardium that may result when a patient with any form of acute pericarditis is treated with anticoagulants. The three principal features of treating tamponade are elevation of intracardiac pressures, limitation of ventricular filling in diastole, and reduction of cardiac output. The amount of pericardial fluid necessary to produce this critical state may be as small as 200 mL when the fluid develops rapidly, or over 2000 mL in slowly developing effusions when the pericardium has had the opportunity to stretch and adapt to the increasing volume of fluid.

The classic findings of falling arterial pressure, rising venous pressure, and a small, quiet heart with faint heart sounds usually are seen only with severe, acute tamponade. Tamponade may also develop more slowly, and the clinical manifestations resemble those of heart failure, including dyspnea, orthopnea, hepatic engorgement, and jugular venous hypertension. Tamponade should be considered in any patient with hypotension and elevation of jugular venous pressure with a prominent x descent and attenuated y descents. A reduction in the amplitude of the QRS complexes and electrical alternans of the ECG should further raise the suspicion of tamponade. Since immediate treatment of tamponade may be life-saving, prompt measures to establish the diagnosis—especially echocardiography sometimes followed by cardiac catheterization—should be undertaken. When measured, the pericardial pressure is elevated and equal to the right atrial pressure. There is "equalization" of pressures such that the pulmonary artery wedge is equal or close to right atrial, right ventricular, and pulmonary artery diastolic pressures. In an emergency, pericardiocentesis may be carried out without cardiac catheterization but is preferably done after confirmation by echocardiography. A rapid infusion of saline increases intracardiac pressures, which in an extreme emergency will afford some temporary relief until definitive treatment can be started.

The best bedside diagnostic technique for identifying pericardial effusion is echocardiography, which is a sensitive, specific, and a noninvasive test that can estimate the quantity and location of pericardial fluid. On two-dimensional transthoracic echocardiography, small pericardial effusions produce a relatively echo-free space between the posterior pericardium and the left ventricular epicardium, whereas larger effusions show as a space between the anterior right ventricle and the parietal pericardium that circumvents the heart with larger effusions. The heart may swing freely within the pericardial sac when the effusion is large, which may be associated with electrical alternans (an alternating small and large QRS) when the to-and-fro motion is severe. With tamponade, inspiration increases the right ventricular diameter while decreasing left ventricular diameter and the mitral valve opening. However, the right ventricular cavity is reduced in late diastole by an exaggerated inward

TABLE 35-1 **Etiology of Pericarditis/Pericardial Effusion**

Infectious
Viral, pyogenic, tuberculous, mycotic
Other infections (syphilitic, parasitic)
Noninfectious
Myocardial infarction, uremia, neoplasia, myxedema
Chylopericardium, trauma, aortic aneurysm, postirradiation
Familial Mediterranean fever, sarcoidosis
Hypersensitivity or autoimmunity
Rheumatic fever
Collagen vascular disease (SLE, rheumatoid arthritis, systemic sclerosis)
Drug-induced (procainamide, hydralazine)
Postcardiac injury (Dressler's syndrome, postpericardotomy syndrome)

motion (collapse) of its free wall and that of the right atrium, which are echocardiographic findings of tamponade.

Pericardial effusion nearly always has the characteristics of an exudate. Bloody pericardial fluid is commonly owing to tuberculosis or tumor, but may also occur in rheumatic fever, post-cardiac injury, post-myocardial infarction (especially if anticoagulants are given), and uremic pericarditis. Table 35-1 lists the more common causes of pericarditis and pericardial effusions. Pericardiocentesis usually yields a serous pericardial exudate that rarely establishes the diagnosis; however, it often relieves tamponade caused by viral, idiopathic, neoplastic, hypothyroid, and uremic effusions. A pericardial window biopsy is best for diagnosing tuberculosis but may also be necessary to treat recurrent effusions causing tamponade. If pericardiocentesis fluid is diagnostic in acute pericardial effusion in an otherwise normal person, it usually yields malignant cytology.

Our patient underwent pericardiocentesis with removal of 800 mL of hemorrhagic pericardial fluid that was positive for antinuclear antibodies (ANA). After the pericardiocentesis, the patient developed a pericardial friction rub and chest pain that was treated with indomethacin. Blood tests for anti-Ro (Sjogren's syndrome antigen A [SSA]), and anti-La (SSB), anti-Sm, and anti-ribonucleoprotein (anti-RNP) were negative, but tests for antibodies to double-stranded DNA and diffuse ANA (>1:320) were positive. C4 was normal and C3 was low. Systemic lupus erythematosus was diagnosed on the basis of four of 11 American College of Rheumatology criteria: positive ANA, serositis (pericarditis), arthritis, and oral ulcers.

Cardiac pathology is common with systemic lupus erythematosus. This includes pericarditis with or without effusion, myocarditis or cardiomyopathy that sometimes involves the conduction system, and myocardial infarction from coronary arteritis or more often from atherosclerosis. Endocardial involvement in SLE may induce thromboembolism and infective or noninfective (Libman-Sacks) endocarditis that may produce valve lesions requiring surgery. However, the most common cardiovascular disease in SLE is pericarditis.

Connective tissue diseases such as SLE not uncommonly cause acute or constrictive pericarditis with or without effusions, although cardiac tamponade is rare. Symptoms may be insidious or may present suddenly and progress rapidly. Pericarditis is clinically apparent in about 30 percent of patients with SLE, but is found by echocardiography in about 50 percent and on autopsy in more than 80 percent of patients with SLE. However, because pericarditis frequently occurs without effusion or pericardial thickening, the echocardiogram can fail to disclose evidence of pericardial disease, even when classic auscultatory findings are present. There have been few reports of tamponade presenting as the initial manifestation of SLE. It is estimated to occur in only about 1 percent of patients early in their course but eventually occurs in about 4 percent of adults with SLE, particularly younger adults. In children with SLE, pericardial tamponade has been reported to occur from as little as 150 mL of pericardial fluid.

Therapy is generally unnecessary for asymptomatic and hemodynamically insignificant pericardial effusions. Treatment for symptomatic patients includes the use of nonsteroidal anti-inflammatory drugs, with or without corticosteroids. For pericardial tamponade, treatment is removal of the pericardial fluid by pericardiocentesis in sufficient quantities to lower the pericardial pressure toward normal followed by nonsteroidal anti-inflammatory drugs or corticosteroids. Occasionally, resection of the pericardium is required when chronic constrictive pericarditis is present. In most cases, acute pericarditis is self-limited and treatment is primarily symptomatic, using nonsteroidal anti-inflammatory drugs to relieve pain.

Our patient was treated with pericardiocentesis for her tamponade and placed on corticosteroid therapy. Five weeks after the patient's initial presentation, she had clinically improved and her follow-up echocardiogram showed only a small amount of residual effusion.

 CLINICAL PEARLS

- Suspect pericardial tamponade in a patient with hypotension and elevation of jugular venous pressure with prominent x descents and attenuated y descents.
- Echocardiography should be done promptly when the tamponade is suspected because immediate treatment may be life-saving.
- Pericarditis is the most common cardiac manifestation of SLE. Mild pericarditis usually responds to nonsteroidal anti-inflammatory drugs.
- Pericardial disorders can occur in various connective tissue diseases and rarely are fatal.
- About 4 percent of adults with SLE have cardiac tamponade, which is the first clinical manifestation in 1 percent.
- Pericardial tamponade owing to SLE is treated with pericardiocentesis and corticosteroids.

🌢 Cardiac tamponade must be treated emergently if a patient suddenly deteriorates.

REFERENCES

1. Langley RL, Treadwell EL. Cardiac tamponade and pericardial disorders in connective tissue diseases: case report and literature review. *J Natl Med Assoc* 1994;86:149–153.
2. O'Rourke RA. Antiphospholipid antibodies: a marker of lupus carditis? *Circulation* 1990;82(2):636–638.
3. Carette S. Cardiopulmonary manifestations of systemic lupus erythematosus. *Rheum Dis Clin North Am* 1988;14(1):135–147.
4. Crozier IG, et al. Cardiac involvement in systemic lupus erythematosus detected by echocardiography. *Am J Cardiol* 1990;65(16): 1145–1148.
5. Gulati S, Kumar L. Cardiac tamponade as an initial manifestation of systemic lupus erythematosus in early childhood. *Ann Rheum Dis* 1992;51(2):279–280.

43-YEAR-OLD MAN WITH BACK PAIN

A 43-year-old man with a history of idiopathic spontaneous pneumothorax and sleep apnea presented to the emergency department with an 18-hour history of sharp, mid-scapular back pain. It developed acutely the prior evening while he was attending a local high school sporting event, and persisted despite his taking non-steroidal anti-inflammatory agents. He denied respiratory complaints, a positional component to the pain, or syncope. He also denied any previous cardiovascular problems. Medications that he took regularly were an H_2 antagonist and a benzodiazepine preparation for sleep. He was married, had two children, and did not drink alcohol or smoke tobacco.

PHYSICAL EXAMINATION

VITAL SIGNS: Temperature, 98.6°F (36.9°C); pulse, 84; respiration, 16; blood pressure, 168/101 mmHg (left arm); 168/98 (right arm)
GENERAL: Marfanoid, acutely ill, and apprehensive
HEENT: Normal
NECK: No lymphadenopathy or thyromegaly
LUNGS: Clear
CARDIAC: Regular rate and rhythm without murmurs, rubs, or gallops
ABDOMEN: Soft, normoactive bowel sounds; no hepatosplenomegaly
EXTREMITIES: No cyanosis or edema; joint laxity
NEUROLOGIC: Deep tendon reflexes 2+; normal strength and sensation throughout

LABORATORY FINDINGS

WBC, 13.8 K/μL (normal differential); Hb, 14.9 g/dL; platelets, 354 K/μL; electrolytes, glucose, urea nitrogen, creatinine, and prothrombin time were normal; arterial blood gas measurements on room air: ph, 7.46; P_{CO_2}, 36 mmHg; P_{O_2}, 82 mmHg; CO_2, 23 mEq/L; O_2 saturation, 98%; creatine kinase, 215 IU/L (MB isoform 2.0); ECG: sinus tachycardia, left anterior fasicular block; chest x-ray and CT scan shown in the following (Figs. 36-1 and 36-2).

What is the most likely cause of this patient's symptoms?

This patient has an aortic dissection. Back pain in an acutely ill patient with an apparent connective tissue disease should raise a strong suspicion

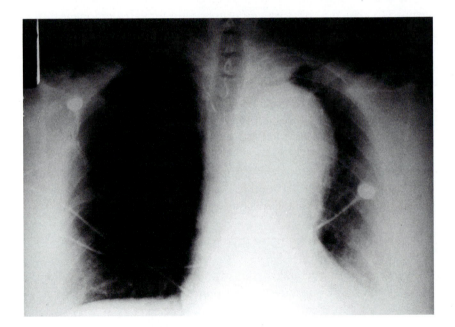

Figure 36-1
PA chest x-ray.

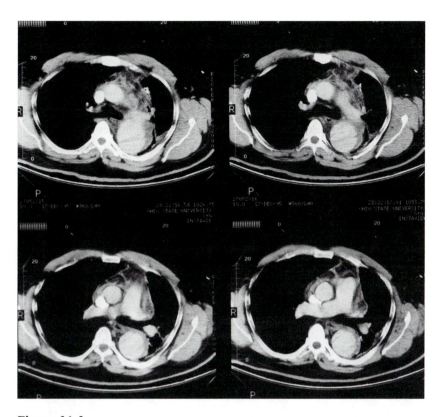

Figure 36-2
CT scan of the chest.

of aortic dissection. The chest x-ray in this patient shows a widened mediastinum that suggests aortic disease and the chest and abdominal CT scans revealed an aortic dissection. A transesophageal echocardiogram (TEE), done to rule out involvement of the proximal aorta and aortic root was normal.

Aortic dissection is a highly lethal condition that strikes thousands of people without warning each year. It is under-reported because many patients whose sudden death is caused by dissection are incorrectly diagnosed as having a "heart attack." Most aortic dissections occur in hypertensive, middle-aged, or elderly patients. Congenital abnormalities associated with it include Marfan syndrome (as in this patient), Turner's syndrome, Ehlers-Danlos syndrome, bicuspid aortic valve, coarctation of the aorta, and osteogenesis imperfecta. When aortic dissection occurs in tients with descending aortic dissection do not have aortic insufficiency or pulse deficits. Other presentations are: (1) heart failure caused by acute aortic insufficiency; (2) acute myocardial infarction, seen in 1 to 2 percent of proximal dissections in which the right coronary artery is most commonly involved; (3) syncope owing to aortic arch involvement or cardiac tamponade; and (4) neurologic syndromes such as CVA, ischemic peripheral neuropathy, and parapareses or paraplegia. The patient often appears to be in shock, but the blood pressure is usually high. Hypertension exists in up to 90 percent of patients with, and is the most important predisposing factor leading to, dissection.

The natural history of untreated acute aortic dissection is dismal. Approximately 50 percent of patients with untreated aortic dissection are dead within 48 hours. Because the mortality rate climbs each hour following an untreated acute dissection, one must continue to consider the diagnosis, even when the initial evaluation of a patient with acute chest or back pain fails to confirm a dissection. The most important factor leading to a correct diagnosis is often a high degree of clinical suspicion.

Although a chest x-ray often provides important clues, it rarely provides evidence for a definitive diagnosis; moreover, aortic dissection should not be excluded by a normal chest x-ray. In suspected dissection, one should proceed immediately with a definitive diagnostic test, either TEE, CT with contrast, or MRI, whichever can be performed most rapidly and reliably (Table 36-1). In most cases this will be a transesophageal echocardiogram or CT scan with contrast. A prompt and reliable diagnosis is imperative to reduce the early mortality associated with this condition.

The initial goal of treatment is to control the patient's pain and reduce the systolic blood pressure to the lowest level that will sustain adequate organ perfusion. This includes aggressive reduction of blood pressure and left ventricular contractility with a β-adrenergic blocking agent and sodium nitroprusside or an alternative vasodilator, maneuvers that reduce progression of the dissection. Immediate transfer to a tertiary facility with cardiothoracic surgical consultation is imperative. Patients with an ascending aortic dissection should be considered for immediate surgical repair. The surgical mortality rate for patients with ascending aortic dissection treated in centers with experienced surgeons is 7 to 20 percent. The management of descending aortic dissection also is prompt blood pressure control and surgical consultation. The operative morbidity and mortality for acute distal dissection is no better than with medical therapy alone. Therefore, most patients with acute distal dissection are treated

TABLE 36-1   Diagnostic Studies
for Aortic Dissection

CLINIAL FEATURES	AORTOG-RAPHY	COMPUTED TOMOG-RAPHY	MAGNETIC RESONANCE IMAGING	TRANS-ESOPHAGEAL ECHOCARDI-OGRAPHY
Sensitivity	86–100%	83–100%★	95–100%★	95–100%
Specificity	94%	94%	95–100%	80–98%
Need for contrast	Yes	Yes	No	No
Suitability in unstable patients	Yes	Yes	No	Yes
Diagnosis of branch occlusion	Yes	No	Yes	Yes★
Diagnosis of pericardial fluid	No	Yes	Yes	Yes
Diagnosis of aortic insufficiency	Yes	No	Yes	Yes
Diagnosis of intimal flap	Yes	Yes	Yes	Yes
Diagnosis of false lumen	Yes	Yes	Yes	Yes
Diagnosis of thrombosis	Yes	Yes	Yes	Yes
Assessment of coronary artery disease	Yes	No	No	Yes★
Invasive	Yes	No	No	Minimally
Intraoperative repair guidance	No	No	No	No

★Proximal portion only.
Adapted from *The Journal of Critical Illness*, vol 7, no 7, July 1992.

49-YEAR-OLD WOMAN WITH CHEST PAIN

A 49-year-old woman with a history of hypothyroidism and depression presented to the emergency department with a 12-hour history of substernal, pressure-like chest pain. The pain developed acutely while at home and persisted despite her taking non-steroidal anti-inflammatory agents. It was associated with nausea, dizziness, and shortness of breath. She had undergone an exploratory laparotomy for ovarian cyst removal 7 days prior to her admission. Medications on admission included levothyroxine and fluoxetine. She was married and had no children, and admitted to occasional alcohol use and smoking approximately 5 cigarettes a day.

PHYSICAL EXAMINATION

VITAL SIGNS: Temperature, 98.6°F (36.9°C); pulse, 97; respiration, 24; blood pressure, 145/90 mmHg
GENERAL: Obese, slightly tachypneic
HEENT: Normal
NECK: No lymphadenopathy or thyromegaly
LUNGS: Clear
CARDIAC: Regular rate and rhythm without murmurs, rubs, or gallops
ABDOMEN: Soft, normoactive bowel sounds; no hepatosplenomegaly
EXTREMITIES: No cyanosis, edema, or swelling
NEUROLOGIC: Deep tendon reflexes 2+; normal strength and sensation throughout

LABORATORY FINDINGS

WBC, 10.2 K/μL (normal differential); Hb, 14.9 g/dL, platelets, 354 K/μL; Electrolytes, glucose, urea nitrogen, creatinine, and prothrombin time, normal; Arterial blood gas measurements on room air: pH, 7.46; P_{CO_2}, 33 mmHg; P_{O_2}, 60 mmHg; bicarbonate, 24 mEq/L; O_2 saturation, 90%; creatine kinase, 42 IU/L; ECG, sinus rhythm; chest x-ray: shown in the following (Fig. 37-1).

What is the likely diagnosis and how should this patient be treated?

The patient has had a pulmonary embolus. Chest pain in a young woman with a recent history of abdominal or pelvic surgery should raise a high suspicion for pulmonary embolus. The arterial blood gas shows an increased alveolar-arterial gradient and the chest x-ray shows blunting of

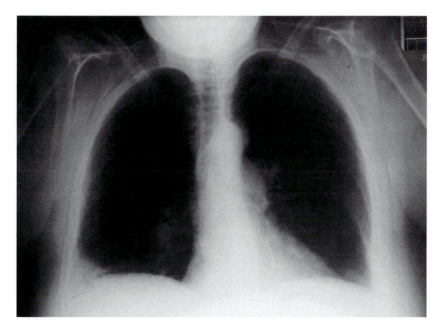

Figure 37-1
PA chest x-ray.

the right costophrenic angle. Both of these findings, especially with an ECG and cardiac enzymes that provide no evidence of cardiac ischemia, should result in a high clinical suspicion for pulmonary embolus. A ventilation/perfusion lung scan was performed that showed a large perfusion defect in the right lower lobe, interpreted as high probability for pulmonary embolus.

Pulmonary embolism (PE) is a leading cause of morbidity and mortality and can occur as a complication of many clinical conditions. Epidemiologic surveys indicate that pulmonary embolism is responsible for more than 100,000 deaths in the United States annually. The disease, however, is most often clinically silent with PE being unsuspected in 70 to 80 percent of the patients whose embolus is diagnosed at autopsy. PE may be the most common preventable cause of hospital death. Despite advances in its diagnosis and prophylaxis, the incidence of PE does not appear to be decreasing. This is probably explained by medical advances such as the higher survival rates of trauma patients, an increase in the number of open-heart and orthopedic replacement procedures and the wide-spread use of indwelling catheters. Autopsy and clinical studies have shown the risk of developing a PE extends for about 1 month beyond the period of hospitalization. Awareness of this prolonged risk is especially important as more same-day surgery is undertaken and as the length of hospital stays for various operations is shortened. Since preventing PE is far easier and more cost effective than its diagnosis and treatment, deep venous thrombosis prophylaxis is often indicated after hospital discharge.

More than 95 percent of pulmonary emboli arise from thrombi in the deep venous system of the lower extremities and pelvis; with the most common source being the larger veins (popliteal vein and above). The risk of deep venous thrombosis is best assessed by recognizing the presence of known clinical risk factors. Conditions predisposing to a high risk of venous thromboembolism include any surgical procedure requiring general anesthesia; the postpartum period; left and right ventricular failure; fractures, injuries, or surgical procedures involving the lower extremities; chronic venous insufficiency; prolonged bed rest; malignancy; obesity, and the use of estrogens. Other predisposing factors are a previous history of venous thrombosis; a family history of venous thrombosis; or a history of a known congenital or acquired aberration in hemostatic mechanisms that leads to a hypercoagulable state (protein C and S deficiencies, Factor V Leiden mutation, antithrombin III deficiency, antiphospholipid antibodies, dysfibrinogenemia, myeloproliferative disorders and hyperviscosity syndromes). In many patients, multiple risk factors are present and they are cumulative. Awareness of these risk factors for venous thromboembolism—and its subsequent complication, pulmonary embolism—and the clinical settings in which the risk factors occur is important in the successful application of prophylaxis.

The most common symptoms and signs of PE are nonspecific: dyspnea, tachypnea, chest pain, or tachycardia. Patients with severe chest pain or hemoptysis usually have an anatomically small embolus near the periphery of the lung where innervation is greatest and where pulmonary infarction is most likely to occur, mainly because of a dearth of collateral bronchial circulation. Patients with life-threatening PE are more apt to exhibit dyspnea, syncope, or cyanosis. PE should be suspected in hypotensive patients who have predisposing factors for, or clinical evidence of, venous thrombosis. The suspicion is heightened when there is evidence of acute cor pulmonale (acute right ventricular enlargement or failure) such as distended neck veins, an S_3 gallop, a right ventricular heave, tachycardia, or tachypnea. Embolism is particularly likely if there is electrocardiographic evidence of acute cor pulmonale manifested by a new right axis deviation, new incomplete right bundle branch block, or right ventricular ischemia. Arterial hypoxemia is a common although not universal consequence of PE. A widened alveolar-arterial gradient can be seen, but a normal gradient and a normal Pao_2 does not exclude the diagnosis of PE.

Many patients with PE have no ultrasonographic or venographic evidence of deep vein thrombosis in the leg. Accordingly, when this happens, patients should nonetheless have further evaluation if the clinical suspicion of PE is high. The chest x-ray may show a parenchymal infiltrate or evidence of a pleural effusion if infarction has occurred; the infiltrates typically abut the pleura and usually appear 12 to 24 hours after the embolism has occurred. However, a normal chest x-ray does not rule out the diagnosis. Ventilation-perfusion lung scanning is the principal diagnostic test. The scan is diagnostically most useful when it is either clearly normal or shows a high-probability pattern suggesting PE. Intermediate- or low-probability scans with high clinical suspicion do not exclude the condition. Only a completely normal lung scan rules out the diagnosis. For example, when the clinical suspicion of PE is intermediate (around 50 percent) and the lung scan is interpreted as showing an intermediate probability of PE, the likelihood of finding angiographic evidence of embolism is almost 30 percent; however, if the clinical suspicion is high (around 90 percent) and the lung scan has a low probability of PE, the likelihood of finding an embolism at angiography is nevertheless about

40 percent (Table 37-1). Thus, the patient usually should undergo pulmonary angiography when the clinical suspicion is high but the probability of PE according to the lung scan is low or intermediate.

The most reliable diagnostic feature on angiography is a constant intraluminal filling defect seen in more than one projection. Pulmonary angiography can almost always be accomplished safely if selective angiography is performed, using the perfusion lung scan as a map for the angiographer, and if a low osmolar contrast agent is used to minimize the transient hypotension, heat sensation, and coughing that often occur with conventional radiocontrast agents. For hemodynamically unstable patients, echocardiography performed at the bedside may suggest PE if the following findings are present: RV dilation and hypokinesis, bowing of the interventricular septum into the left ventricle, tricuspid regurgitation, and preserved left ventricular function. Echocardiography can also help exclude other life-threatening conditions such as ventricular septal rupture, aortic dissection, and pericardial tamponade that may be considered in the differential diagnosis.

Anticoagulation therapy is the cornerstone treatment for PE. When embolism is strongly suspected on clinical grounds, treatment should be initiated while the diagnostic evaluation is being performed. Therapy begins with heparin given by intravenous bolus followed by its continuous infusion. The therapeutic target is a partial thromboplastin time (PTT) of 1.5 to 2.5 times control. Treatment with heparin should be continued for 5 to 10 days and oral anticoagulation should be overlapped with heparin for 4 to 5 days. For many patients, heparin and warfarin therapy can be

TABLE 37-1   Clinical Probability of PE

Lung Scan Probability of PE	High (%) (80–100%)	Medium (%) (20–79%)	Low (%) (0–19%)
High probability	96	88	56
Intermediate probability	66	28	16
Low probability	40	16	4
Normal	0	6	2

Modified from The PIOPED investigators: Value of the ventilation/perfusion scan in acute pulmonary embolism. *JAMA* 1990; 263:2753–2759.

started together and heparin discontinued on day 5 or 6 if the prothrombin time (PT) is therapeutic (INR of 2.0–3.0). For a massive PE, a longer period of heparin therapy may be considered. Recently, the administration of low-molecular-weight heparin has been shown to be as safe and effective as administration of unfractionated heparin, even when treating hemodynamically stable PE. Long-term oral anticoagulant therapy should be continued for at least 3 months to prolong the prothrombin time to an INR of 2.0 to 3.0. When oral anticoagulants are either contraindicated or inconvenient, adjusted-dose heparin therapy should be given to prolong the PTT to 1.5 to 2.5 times control. Alternatively, low-molecular-weight heparin can be used in place of unfractionated heparin. Patients with recurrent thromboembolism or a continuing risk factor, such as the hemostatic abnormalities noted in the preceding should be treated indefinitely.

Thrombolytic therapy for pulmonary embolism is highly individualized based on the patients' clinical status. There is broad consensus in the United States that thrombolysis is indicated for hypotensive patients who have suffered a PE, but controversy remains for the role of thrombolytic therapy for hemodynamically stable patients. However, it may be a very useful adjunct to heparin for hemodynamically stable patients who have echocardiographic evidence of RV dysfunction, a large PE, or extensive deep vein thrombosis. The contraindications to thrombolysis are the same as those for acute myocardial infarction. Rarely, surgical pulmonary embolectomy should be considered in patients with an acute, massive PE that has not responded to thrombolytic therapy or when there is an absolute contraindication to the thrombolytic agents. Another potential indication for embolectomy is chronic pulmonary hypertension owing to chronic pulmonary thromboembolic disease.

Our patient was treated with intravenous heparin and started on warfarin the second hospital day. She was discharged on hospital day 5 after therapeutic anticoagulation was achieved on warfarin. She was treated for 3 months with warfarin therapy with an INR between 2.0 and 3.0.

 ## CLINICAL PEARLS

- Pulmonary embolism may be the most preventable cause of hospital death.
- Prophylaxis for thromboembolism is underused and should be guided by an awareness and assessment of known risk factors for PE.

- A normal Pa_{O_2} and normal alveolar-arterial gradient does not exclude the diagnosis of PE.
- Clinical assessment combined with ventilation–perfusion lung scan is the principal way to determine the likelihood of PE.
- Treatment with heparin should be initiated immediately and should not await diagnostic confirmation when there is a strong clinical suspicion of PE.
- Once PE is confirmed treatment should continued for at least 3 months.

REFERENCES

1. Hyers TM, Hull RD, Weg JG. Antithrombotic therapy for venous thromboembolic disease. Fourth ACCP Consensus Conference on Antithrombotic Therapy. *Chest* 1995; 108:335S–351S.
2. The PIOPED Investigators. Value of the ventilation/perfusion scan in acute pulmonary embolism. *JAMA* 1990; 263:2753–2759.
3. Stein PD, Goldhaber SZ, Henry JW. Alveolar-arterial oxygen gradient in the assessment of acute pulmonary embolism. *Chest* 1995; 107: 139–143.
4. Goldhaber SZ. Advances in treating pulmonary embolism. *Prim Cardiol* 1994; 20:15–21.
5. Koopman MM, Prandoni P, Piovella P, et al. Treatment of venous thrombosis with intravenous unfractionated heparin administered in the hospital compared with subcutaneous low-molecular-weight heparin administered at home. *NEJM* 1996; 334(11):682–687.

50-YEAR-OLD WOMAN WITH BREAST CANCER AND THROMBOCYTOPENIA

A 50-year-old woman with breast cancer was admitted to the Bone Marrow Transplant Unit for an autologous peripheral stem cell transplant. Eight months earlier she had undergone a modified radical left mastectomy for a poorly differentiated invasive ductal carcinoma that was positive for estrogen and progesterone receptors and had metastasized to 13 axillary lymph nodes. Postoperatively, her CT and bone scans were unremarkable and she was treated with four courses of Adriamycin and Cytoxan, followed by two courses each of Taxotere and Taxol. She was then enrolled in a clinical study of autologous bone marrow transplantation with peripheral stem cells. According to the study protocol, Hickman and Permacath catheters were placed 1 month prior to transplant and after an adequate number of stem cells had been collected she was scheduled for transplantation. Six days prior to transplantation she was admitted to the hospital and a regimen of Cytoxan, carboplatin, and thiotepa was started and her platelet count dropped accordingly. However, following the transplant her platelets remained low despite multiple HLA-matched transfusions and a return to normal of her red and white blood cell counts. All potential offending medications were withheld but her thrombocytopenia did not improve.

PHYSICAL EXAMINATION

VITAL SIGNS: Temperature, 98.4°F (36.8°C); pulse, 83; respiration, 18; blood pressure, 124/82 mmHg

GENERAL: Otherwise well appearing
HEENT: Palatal petechiae
NECK: No thyromegaly
LUNGS: Clear
CARDIAC: Normal
ABDOMEN: Normal bowel sounds, soft, non-tender; no hepatospleno-
    megaly
EXTREMITIES: No edema
SKIN: Bilateral lower extremity petechiae

LABORATORY FINDINGS

WBC, 7.4 K/μL (67% segmented neutrophils, 22% lymphocytes); Hb,
11.1 g/dL (MCV 81 fl); platelets, 2 K/μL; mean platelet volume, 11.2 fl
(normal, 6.2–10.6); peripheral blood smear: no platelet clumping, no
schistocytes; electrolytes, blood urea nitrogen, and creatinine, normal;
lactate dehydrogenase, 732 U/L (normal, 0–625); activated partial thromboplastin time and prothrombin time, normal; platelet-associated IgG and
IgM antibody, negative.

What is the likely cause of this patient's thrombocytopenia?

This patient has heparin-induced thrombocytopenia (HIT). Approximately 48 hours after all heparin (including IV flushes) was discontinued
her platelet count rapidly rose to over 150,000. Heparin-induced anti-
platelet antibodies found in her serum confirmed the diagnosis.

Decreased platelet production, their accelerated destruction (immunologic or other), or their sequestration in the spleen or a combination of
these events may cause thrombocytopenia, defined as a platelet count of
less than 150,000. These broad diagnostic categories may be distinguished
by a careful clinical evaluation that attempts to differentiate hereditary and
acquired platelet disorders. A history of excessive bleeding after surgical
or dental procedures, or of recurrent petechiae, the clinical hallmark of
thrombocytopenia, in the buccal mucosa or at sites of increased intra-

vascular pressure such as the lower extremities suggests a longstanding problem. The physical examination may disclose an enlarged spleen, suggesting secondary thrombocytopenia, or may reveal generalized lymph node enlargement caused by other hematologic disorders or malignancies. The peripheral blood smear should be examined for the size and number of platelets and for evidence of platelet clumping or other blood cell line abnormalities. In vitro platelet clumping caused by the anticoagulant EDTA used in blood collection tubes may cause pseudothrombocytopenia. The mean platelet volume (MPV) may be diagnostically helpful: Immature platelets have large volumes as a result of their rapid turnover or the production of dysplastic platelets, whereas low platelet volumes suggest prolonged platelet turnover. An abdominal CT, if necessary, can confirm a bedside diagnosis of splenomegaly. Assessment of bone marrow cellularity and morphology in an aspirate or biopsy specimen is often necessary. With this information, one can systematically approach the differential diagnosis of thrombocytopenia (Table 38-1).

Medications are a common cause of thrombocytopenia. They have either a myelosuppressive effect, typified by thiazide diuretics and ethanol, or more commonly an immunologic effect, typified by quinidine and heparin. Drug-antibody complexes often secondarily involve platelets, which in effect become innocent bystanders that are destroyed. Removal or treatment of the inciting cause may reverse the thrombocytopenia.

Another common and often overlooked cause of thrombocytopenia in the hospitalized patient is heparin-induced thrombocytopenia, which is part of the spectrum of the heparin-induced thrombotic thrombocytopenia syndrome. The incidence of HIT in most prospective studies varies from 1 to 5 percent. The thrombocytopenia is usually mild (platelet count >50,000), and typically develops 6 to 10 days after administration is initiated.

Heparin interacts with platelets to produce thrombocytopenia in two ways. The first, termed *type 1 heparin-associated thrombocytopenia*, occurs when heparin binds to specific platelet receptors, inducing platelet activation and destruction. This is a dose-dependent effect that is not mediated by an immune mechanism and rarely leads to significant thrombocytopenia. It is often unrecognized, but may occur in up to 30 percent of patients receiving intravenous heparin.

The second heparin-platelet interaction, termed *type 2 heparin-associated thrombocytopenia*, is an immune-mediated process that typically results in severe thrombocytopenia. In this case, heparin binds to platelet factor 4 (PF4), producing an immunologically active complex that provokes

TABLE 38-1   Major Causes of
Thrombocytopenia

Decreased platelet production
    Aplastic anemia
    Leukemia
    Iatrogenic myelosuppression
    B_{12}/folate deficiency
Increased platelet destruction
    Nonimmune-mediated
        Disseminated intravascular coagulation (DIC)
        Heart-lung bypass
        Thrombotic thrombocytopenic purpura (TTP)
    Immune-mediated
        Drug-induced (penicillin, sulfa)
        Post-transfusion purpura
        Idiopathic thrombocytopenic purpura (ITP)
Hypersplenism
    Cirrhosis
    Infiltrative diseases

Adapted from Schafer AJ, Thrombocytopenia and Disorders of Platelet Function. Internal Medicine. Stein JH, (ed.) Mosby, St. Louis, p. 799.

antibody formation. The antibody in turn binds with the heparin–PF4 complex on platelet membranes, activating the platelets and leading to their destruction. The resulting immune-mediated platelet aggregates can form in situ thrombosis ("white clot syndrome"). The dose and route of heparin administration are not related to this cascade of events, which can produce antibodies within 5 days of exposure to subcutaneous heparin or intravenous heparin flushes alone. Compounding the problem, PF4 may also form complexes with endothelial-bound heparin that cross-react with the platelet antibodies. This can lead to endothelial damage, which, if extensive, may induce an apparent clinical paradox: thrombosis with thrombocytopenia and disseminated intravascular coagulation (DIC).

Up to one-third of patients with heparin antibodies develop a thrombotic complication, including deep venous thrombosis, pulmonary embolism, myocardial infarction, cerebrovascular accident, skin necrosis, and peripheral arterial occlusion. Thrombosis occurring during heparin therapy is often misdiagnosed as a treatment failure rather than a complication from HIT. It should be suspected among those at especially high risk: the elderly, patients who experience an early drop in platelets with heparin therapy, or in patients following cardiothoracic surgery.

Treatment consists of stopping the heparin. Intravenous IgG may be helpful but its indications are not well established. Patients with thrombi should receive alternative forms of anticoagulation, although unfortunately the low-molecular-weight heparins currently available in the United States almost always cross-react with the heparin antibody and thus are not useful in this situation. On the other hand, ancrod or a direct-acting antithrombin (hirudin) or low-molecular-weight heparinoids (danaparoid sodium) appear to be safe and effective in small trials. It is especially important to know that warfarin is ineffective and may be potentially dangerous in acute HIT.

Our patient did not develop a thrombotic complication. Simply stopping all forms of heparin corrected her thrombocytopenia and prevented its devastating consequences. She remains in remission 6 months following bone marrow transplantation.

 ## CLINICAL PEARLS

- Heparin-induced thrombocytopenia (HIT) develops in up to 5 percent of patients receiving heparin.
- HIT is often mild and easily unrecognized, but about one-third are severe, life-threatening, and associated with thrombotic complications.
- HIT with thrombosis should be suspected in the elderly, when thrombocytopenia occurs shortly after starting heparin, and after cardiothoracic surgery.
- HIT can be complicated by either arterial or venous thrombosis. HIT and thrombi may be treated with ancrod, hirudin, or danaparoid sodium
- Neither the low-molecular-weight heparins presently available in the United States nor warfarin should be used to treat HIT with thrombi.

REFERENCES

1. Warkentin TE, Chong BH, Greinacher A. Heparin-induced thrombocytopenia: Towards consensus. *Thromb Hemostas* 1998; 79:1–7.
2. Nand S, Wong W, Yuen B, et al. *Am J Hematol*, 1997; 56(1):12–16.
3. Warkentin TE, Levine MN, Hirsch J, et al. Heparin-induced thrombocytopenia in patients treated with low-molecular-weight heparin or unfractionated heparin. *N Engl J Med* 1995; 332:1330–1335.
4. Kelton JG, Warkentin TE. Heparin-induced thrombocytopenia: Diagnosis, natural history, and treatment options. *Postgrad Med* 1998; 103:169–178.

50-YEAR-OLD WOMAN
WITH HYPOKALEMIA

A 50-year-old woman with a history of type 2 diabetes mellitus, new onset hypertension, and recently diagnosed pancreatic cancer; presented to the hospital with a 2-day history of nausea, vomiting, abdominal pain, malaise, and fatigue. She described the abdominal pain as achy in nature, diffuse, and constant without relation to food or position. Four months prior she had been diagnosed with pancreatic cancer with liver metastasis. Laparoscopic liver biopsy at that time was consistent with adenocarcinoma. She underwent 12 palliative external-beam radiation treatments as well as chemotherapy that relieved her abdominal pain. Follow-up abdominal CT scan demonstrated a decrease in primary tumor size but an increase in the size and number of liver metastases. She denied any fevers, chills, visual changes, or headaches. Medications at the time of admission included clonidine, insulin, glyburide, fentanyl patch, and stool softeners. Her family history and social history were unremarkable.

PHYSICAL EXAMINATION

VITAL SIGNS: Temperature, 98.6°F (36.9°C); pulse, 84; respiration, 16; blood pressure, 116/69 mmHg
GENERAL: Tall, thin woman who appeared irritable and anxious
HEENT: Dry mucous membranes, otherwise normal
NECK: No lymphadenopathy or thyromegaly
LUNGS: Clear
CARDIAC: Regular rate and rhythm without murmurs, rubs, or gallops
ABDOMEN: Decreased bowel sounds; diffusely tender to palpation especially in the RUQ; soft, nondistended; firm liver edge palpated 3 cm below the rib margin

consistent with an adenoma (not shown). The suppressed aldosterone, increased cortisol, and remarkably high ACTH levels indicate that this patient has an ectopic ACTH syndrome, which typically does not give a cushingoid appearance. The ectopic source of ACTH production was her pancreatic tumor, not the adrenal adenoma that was an incidental and possibly misleading finding.

Cushing originally described a syndrome of truncal obesity with thin extremities, moon facies, hypertension, fatigability, amenorrhea, hirsutism, fragile skin, purple abdominal striae, edema, glucosuria, and osteoporosis. Its most common cause is exogenous administration of corticosteroids. Endogenous Cushing syndrome is due to increased production of cortisol by the adrenal gland. Most are the result of bilateral adrenocortical hyperplasia caused by hypersecretion of pituitary ACTH or its production by nonendocrine tumors. Most have ACTH-secreting pituitary microadenomas (<10 mm; 50 percent are 5 mm or less), but a macroadenoma (>10 mm) of the pituitary or diffuse hyperplasia of the corticotropic cells may also cause the syndrome, which is termed Cushing disease when it is caused by an ACTH-producing pituitary tumor or hyperplasia.

Nonendocrine tumors may cause bilateral adrenal hyperplasia by secreting polypeptides that are biologically, chemically, and immunologically indistinguishable from ACTH or corticotropin-releasing hormone (CRH). Ectopic CRH production causes clinical and radiographic features that are indistinguishable from those produced by the hypersecretion of pituitary ACTH in Cushing disease, except that the typical cushingoid appearance is usually absent, whereas hypokalemic alkalosis and glucose intolerance are prominent features. Typically patients have severe muscle weakness and weight loss, hyperpigmentation owing to the high ACTH levels and diabetes mellitus resulting from profound hypokalemia. Most ectopic ACTH-producing tumors are caused by primitive small cell (oat cell) bronchogenic carcinomas or by tumors of the thymus, pancreas, or ovary, medullary thyroid carcinoma or bronchial adenomas. (Table 39-1). The onset of ectopic ACTH syndrome may be sudden, particularly with oat cell lung carcinoma, accounting for the absence of classic physical findings of Cushing syndrome; however, the clinical course with carcinoid tumors, medullary thyroid carcinoma, or pheochromocytoma is longer and typical cushingoid features may be present.

Diagnostic evaluation centers on locating the source of ACTH hypersecretion. Unlike Cushing disease, ectopic ACTH syndrome afflicts

TABLE 39-1   **Causes of Ectopic ACTH
Syndrome**

Small-cell lung carcinoma (majority of clinically apparent)
Carcinoid
    Lung, gastric, thymus ovary, pancreas, ileal, kidney
    Bronchial carcinoid (majority in radiologically occult)
Neuroendocrine carcinoma
Islet-cell pancreas
Medullary thyroid carcinoma
Pheochromocytoma
Paraganglioma
Nephroblastoma
Adenocarcinoma of colon, esophagus, lung ovary, breast, ileum
Squamous-cell carcinoma of larynx, cervix
Myeloblastic leukemia
Inflammatory tissue

both sexes with equal frequency. Aldosterone levels are generally normal, and patients often have massive hypercortisolism (urine free cortisol >1500 μg/24 h) and very high plasma ACTH levels (>200 pg/mL). Although ACTH secretion typically can be suppressed by dexamethasone in pituitary Cushing but not the ectopic ACTH syndrome, this test does not reliably differentiate the two. The ovine CRH (oCRH) test is more reliable in this regard. In Cushing disease the pituitary is responsive to oCRH and serum ACTH levels rise in response to it, whereas most ectopic ACTH-producing tumors fail to respond.

Radiographic evaluation of the pituitary and adrenal glands offers limited information to differentiate pituitary Cushing from the ectopic ACTH syndrome. Regardless of the source of ACTH, the adrenal glands usually show significant bilateral enlargement, but occasionally will demonstrate unilateral or bilateral masses. The diagnostic challenge lies in identifying an occult tumor causing the ectopic ACTH syndrome, as failure to differentiate it from pituitary Cushing disease may lead to unnecessary pituitary surgery. Finding features on CT scan or MRI that are consistent with a pituitary microadenoma does not prove Cushing disease. Patients with ectopic CRH-secreting tumors are as likely to have an abnormal imaging scan of the pituitary as are patients with pituitary ACTH-dependent Cushing syndrome. Bilateral inferior petrosal sinus ACTH sampling with CRH stimulation is the most reliable method to determine the source of ACTH hypersecretion. Demonstrating a gradient between the ACTH level in the petrosal sinus and peripheral blood localizes the source of ACTH overproduction to the pituitary gland but does not distinguish pituitary-dependent adrenal hyperplasia from pituitary hyperplasia secondary to a tumor producing CRH. Serum CRH levels should be measured in the peripheral blood prior to petrosal sinus sampling. Octreotide scanning may locate the ectopic tumor. If the tumor is not visualized with octreotide and if it produces no other hormones, there is no other reliable test available to make the distinction between ectopic CRH and pituitary Cushing disease. This remains an important and unsolved diagnostic dilemma.

Treatment of ectopic ACTH syndrome should be directed at the neoplasm causing it along with prompt correction of electrolyte abnormalities and treatment of the hypercortisolemia, which may cause significant immunosuppression. Opportunistic infections are common in the ectopic ACTH syndrome and patients with urine free cortisol levels >2000 μg/24 h should be evaluated for *Pneumocystis* pneumonia since this association is common. Surgical resection of the neoplasm is the treatment of choice for ectopic ACTH syndrome but often is incomplete. Medical therapy may be employed if the neoplasm is inoperative or while waiting for surgery. Ketoconazole is a potent inhibitor of adrenal steroid biosynthesis through the cytochrome P_{450} system, and can cause a "chemical adrenalectomy" by the administration of 600 to 1200 mg/day. In addition, mitotane or blockers of steroid synthesis (aminoglutethimide and metyrapone) have been effective either alone or in combination. More recently, somatostatin analogues have also been used effectively. Hypoadrenalism is a risk with all these agents, and replacement steroids may be required. The prognosis with this syndrome is closely related to that of the underlying neoplasm.

Our patient's hypokalemia was treated with potassium replacement and ketoconazole was given to treat her hypercortisolemia, which improved her electrolyte status and she improved clinically. Unfortunately, several weeks after her discharge from the hospital she died from metastatic pancreatic cancer.

CLINICAL PEARLS

- A chloride-resistant metabolic alkalosis with hypertension and hypokalemia should initiate an investigation for excess mineralocorticoid activity.
- Ectopic ACTH syndrome usually presents without physical findings of Cushing syndrome.
- Occult ectopic ACTH syndrome must be differentiated from pituitary Cushing disease to avoid unnecessary pituitary surgery.
- Pituitary and adrenal gland radiographic evaluations usually do not differentiate ectopic ACTH from pituitary Cushing disease.
- Opportunistic infections are associated with the massive hypercortisolemia of ectopic ACTH syndrome.
- Treatment of ectopic ACTH syndrome includes correction of electrolyte abnormalities, pharmacologic inhibition of steroid biosynthesis, and surgical resection of the tumor if possible.

REFERENCES

1. Findling JW, Raff H. Ectopic adrenocorticotropic hormone, in *Endocrine Tumors*, Mazzaferri EL, Samaan NA (eds). Boston, Blackwell Scientific, 1993, pp 554–566.
2. Zhu L, Domenico DR, Howard JM. Metastatic pancreatic neuroendocrine carcinoma causing Cushing syndrome. ACTH secretion by metastases 3 years after resection of nonfunctioning primary cancer. *Int J Pancreatol* 1996; 19(3):205–208.
3. Tsigos C, Chrousos GP. Differential diagnosis and management of Cushing's syndrome. *Annu Rev Med* 1996; 47:443–461.
4. Meier CA, Biller BM. Clinical and biochemical evaluation of Cushing's syndrome. *Endocrinol Metab Clin NA* 1997; 26(4):741–762.
5. Wajchenberg BL, Mendonca B, et al. Ectopic ACTH syndrome. *J Ster Biochem Mol Biol* 1995; 53(1–6):139–151.

48-YEAR-OLD WOMAN WITH MYALGIAS AND WEAKNESS

A 48-year-old woman presented to the emergency department with complaints of muscle weakness, fatigue, and pain in her arms and legs for the past 3 to 4 days. She noted that her urine had become a dark "cola" color for the past 2 days prior to admission. She had experienced similar episodes with similar symptoms in the past, usually preceded by heavy exertion. Lifting heavy objects while helping a friend move furniture preceded this most recent episode. Past medical history was significant for essential hypertension and her family history was positive for her mother having a similar problem with episodic weakness and muscle pain. She denied the use of tobacco or alcohol and was not taking any prescription or over-the-counter medications.

PHYSICAL EXAMINATION

VITAL SIGNS: Temperature, 98.6°F (36.9°C); pulse, 100; respiration, 18; blood pressure, 160/90 mmHg

GENERAL: Alert; mild discomfort on moving

HEENT: Normal

NECK: No lymphadenopathy or thyromegaly

LUNGS: Clear

CARDIAC: Slightly tachycardic; regular rate and rhythm without murmurs, rubs, or gallops

ABDOMEN: Soft, normoactive bowel sounds; no hepatosplenomegaly

EXTREMITIES: No cyanosis or edema, pain, on palpation of muscle groups—worse proximally

NEUROLOGIC: Deep tendon reflexes 2+; normal sensation throughout, normal strength throughout with precipitation of pain by resistance movements

LABORATORY FINDINGS

WBC, 10.8 K/μL (normal differential); Hb, 14.9 g/dL; platelets, 354 K/μL; electrolytes: sodium, 140 mEq/L; potassium, 6.0 mEq/L; chloride, 101 mEq/L; bicarbonate, 19 mEq/L; bun, 47 mg/dL; creatinine, 2.2 mg/dL; glucose, 120 mg/dL; anion gap, 20 mEq/L (normal, <12 mEq/L); creatine kinase, 175,000 U/L (normal 30–170 U/L); urinalysis, pH, 8.0; positive for myoglobin and hemoglobin; urine sediment: few coarse granular casts

What is the likely diagnosis and how should this patient be treated?

This patient has rhabdomyolysis with myoglobin-induced acute tubular necrosis (ATN). From the history and clinical presentation one should suspect a skeletal muscle or glycogen storage disorder as the etiology of the patient's rhabdomyolysis. Other metabolic myopathies (endocrine-, nutritional-, or electrolyte-induced) could also account for the patient's rhabdomyolysis, but the positive family history and episodic nature of her symptoms with physical exertion strongly suggest a glycogen storage disorder, which in this case is myophosphorylase deficiency or McArdle's disease.

The glycogen storage diseases are a group of genetic disorders involving abnormalities in the pathways for the storage and utilization of glycogen that normally maintain blood sugar levels and provide energy. Some forms are not associated with actual increases in glycogen content in tissues because the metabolic pathways involved in glycogen synthesis differ among tissues. For example, certain reactions are active in the liver but trivial or absent in muscle and different genes in muscle and liver encode similar enzyme functions. The clinical manifestations, diagnostic criteria, and therapy for glycogen storage diseases are based on the metabolic pathways involved (Table 40-1).

According to this schema, two broad categories of disease can be delineated: those with a *hepatic-hypoglycemic* pathophysiology and those with a *muscle-energy* pathophysiology. Diseases with individualized pathophysiology also occur. Some designate these disorders by the specific enzyme or

TABLE 40-1   Glycogen Storage Diseases

Type	Basic Defect/Enzyme Deficiency	Primary Organ Involved
Hepatic-hypoglycemic disorders		
Ia (von Gierke)	Glucose-6 phosphatase	Liver
Ib	Glucose-6-phosphate Microsomal translocase	Liver
III (Cori)	Debrancher enzyme	Liver, skeletal muscle, heart
VI (Hers)	Liver phosphorylase	Liver
VIII (formerly VIb or IX)	Liver phosphorylase b kinase	Liver, skeletal muscle
Muscle-energy disorders		
V (McArdle)	Muscle phosphorylase	Skeletal muscle
VII	Muscle phosphofructo-kinase	Skeletal muscle, Red blood cells (RBCs)
Disorders with individual pathophysiology		
II (Pompe)	Lysosomal gluco-sidase	Skeletal muscle, heart
IV (Anderson)	Brancher enzyme	Skeletal muscle, liver

protein deficiency; however, the Roman numeral designation for types I through VII is in widespread use. Eponyms are of historical interest.

The *hepatic-hypoglycemic* disorders can be subdivided into those that elevate and those that decrease glucose-6-phosphate and its metabolites. This is why increased glycolysis and lactic acidosis occur in type I disease but not in other forms of hepatic-hypoglycemic disease (see Table 40-1). Likewise, various forms of type I disease are distinct because gluconeogenesis, galactose, and fructose cannot contribute effectively to the maintenance of blood sugar, in contrast to the other forms of hepatic-hypoglycemic disease. Dietary therapy with frequent feeding, which is a rational approach to the hepatic-hypoglycemic disorders, is tailored to reduce protein and to eliminate sources of galactose and fructose in type I disease.

The *muscle-energy* disorders include phosphorylase deficiency (type V or McArdle's disease), and phosphofructokinase and phosphoglycerate mutase deficiencies. The clinical picture is one of muscle pain, myoglobinuria, and elevation of muscle enzymes in the serum following vigorous exercise. Interrupting the pathway from glycogen to lactate with an accompanying failure to oxidize NADH is the unifying theme in these disorders. Thus, the failure of blood lactate to increase in response to exercise is a useful diagnostic test for the muscle-energy deficiency disorders. Pumping a pressure cuff above arterial pressure while the ischemic hand is exercised to a maximum effort is the ischemic exercise test that is of particular use in the initial evaluation. After the pressure cuff is released, blood is drawn from the other arm at 2, 5, 10, 20, and 30 minutes for measurement of lactate and pyruvate, muscle enzymes, and myoglobin. With a positive test, lactate levels do not rise, whereas serum creatine kinase is elevated.

Myophosphorylase Deficiency, Type V, McArdle's Disease

Myophosphorylase deficiency, or McArdle's disease, is uncommon. It is a hereditary metabolic myopathy transmitted as an autosomal recessive disorder. The specific enzyme defect has been localized to chromosome 11 and is increased in frequency in men. Symptoms of pain and cramping after exercise can present in childhood; however, the majority become manifest during the second or third decade of life. These individuals are well at rest and tolerate low levels of activity when lipids (free fatty acids) are being utilized as the major source of energy. Symptoms develop after increased activity of higher intensity when carbohydrate becomes the major source of energy. Affected individuals are otherwise healthy, without evidence of hepatic, cardiac, or metabolic disturbance. Performance of an ischemic exercise test usually causes painful cramping, which is helpful diagnostically. Blood lactate does not rise, whereas serum creatine phosphokinase, which is usually elevated at rest, rises substantially after strenuous exercise. Documenting elevated glycogen content and reduced myophosphorylase activity in biopsied muscle tissue confirm the diagnosis of McArdle's disease. The glycogen is usually deposited in subsarcolemmal regions of the muscle, which is not, however, specific for McArdle's disease. Demonstrating the enzyme deficiency is the only way to make the diagnosis.

The complications of McArdle's disease relate mainly to the development of rhabdomyolysis and ATN. Increased levels of muscle enzymes and myoglobinuria usually occur simultaneously with the symptoms of muscle pain and cramping. There is some evidence that recurrent and frequent episodes of ATN in these individuals may lead to the development of chronic interstitial nephritis. Muscle necrosis can also cause hyperuricemia, hypocalcemia and hyperkalemia. Mental clouding, syncope, and seizures can occur during prolonged exercise as the result of a respiratory alkalosis caused by an appropriate increase in minute ventilation without the usual concomitant metabolic acidosis. Another complicating factor is that many episodes of pain and cramping go undiagnosed and are not evaluated because the patient does not seek medical attention. These patients need to be educated about their disease process and how to avoid serious complications.

Management of myophosphorylase deficiency requires the avoidance of strenuous exercise. Individuals can be educated on how to perform brief periods of exercise or strenuous activity that does not induce rhabdomyolysis. Dietary modification that attempts to bypass the metabolic block and provide substrate for energy has not been very successful. Glucose or fructose ingestion prior to exercise may reduce symptoms. Research using adenovirus-mediated delivery into myocytes of myophosphorylase is still experimental.

Our patient was treated for her rhabdomyolysis with intravenous fluids and alkalinization of her urine in an attempt to prevent toxic tubular injury. Her serum creatinine decreased to 1.5 mg/dL at the time of her discharge from the hospital and her skeletal muscle biopsy was consistent with myophosphorylase deficiency. She was educated about her disease and instructed to avoid strenuous exercise and to follow-up closely with her physician.

    # CLINICAL PEARLS

- Myalgias and muscle weakness *only* associated with exertion should raise the suspicion of a glycogen storage disease.
- Myalgias and a change in urine color should raise the concern for pigment-induced (myoglobin and/or hemoglobin) renal injury.
- Glycogen storage diseases are genetic disorders involving the pathways for storage of glycogen.
- Hepatic glycogen storage disorders cause hypoglycemia, whereas muscle glycogen storage disorders induce muscle pain and cramping.
- The *ischemic exercise test* is useful in the diagnosis of muscle-energy deficiency disorders by demonstrating a *lack* of lactate rise following anaerobic exercise.
- The treatment for McArdle's disease is mainly the avoidance of vigorous exercise.

REFERENCES

1. Lewis SF, Haller RG. The pathophysiology of McArdle's disease: clues to regulation in exercise and fatigue. *J Appl Physiol* 1986; 61(2): 391–401.
2. Lubran MM. McArdle's disease: a review. *Ann Clin Lab Sci* 1975; 5(2):115–122.
3. Taylor RG, Lieberman JS. Ischemic exercise test: failure to detect partial expression of McArdle's disease. *Muscle Nerve* 1987; 10(6): 546–551.
4. Beynon RJ, Bartam C. Interrelationships between metabolism of glycogen phosphorylase and pyridoxal phosphate: implications in McArdle's disease. *Adv Food Nutr Res* 1996; 40:135–147.
5. Isselbacher KJ, Braunwald E, Wilson JD, et al. *Harrison's Principles of Internal Medicine*, 13th ed. New York, McGraw-Hill, 1994, pp. 2099–2105.

23-YEAR-OLD MAN WITH MALAISE AND WEIGHT LOSS

A 23-year-old man with no previous medical history presented to the emergency department with increasing malaise, intermittent fevers, and a 30-pound weight loss over the past 6 to 8 weeks. The patient had been well prior to these complaints, and his recent past medical history was only significant for a dental abscess that had developed from neglected dental caries. Three months prior to presentation he had this dental abscess incised and drained and was placed on a short course of antibiotic therapy. His review of systems was positive for occasional night sweats. He denied chest pain, shortness of breath, syncope or presyncope, abdominal pain, or change in bowel or bladder habits. He was taking no medication, lived alone, and had no known recent contacts with anyone who was ill. His family history was unremarkable. His social history was negative for tobacco, alcohol, or other illicit drug use.

PHYSICAL EXAMINATION

VITAL SIGNS: Temperature, 98.6°F (36.9°C); pulse, 80; respiration, 18; bp, 138/78 mmHg

GENERAL: Ill-appearing, no acute distress

HEENT: Dry mucous membranes, poor dentition, otherwise normal

NECK: No lymphadenopathy or thyromegaly

LUNGS: Clear

CARDIAC: Regular rate and rhythm; normal S1 and S2; 3/6 harsh, systolic ejection murmur that radiated to both carotids; 2/6 early diastolic blowing murmur over the LUSB radiating to the apex

ABDOMEN: Soft, normoactive bowel sounds, nondistended, no hepatosplenomegaly

EXTREMITIES: No cyanosis, clubbing, or edema

NEUROLOGIC: Cranial nerves intact; deep tendon reflexes 2+; normal strength and sensation throughout

LABORATORY FINDINGS

WBC, 6.7 K/μL (normal differential); Hb, 11.7 g/dL; platelets, 168 K/μL; electrolytes: sodium, 140 mEq/L; potassium, 4.1 mEq/L; chloride, 94 mEq/L; bicarbonate, 28 mEq/L; bun, 18 mg/dL; creatinine, 1.4 mg/dL; glucose, 168 mg/dL; urinalysis: pH, 8.0; no active urine sediment; ECG: normal; chest x-ray: unremarkable; transthoracic echocardiogram is shown in Figures 41-1 and 41-2.

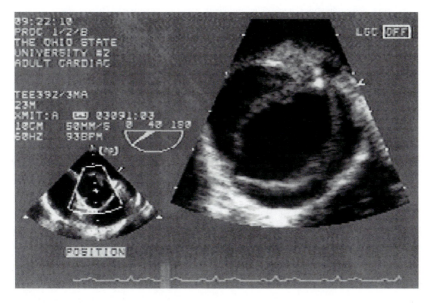

Figure 41-1
Aortic valve as seen by transthoracic echocardiogram.

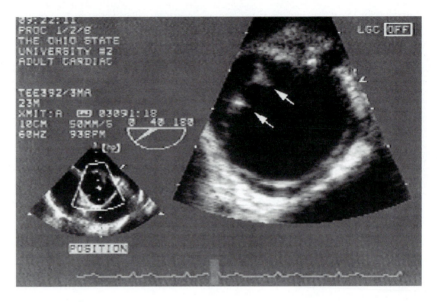

Figure 41-2
Aortic valve as seen by transthoracic echocardiogram.

What is the likely diagnosis and how should this patient be treated?

This patient has endocarditis. His physical examination is consistent with aortic valve stenosis and insufficiency. The transthoracic echocardiogram shows a bicuspid aortic valve with evidence of valvular vegetations (see Figs. 41-1 and 41-2). The patient had never been told that he had a heart murmur, and thus was never educated about antimicrobial prophylaxis for a bicuspid aortic valve. He developed symptoms about 4 weeks after having had a dental abscess incised and drained.

Infective endocarditis (IE) is a disease in which the infective organisms invade the endothelial lining of the heart. The infection may involve the valvular leaflets, chordae tendineae, mitral and aortic rings, ventricular endocardium, and endothelial lining of the great arteries involved with coarctation of the aorta or a patent ductus arteriosus. Pelletieri and Petersdorf first established the criteria for the diagnosis of IE in 1977. Von Reyn and associates subsequently modified these criteria in 1981, proposing four diagnostic categories: definite, probable, possible, and rejected. Durack and colleagues from Duke University have published more recent criteria that are helpful in making a definitive diagnosis of IE (Table 41-1). The Duke group has proposed major and minor criteria for making a clinical diagnosis of IE with two major, or one major plus three minor, or five minor criteria to establish a diagnosis. Persistent bacteremia with organisms typical for endocarditis and an oscillating mass by echocardiography on a valve make a clinically definitive diagnosis of IE (two major criteria). An echocardiogram is frequently positive with the clinical syndrome of IE, but a negative echocardiogram does not rule out the diagnosis.

TABLE 41-1   Duke Criteria for Clinical Diagnosis of Infective Endocarditis

Major Criteria
Persistently positive blood cultures:
    Typical organisms for endocarditis
    Persistent bacteremia: >2 positive cultures separated by at least
                            12 hours, or
                            >3 positive cultures at least 1 hour apart,
                            or if >4 cultures are drawn—70% samples
                            positive
Evidence of endocardial involvement
    Positive echocardiogram—vegetation, abscess, valve perforation
    New valvular regurgitation
Minor Criteria
Predisposing heart condition
Fever
Vascular phenomena
Immunologic phenomena
Positive blood cultures—not meeting major criteria
Echocardiogram—not meeting major criteria
Diagnosis
Two major criteria, or
One major plus three minor criteria, or
Five minor criteria

Infective endocarditis usually develops in individuals with underlying structural cardiac defects who develop bacteremia with organisms likely to cause endocarditis. Bacteremia may occur spontaneously or may complicate a focal infection (e.g., urinary tract infection, pneumonia, or cellulitis). Some surgical and dental procedures and instrumentations involving mucosal surfaces or contaminated tissue can cause transient bacteremia that rarely persists for more than 15 minutes. Blood-borne bacteria may lodge on damaged or abnormal heart valves or on the endocardium or the endothelium near anatomic defects, resulting in bacterial endocarditis or endarteritis. Although transient bacteremia is common following many invasive procedures, only certain bacteria commonly cause endocarditis. It is not always possible to predict which patients will develop this infection or what procedure will be responsible for it.

The predominant underlying lesion with IE in the past was rheumatic heart disease, which now afflicts no more than 30 percent of the adults with IE. Recent studies have found that mitral valve prolapse with regurgitation is the most frequent lesion and degenerative lesions of aortic and mitral valves, congenital heart disease, and rheumatic heart disease account for the rest. The risk of developing IE with mitral valve prolapse is strongly correlated with the severity of valvular thickening and redundancy as detected by echocardiography. These findings have been noted in more than 90 percent of the cases of mitral valve prolapse associated with endocarditis. Congenital heart disease underlies the infection in up to 20 percent of patients with IE. The most common predisposing congenital lesions include patent ductus arteriosus, ventricular septal defect, bicuspid aortic valve, coarctation of the aorta, tetralogy of Fallot, and ruptured aneurysms of the sinus of Valsalva. IE also occurs with hypertrophic obstructive cardiomyopathy, particularly on the subaortic endocardium of the hypertrophied septum.

Animal models of IE have provided useful information about its pathophysiology, natural history, treatment, and prevention. It is now known that IE results from a complex interaction between damaged vascular endothelium, local hemodynamic abnormalities, circulating bacteria, and local and systemic host defenses. Undamaged cardiac valves are resistant to bacterial attachment and infection. Constant trauma to the endothelial lining of the heart is produced by the abnormal hemodynamics resulting from valvular or congenital cardiac lesions. A damaged endothelium is an important inducer of thrombogenesis, which helps form a nonbacterial thrombotic endocardial (NBTE) lesion. Bacteria colonize NBTE lesions, forming infective vegetations. Endogenous bacteria gain a portal of entry into the blood from a loss of skin or mucosal integrity from trauma or manipulation of the oropharynx or of the gastrointestinal or genitourinary tracts. The infected vegetation constantly discharges bacteria into the circulation, thus producing persistent bacteremia, which results in fever, weight loss, fatigue, anemia, and metastatic infections. Persistent bacteremia stimulates the host's humoral and cellular immune systems, which form circulating immune complexes that are probably responsible for the skin manifestations of IE, including petechiae and Osler's nodes, and also the arthritis, glomerulonephritis, and positive rheumatoid factor.

IE can be caused by a wide variety of microorganisms; however, streptococci and staphylococci cause most cases, which can be further classified according to their occurrence on a native or prosthetic valve or with intravenous drug use. The majority of native valve endocarditis (NVE) cases are caused by *Streptococcus viridans* (50%) and *Staphylococcus aureus* (20%). The predominant organism with intravenous drug abuse is *S. aureus*, which accounts for 80 percent of cases with tricuspid valve infection. Prosthetic valve endocarditis (PVE) occurs in up to 4 percent of patients with prosthetic heart valves. It is classified as early PVE if it occurs within 2 months of surgery or late PVE if it occurs more than 2 months after a cardiac operation. Early PVE is thought to be owing to intraoperative contamination with nosocomial bacteria, particularly *Staphylococcus epidermidis*. With increasing surgical experience and perioperative antibiotic prophylaxis, early PVE has become less common and currently accounts for fewer than 10 percent of the PVE cases. Late-onset PVE still continues to be a significant problem and is caused by the same organisms that cause NVE.

The diagnosis of IE should be suspected in any patient with unexplained fever and multisystem disease. The onset may be acute, as highly invasive organisms infect an otherwise normal valve, causing the sudden onset of rigors, high fevers, new or changing heart murmurs, septic emboli to any organ, pyogenic arthritis, and petechial lesions of the skin and mucosa. The clinical picture of IE also may be subacute (SBE) or chronic. This occurs when less invasive endogenous organisms infect preexisting heart lesions and become manifest over several weeks to months, during which low-grade fever, changing heart murmurs, anorexia, embolic phenomena, renal manifestations, weight loss, and anemia and splenomegaly are common features. Heart valve leaflets may be perforated or destroyed, causing regurgitation, which is more common with acute IE. The infection can spread to surrounding structures and produce ring abscesses and mycotic aneurysms. Ring abscesses can produce heart block. Septic embolus to the coronary artery may cause a septic myocardial infarction.

Right-sided endocarditis may cause pulmonary infiltrates from septic lung emboli. Septic pericarditis is uncommon, occurring predominantly with acute IE from *S. aureus* infections. Exudative pleural effusions may also be observed.

A variety of skin and peripheral manifestations have been described in IE, particularly SBE. Petechiae occur in long-standing infection and are found on conjunctivae, buccal mucosa, and extremities. Splinter hemorrhages appear as dark streaks beneath the fingernails or toenails at the base of the nail. Splinter hemorrhages and petechiae result from increased capillary permeability owing to local vasculitis or microemboli. Osler's nodes, which are seen in SBE, are tender nodules that develop in the pulp of the digits as the result of immunologically mediated vasculitis. Janeway lesions are nontender, hemorrhagic macules on the palms or soles of patients with acute IE, particularly that caused by *S. aureus*. They are infrequently noted and are believed to be owing to septic emboli. Roth spots are oval-shaped hemorrhages in the retina with a pale center that are highly suggestive of IE but occur with other disorders. Emboli to the major systemic vessels may cause signs and symptoms of stroke and ischemia of the extremities. Mycotic aneurysms, which are infrequently observed, are believed to be owing to septic emboli to the vasa vasorum or direct infection of the arterial wall. Aneurysms may form in any vessel but are more frequent in cerebral arteries, the abdominal aorta, and sinus of Valsalva, coronary artery, and extremity arteries. Emboli to the renal artery may cause segmental infarction of the kidney, hematuria, flank pain, and hypertension. Focal and diffuse glomerulonephritis may occur from the deposition of circulating immune complexes on the glomerular basement membrane.

Antibiotic therapy and cardiac surgery (repair or replacement of the infected valve in selected patients) have completely changed the outlook of patients with IE. Antibiotic therapy generally can be started empirically after drawing three blood cultures in the first 3 to 4 hours in a patient with suspected endocarditis. Therapy for acute endocarditis should be started promptly because delay results in further valvular damage and abscess formation. Both minimal inhibitory concentrations (MIC) and minimal bactericidal concentrations (MBC) of different antibiotics to the organism should guide the selection of antibiotics. The prognosis of patients with IE has improved since the introduction of antibiotics and susceptibility testing. Mortality, however, remains high when there is significant valvular damage and hemodynamic instability, ring abscesses, and refractory bacteremia. With advances in cardiac surgical techniques, valve replacement surgery has become a safe and effective form of therapy for active IE. A multidisciplinary approach is necessary for decision making regarding surgery with input from cardiology, thoracic surgery, and infectious disease services. Surgical treatment is indicated during the acute phase of endocarditis in the presence of refractory heart failure, persistent sepsis, recurrent emboli, annular abscess, mycotic aneurysms, and intracardiac fistulae. Prosthetic valve endocarditis is associated with higher morbidity and mortality. Endocarditis of bioprosthetic valves should be initially managed with antibiotics and not surgery, unless echocardiography shows major valve dysfunction. Infection of the mechanical valves generally involves the sewing ring and causes perivalvular regurgitation and more frequently requires surgical intervention.

There are currently no randomized and carefully controlled trials to definitively establish that antibiotic prophylaxis protects against endocarditis during bacteremia-inducing procedures when underlying structural heart disease exists. Further, most cases of endocarditis are not attributable to an invasive procedure. Nonetheless, certain cardiac conditions are associated with endocarditis more often than others, and the use of prophylactic antibiotics is recommended to prevent IE in high-risk patients undergoing certain procedures. People at risk of IE should maintain the best possible oral health to reduce the potential for bacteremia. The recently updated recommendations of the American Heart Association (AHA) stratify cardiac conditions into high- and moderate-risk categories based on the potential outcome if endocarditis occurs. Those at highest risk have prosthetic heart valves, a previous history of endocarditis, complex cyanotic congenital heart disease, or surgically constructed systemic pulmonary shunts or conduits. Those at moderate-risk have patent ductus arteriosus, ventricular septal defect, coarctation of the aorta, bicuspid aortic valve, acquired valvular dysfunction (e.g., rheumatic heart disease or collagen vascular disease), or hypertrophic cardiomyopathy. Mitral valve prolapse (MVP) is common but the need for prophylaxis with this condition is controversial. The AHA recommends prophylaxis be given to those with MVP and regurgitation, or when it is not known if regurgitation is present and the procedure must be done before further evaluation can be completed. If regurgitation is not present, then the prophylaxis is not recommended.

Bacteremias commonly occur during normal activities such as routine tooth brushing or chewing. Prophylaxis is recommended for procedures known to induce bacteremias with organisms commonly associated with endocarditis. Antibiotic prophylaxis is recommended for at-risk patients undergoing dental and oral procedures associated with bleeding from hard or soft tissues, periodontal surgery, scaling, and professional teeth cleaning. Surgical procedures involving the respiratory, gastrointestinal, and genitourinary tracts may lead to bacteremia, and antibiotic prophylaxis is generally recommended for those that have a high likelihood of causing mucosal damage.

Prophylaxis is most effective when given perioperatively in dosages that are sufficient to assure adequate antibiotic concentrations in the serum during and after the procedure. The recently updated AHA guidelines recommend one dose of antibiotic 1 hour before the procedure and none 6 hours thereafter. This is based on recent comparisons that show that the pre-procedure dose results in adequate serum levels for several hours, making a second dose unnecessary.

Our patient was treated with antibiotic therapy for 6 weeks and clinically improved. He remained afebrile and asymptomatic when antibiotics were stopped. He is currently being followed closely for his bicuspid aortic valve and the timing and need for valve replacement. He has been educated about the use of prophylaxis.

 ## CLINICAL PEARLS

- Infective endocarditis (IE) usually develops when focal infections or procedures produce bacteremia that colonizes existing structural cardiac defects.
- Mitral valve prolapse, especially with thickened, redundant leaflets, is the most common underlying lesion in IE.
- Bacteria that cause IE gain access to the blood as a result of a loss of skin or mucosal integrity of the oropharynx or gastrointestinal or genitourinary tracts.
- Septic emboli are more common with acute IE, whereas subacute IE causes deposition of circulating immune complexes in the skin and other organs.
- Antibiotics and surgery have improved the outcome of IE, but decisions regarding the need and timing of surgery require a multidisciplinary approach.
- The AHA recommends antibiotic prophylaxis 1 hour prior to invasive procedures for patients at high- or moderate-risk of developing IE.

REFERENCES

1. Bansal RC. Infective endocarditis. *Med Clin North Am* 1995;79(5): 1205–1240.
2. Dajani AS, Taubert KA, Wilson W, et al. Prevention of bacterial endocarditis. Recommendations by the American Heart Association. *JAMA* 1997;277:1794–1801.
3. Dajani AS, Taubert KA, Wilson W, et al. Prevention of bacterial endocarditis. Recommendations by the American Heart Association. *Circulation* 1997;96:358–366.
4. Moon MR, Stinson EB, Miller DC. Surgical treatment of endocarditis. *Progr Cardiovasc Dis* 1997;40(3):239–264.
5. Durack DT. Prevention of infective endocarditis. *N Engl J Med* 1995;332(1):38–44.
6. Kubak BM, Nimmagadda AP, Holt CD. Advances in medical and antibiotic management of infective endocarditis. *Cardiol Clin* 1996; 14(3):405–436.

81-YEAR-OLD MAN WITH ABDOMINAL PAIN, JAUNDICE, AND WEIGHT LOSS

An 81-year-old man with a history of hypertension, coronary artery disease, BPH, and gout presented with a 1-week history of abdominal pain and jaundice associated with 2 months of anorexia and a 30-pound weight loss. He had been experiencing midepigastric abdominal pain associated with abdominal bloating that was worse after eating. He also had a constant vague right upper quadrant pain and loose stools that intermittently appeared clay-colored without nausea and vomiting. He had no history of hepatobiliary disease or inflammatory bowel disease and denied fevers, chills, chest pain, shortness of breath, or risk factors for hepatitis such as prior blood transfusions. His regular medications included allopurinol, terazosin, furosemide, nitroglycerin patch, and aspirin. He never smoked and used alcohol only on occasion.

PHYSICAL EXAMINATION

VITAL SIGNS: Temperature, 97°F (36°C); pulse, 56; respiration, 14; bp, 176/78 mmHg

GENERAL: Age-appropriate, emaciated male

HEENT: Eyes: scleral icterus

MOUTH: Jaundice of the lingual frenulum

NECK: No lymphadenopathy or thyromegaly

LUNGS: Clear

CARDIAC: Normal

ABDOMEN: Normal bowel sounds, distended but soft with right upper
quadrant tenderness; liver span by percussion 10 cm in the mid-
clavicular line, no splenomegaly; negative Murphy's sign
RECTAL: Guaiac negative
EXTREMITIES: No edema
NEUROLOGIC: No focal deficits, normal strength
SKIN: Jaundice, no telangiectasias

LABORATORY FINDINGS

WBC, 5.8 K/μL (normal differential); Hb, 12.4 g/dL; platelets
276 K/μL; electrolytes, urea nitrogen, and creatinine, normal; AST,
130 U/L (normal, 0–60); ALT, 126 U/L (normal, 0–60); Alk phos, 532
U/L (normal, 0–110); GGT, 472 U/L (normal, 5–85); LDH, 1,232 U/L
(normal, 0–625); total bilirubin, 9.4 mg/dL (normal, 0–1.5); direct bilirubin, 9.0 mg/dL (normal, 0–0.3); prothrombin and partial thromboplastin
time, normal; amylase and lipase, were normal. Acute abdominal series
revealed a nonspecific bowel gas pattern. Right upper quadrant ultrasound demonstrated a large stone in the gallbladder with intrahepatic biliary duct dilation. Endoscopic retrograde cholangiopancreatography
(ERCP) is shown in Fig. 42-1.

What is the likely diagnosis and how should this patient be treated?

This patient has cholangiocarcinoma, commonly termed a Klatskin's
tumor. The ERCP demonstrates intrahepatic biliary duct dilation with
severe narrowing of the common hepatic duct at the bifurcation of the
right and left hepatic ducts, characteristic of cholangiocarcinoma.

Jaundice is a term derived from the French word *jaune* for yellow,
which is used to describe the skin discoloration from bilirubin. For many
years it posed a diagnostic dilemma, but our current diagnostic approach
to jaundice is rooted in Osler's characterization of it as either owing to
hepatogenous or hematologic causes.

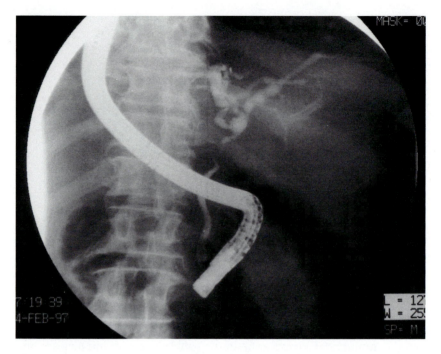

Figure 42-1
Endoscopic retrograde cholangiopancreatography.

Normal bilirubin levels are between 0.3 and 1.0 mg/dL. Hyperbilirubinemia results from an imbalance between the production and clearance of bilirubin, an end product of red blood cell destruction. Jaundice typically is manifest when total bilirubin levels reach 2.0 to 3.0 mg/dL, unless the patient has a dark complexion or edema that masks the jaundice until bilirubin levels rise much higher. Scleral icterus or a yellow tint to the lingual frenulum may be the earliest evidence of jaundice, differentiating it from hypercarotenemia (e.g., from myxedema or excessive carrot ingestion) that discolors the skin but not the sclera or mucosa.

Most of the serum bilirubin derives from red cell destruction in the reticuloendothelial system. This liberates the heme moiety of red blood cells, which is metabolized to biliverdin, then to bilirubin. Serum bilirubin is either in an unconjugated water-insoluble (indirect) form that avidly binds to albumin, or in a conjugated water-soluble (direct) form that is excreted by the kidney. Hepatocytes take up unconjugated bilirubin and oxidatively conjugate its glucuronic acid to bilirubin glucuronide, which is the only form that can be excreted into bile. Any impairment in this rate-limiting step in the hepatic metabolism of bilirubin leads to its efflux into the bloodstream causing hyperbilirubinemia, bilirubinuria, and jaundice.

Determining whether bilirubin is predominantly conjugated or unconjugated is the first step in discerning the etiology of jaundice. Finding bilirubin in the urine indicates that it is conjugated because this is the only form excreted by the kidney. As general guides, when 50 percent or more of the serum bilirubin is conjugated this is probably the primary problem, whereas when 80 percent or more is unconjugated this is more likely the main problem. This distinction provides a working framework for the differential diagnosis (Table 42-1).

Abnormalities in bilirubin metabolism generally occur by three different mechanisms: overproduction, hepatic dysfunction (decreased uptake or impaired conjugation), and decreased excretion. Although this may be a helpful diagnostic paradigm, a patient may have more than one abnormality causing hyperbilirubinemia. A careful history and physical examination and basic laboratory studies usually provide the basis for further diagnostic testing.

Finding unconjugated hyperbilirubinemia suggests a diagnosis of hemolysis or ineffective erythropoiesis, although less common causes are hereditary syndromes (Gilbert's or Crigler-Najjar) or acquired disorders (drugs, sepsis) that produce deficiencies of hepatic glucuronyl transferase, one of the enzymes responsible for the hepatocyte uptake of bilirubin. None of these disorders is typically associated with intrinsic hepatocellular abnormalities.

The cause of conjugated hyperbilirubinemia is usually more evasive than that of unconjugated hyperbilirubinemia, but it most commonly results from hepatocellular injury, cholestasis, or extrahepatic biliary obstruction. Conjugated hyperbilirubinemia is owing to impaired hepatic excretion (Dubin-Johnson syndrome, drugs, hepatocellular dysfunction) or more commonly, extrahepatic biliary obstruction (gallstones, malignancy, sclerosing cholangitis).

Hepatocellular injury raises the serum transaminase levels (AST, ALT) much more than it does other liver enzymes. Patients with this pattern of liver tests should be carefully evaluated for evidence of viral, drug- or toxin-induced hepatitis, hepatic congestion (heart failure, Budd-Chiari syndrome), alcoholic liver disease, or sepsis, and often require liver biopsy to establish the diagnosis. In contrast, cholestatic liver disorders usually preserve hepatocellular function while moderately obstructing the flow of bile. This usually occurs as a consequence of infiltrative or inflammatory

TABLE 42-1   Differential Diagnosis of Jaundice

Unconjugated Hyperbilirubinemia
Overproduction
  Hemolysis
  Ineffective erythropoiesis
Decreased hepatic uptake
  Prolonged fasting
  Sepsis
Decreased bilirubin conjugation
  Hereditary transferase deficiency (e.g., Gilbert's syndrome, Crigler-Najjar syndrome)
  Neonatal jaundice
  Acquired transferase deficiency (e.g., drugs, breast milk, hepatocellular dysfunction)
  Sepsis
Conjugated Hyperbilirubinemia
Impaired hepatic excretion
  Familial or hereditary disorders (e.g., Dubin-Johnson syndrome, Rotor syndrome)
  Acquired disorders (e.g., drugs, hepatocellular dysfunction, sepsis)
Extrahepatic biliary obstruction
  Intraductal obstruction (e.g., gallstones, malignancy, sclerosing cholangitis)
  Extrinsic biliary duct compression (e.g., malignancy, pancreatitis)

Kaplan LM, Isselbacher KJ. Jaundice, in *Harrison's Principles of Internal Medicine*, 14th ed. Fauci AS et al. (eds.). New York, McGraw-Hill, 1998.

processes within the hepatobiliary tree that elevate the serum alkaline phosphatase and conjugated bilirubin levels out of proportion to the transaminase elevations. Extrahepatic obstruction has many causes, but gallstones are far and away the most common. Other less common causes include primary sclerosing cholangitis, biliary strictures, cholangiocarcinoma (Klatskin's tumor), or extrinsic compression of the biliary tree from lymphoma or pancreatic cancer.

Biliary imaging should be done when the patient's presentation suggests cholestasis or extrahepatic biliary obstruction. This may be done with ultrasonography or CT scans that detect extrahepatic biliary duct dilatation with a high degree of accuracy and often identify the source of obstruction (e.g., intrahepatic, portal, or pancreatic masses, or cholelithiasis). However, both techniques often fail to detect intraductal stones (choledocholithiasis). When there is CT or ultrasonographic evidence or a strong suspicion of extrahepatic obstruction, either percutaneous or endoscopic cholangiography usually will identify the site and nature of the obstruction.

Cholangiocarcinoma is primarily a disease of men who are around age 60 at the time of diagnosis. It has a strong association with other bile duct disorders, particularly primary sclerosing cholangitis, which often occurs with ulcerative colitis. Dull, right upper quadrant abdominal pain, jaundice, and weight loss are the typical presenting features of cholangiocarcinoma. A biopsy or cytology specimen may be necessary to identify the tumor, but its radiographic appearance may be so characteristic as to establish the diagnosis. Surgical resection is the only effective treatment of these tumors, but only 25 percent are resectable. Palliative therapy includes biliary stenting, external radiation therapy, and chemotherapy. The overall 5-year survival rate is less than 5 percent.

Our patient had successful placement of a biliary stent and was treated with palliative external radiation therapy. He died 3 months after his diagnosis was established.

 ## CLINICAL PEARLS

- Hyperbilirubinemia results from an imbalance between the production and clearance of bilirubin from the destruction of red blood cells.
- Jaundice does not typically become apparent until the bilirubin level is greater than 2 mg/dL.
- The sclera and lingual frenulum are typically the first areas to demonstrate jaundice and differentiate it from hypercarotenemia.
- Bilirubin is typically found in the urine only with conjugated (direct) hyperbilirubinemia.
- Unconjugated (indirect) hyperbilirubinemia is from overproduction (hemolysis), decreased hepatic uptake (fasting, sepsis), or decreased conjugation (Gilbert's or Crigler-Najjar syndromes).

- Conjugated (direct) hyperbilirubinemia is owing to impaired hepatic bilirubin excretion (Dubin–Johnson syndrome, drugs, and hepatocellular dysfunction) or more commonly to extrahepatic biliary obstruction (usually gallstones, but also malignancy or sclerosing cholangitis).
- Cholangiocarcinoma (Klatskin's tumor) is primarily a disease of middle-aged men that has a 5-year survival rate of less than 5 percent.

REFERENCES

1. Lester R. The pathogenesis of cholestasis: Past and future trends. *Semin Liver Dis* 1993;13:219.
2. Thuluvath PJ, Rai R, Venbrux AC, Yeo CJ. Cholangiocarcinoma: A review. *Gastroenterologist* 1997:5:306–315
3. Sleisenger MH, Fordtran JS, eds. *Gastrointestinal Disease*, 5th ed. Philadelphia, Saunders, 1993.
4. Kaplan LM, Isselbacher KJ. Jaundice, in *Harrison's Principles of Internal Medicine*, 14th ed. Fauci AS et al, (eds.) New York, McGraw-Hill, 1998.

65-YEAR-OLD WOMAN WITH LUNG CANCER AND POLYURIA

A 65-year-old woman was admitted to the hospital with a 1-week history of excessive thirst, polydipsia, nocturia, and polyuria. Three months ago she had undergone pulmonary resection for newly diagnosed adenocarcinoma of the lung without distant metastases. She had received no adjuvant chemotherapy and was recovering from her surgery without difficulty until she developed the symptoms mentioned in the preceding. Micturition had been occurring every 45 to 60 minutes during the day and up to eight times a night; and she had excessive thirst, drinking about 5 to 7 liters of fluid a day with an unusual craving for cold drinks. She denied nausea, weakness, fevers, or fatigue, but her daughter thought that her mother had been intermittently confused over the past week. Her past medical history and family history were otherwise unremarkable, but social history was positive for a 60-pack year tobacco use.

PHYSICAL EXAMINATION

VITAL SIGNS: Temperature, 98.6°F (36.9°C); pulse, 84; respiration, 16; bp, 100/69 mmHg
GENERAL: Thin woman who appeared pale and dehydrated
HEENT: Normal
NECK: No lymphadenopathy or thyromegaly
LUNGS: Left thoracotomy scar; decreased breath sounds with dullness to percussion over the left base; otherwise the lung fields were clear
CARDIAC: Regular rate and rhythm without murmurs, rubs, or gallops
ABDOMEN: Normoactive bowel sounds; soft, nontender with no hepatosplenomegaly

EXTREMITIES: No cyanosis, clubbing, or peripheral edema
INTEGUMENT: Normal
NEUROLOGIC: Cranial nerves intact; deep tendon reflexes 2+; normal
strength and sensation throughout

LABORATORY FINDINGS

WBC, 7.8 K/μL (normal differential); Hb, 10.2 g/dL; MCV, 88 fL; platelets, 300 K/μL; electrolytes: sodium, 145 mEq/L; potassium, 4.0 mEq/L; chloride, 103 mEq/L; bicarbonate, 24 mEq/L; urea nitrogen, 14 mg/dL; creatinine, 1.1 mg/dL; glucose, 90 mg/dL; serum osmolality, 292 mOsm/L; urinalysis: specific gravity, 1.001; glucose, protein, and microscopic: negative; urine osmolality, 75 mOsm/L; chest x-ray with evidence of previous left lower lobectomy, no acute process; ECG: normal. MRI of the brain shown (Fig. 43-1).

What is the likely diagnosis and how should this patient be treated?

This patient has central diabetes insipidus (DI), a term that refers to the passage of a large quantity of dilute urine.

The brain MRI showed several metastatic lesions, one of which involved the hypothalamus and pituitary gland (arrows). The history of polyuria, excessive thirst, and polydipsia, with the preceding laboratory results and a urinary osmolality of 75 mOsm/L should raise the suspicion of diabetes insipidus. Table 43-1 shows the results of a water deprivation test in this patient—confirming the diagnosis of central DI.

The posterior pituitary is composed of the terminal portions of neurons that originate in the supraoptic and paraventricular nuclei of the anterior hypothalamus. Vasopressin (AVP) or antidiuretic hormone (ADH) is synthesized in the magnocellular neurons of the anterior hypothalamus as a prohormone. This precursor molecule is then processed by enzymes that generate AVP, a 10,000-dalton protein, as it moves along the axon of the nerve cell where it is packaged into neurosecretory granules and

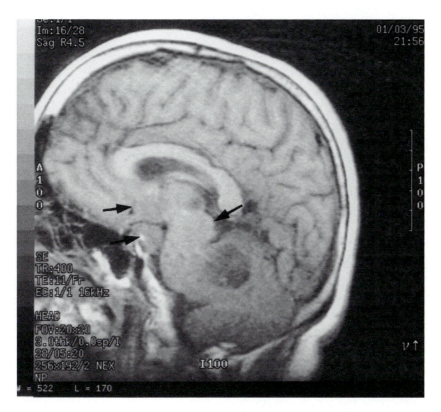

Figure 43-1
MRI of the brain.

TABLE 43-1   Water Deprivation
Test

	URINE OUTPUT (mL/HR)	URINE OSM (mOsm/L)	SERUM OSM (mOsm/L)
Onset of test	200	75	292
Water deprivation	180	80	312
5 units IV vasopressin	100	190	311

stored until its release into the peripheral circulation in response to appropriate stimuli.

Polyuria is a common clinical problem that generally is owing to one of three abnormalities: an osmotic diuresis, resistance to AVP, or deficient AVP secretion. The most common is that caused by glycosuria, a presenting symptom of diabetes mellitus. Excessive water intake and hypotonic polyuria may be owing to a failure of AVP release in response to normal physiologic stimuli (central or neurogenic DI) or a failure of the kidney to respond to AVP (nephrogenic DI). AVP conserves water by concentrating the urine. It binds to a receptor in the distal tubular epithelium of the kidney, mainly in the collecting ducts where it enhances the hydroosmotic flow of water from the renal lumen to the medullary interstitium. This helps maintain the osmolality and volume of body fluids constant.

Deficient release of AVP in response to appropriate stimuli can be caused by lesions at several sites in the physiologic chain that regulates hormone release. Deficiency of AVP (neurogenic or central DI) reflects either functional or structural disease of the supraoptic hypothalamic neurons that secrete the hormone. It also may be owing to genetic defects in the secretion of AVP. Two clues—sudden onset of polyuria and a preference for iced beverages—suggest DI. Neurogenic DI must be distinguished from primary polydipsia because drinking excessively also results in polyuria and suppressed AVP secretion.

There are four major causes of central DI. The first is *neoplastic* or *infiltrative lesions*, mainly of the hypothalamus or pituitary stalk involving the posterior pituitary neurons, which may be involved with pituitary adenomas, craniopharyngiomas, germinomas, pinealomas, metastatic tumors, leukemia, histiocytosis X, and sarcoidosis. These lesions also may cause partial or complete loss of anterior pituitary function.

The second cause is *pituitary* or *hypothalamic surgery*, which can cause DI that is usually associated with anterior hypopituitarism. Surgically induced DI usually develops between 1 and 6 days after surgery and often disappears after a few days. Removal of the posterior pituitary induces permanent DI only if the pituitary stalk is sectioned high enough to induce retrograde degeneration of most neurons of the supraoptic nucleus.

The third major cause is *severe head injury*, which is usually associated with skull fractures that cause DI and is associated with anterior hypopituitarism in about one-sixth of the patients. Spontaneous remissions of traumatic DI may occur even after 6 months, presumably because disrupted axons regenerate within the pituitary stalk.

The fourth is *idiopathic DI*, which usually starts in childhood and is seldom associated with anterior pituitary dysfunction. This is a diagnosis of exclusion that can be made only after a careful search has failed to reveal a cause of AVP deficiency. The presence of anterior hypopituitarism or hyperprolactinemia or radiologic evidence of lesions within or above the sella suggests a causative lesion. The diagnosis of idiopathic DI is made with increasing confidence as the duration of follow-up increases and there are no other findings. In idiopathic DI the number of neurons in the supraoptic and paraventricular nuclei may be decreased and there may be circulating antibodies to hypothalamic nuclei. In rare instances, DI is inherited as an isolated defect or as part of an autosomal recessive syndrome consisting of DI, diabetes mellitus, optic atrophy, and deafness known as the *Wolfram syndrome*.

DI may appear during pregnancy and cease a few days after delivery, or it may commence after parturition in women with Sheehan's syndrome, especially when cortisol deficiency is treated. Mild symptoms of DI may either increase or improve during pregnancy. AVP-resistant DI also may develop during pregnancy, perhaps owing to increased circulating levels of placental vasopressinase; such patients respond to treatment with desmopressin (see the following).

Polyuria, excessive thirst, and polydipsia are almost invariably present in DI. These symptoms are characteristically sudden in onset when the disorder first presents and also when the effects of exogenous vasopressin disappear during long-term therapy. In the most severe cases the urine is pale and its volume is immense (up to 20 L/d), requiring micturition every 15 to 30 minutes throughout the day and night. More frequently, however, urine volume is only modestly increased (2.5–6 L/d), and occasionally it may be less than 2 L/d. Urinary concentration (less than 290 mOsm/L, specific gravity less than 1.010) is below that of the serum in severe cases but may be higher than that of serum (290–600 mOsm/L) in mild DI. If a patient becomes severely dehydrated, however, the urine may become more concentrated as it slowly passes through the collecting tubules.

A slight rise in serum osmolality resulting from hypotonic polyuria stimulates thirst. Large volumes of fluid are imbibed and cold drinks are preferred; patients often go to great trouble to secure cold fluids. Normal function of the thirst center ensures that polydipsia closely matches polyuria and thus dehydration is seldom detectable except by a mild elevation of serum sodium. However, when replenishment of excreted water is inadequate, dehydration may become severe, causing weakness, fever, psychic disturbances, prostration, and death. These features are associated with a rising serum osmolality and serum sodium concentration. Dehydration also can occur during unconsciousness produced by surgical anesthesia, head trauma, or other causes.

The cause of hypotonic polyuria can usually be recognized by a pragmatic clinical approach. Even though stimuli such as nausea, nicotine, hypoglycemia, and hypotension may release AVP, the results are clinically irrelevant. Diagnostic approaches that utilize plasma and urine osmolality determinations are readily available, reliable, and safe, and allow rapid recognition and treatment. Measurements of plasma or urine AVP are expensive and time consuming, and are only occasionally needed when osmolality measurements are inconclusive.

The standard test for evaluating patients for DI is the *water deprivation test*. Comparison of the urinary osmolality after dehydration with that after vasopressin administration is a simple and reliable way of diagnosing DI and differentiating AVP deficiency from other causes of polyuria. The maximal urinary concentrating ability varies among individuals and no absolute lower limit of normal can be defined in patients with nonspecific illness. It is impossible to identify AVP deficiency solely on the urinary osmolality achieved after specified periods of water deprivation. However, if after prolonged dehydration vasopressin administration induces a *further* rise in urinary osmolality, then there is a strong implication that vasopressin deficiency exists. This, however, is a very dangerous means of proving the diagnosis in a patient with clinically overt DI.

During the *water deprivation test*, fluids are withheld long enough to result in stable hourly urinary osmolalities. This is usually associated with a loss in body weight of at least 1 kg. Patients with large urinary volumes should be watched carefully and the test terminated if weight loss exceeds 2 kg or the clinical condition deteriorates. After stability in urinary osmolality is achieved, the patient is given 5 units of aqueous arginine vasopressin or 1 μg desmopressin by subcutaneous injection or 10 μg desmopressin by nasal spray. Plasma osmolality is determined immediately before the administration of vasopressin; urinary osmolality is measured 30 to 60 minutes thereafter.

Interpretation. In those with normal pituitary function, urinary osmolality does not rise more than 9 percent after AVP administration, regardless of the maximal urinary osmolality achieved after dehydration alone. In central DI the rise in urinary osmolality after vasopressin exceeds 9 percent. To ensure adequate dehydration, plasma osmolality before the vasopressin administration should be above 288 mOsm/L. Patients with polyuria from renal diseases, potassium depletion, or nephrogenic DI usually show little rise in urinary osmolality with dehydration and no further rise after vasopressin. Patients with compulsive water drinking (primary polydipsia) often require prolonged water deprivation before plasma osmolality reaches 288 mOsm/L and before a plateau in urinary osmolality is reached; moreover, urinary osmolality rises by less than 9 percent after exogenous vasopressin.

DI can be treated by hormone replacement. As with most peptides, oral administration of vasopressin is ineffective. Aqueous arginine vasopressin administered subcutaneously in doses of 5 to 10 units has only a 3- to 6-hour duration of action and its main use is in the initial management of unconscious patients with acute DI following head trauma or a neurosurgical procedure. Its short duration of action allows recognition of the recovery phase of neurohypophyseal function and minimizes the risk of water intoxication from intravenous fluids. Desmopressin has prolonged antidiuretic activity and is almost completely devoid of pressor effects. When given intranasally in amounts between 10 and 20 μg or by subcutaneous injection, its antidiuretic action usually persists for 12 to 24 hours. This is the drug of choice for most patients with DI. Patients with some residual AVP activity causing partial DI may respond to oral chlorpropamide, clofibrate, or carbamazepine. When antidiuretic therapy is initiated for longstanding DI, excessive drinking may result in serious water intoxication, which must be carefully avoided. Education about drinking according to thirst must be reinforced constantly in some patients. Intake and output of fluids, body weight, serum sodium, and renal function should be closely monitored after the initiation of therapy.

Our patient had central DI secondary to a lung cancer metastasis involving her hypothalamus and pituitary. Her failure to increase urine osmolality following water deprivation and the significant increase in urine osmolality that occurred after AVP confirmed the diagnosis of central DI. She was treated with intranasal desmopressin, which effected an improvement in her symptoms that permitted her to receive radiation therapy for her metastatic disease as an outpatient.

 ## CLINICAL PEARLS

◢ Polyuria is a common clinical problem that generally is owing to an osmotic diuresis, resistance to vasopressin (AVP), or deficient AVP secretion.

- Hypothalamic or pituitary stalk involvement by neoplastic or infiltrative lesions, surgical procedures, or severe head injuries, can cause central diabetes insipidus (DI).
- Idiopathic DI is a diagnosis of exclusion and is rarely an inherited disorder.
- Central DI may occur during pregnancy (owing to vasopressinase) and cease a few days after delivery, or may follow Sheehan's syndrome (postpartum hypopituitarism).
- Polyuria, excessive thirst, and polydipsia are the main clinical characteristics of DI.
- With severe DI, urinary volumes may exceed 20 L/day and dehydration can be life-threatening if the patient is not permitted access to water, has no thirst mechanism, or is unconscious.
- The water deprivation test is the standard test for the diagnosis of DI. With neurogenic (central) DI, urine osmolality rises more than 9 percent from that achieved by dehydration alone.
- Intranasal desmopressin is the treatment of choice for most patients with central DI.

REFERENCES

1. Oiso Y, Iwasaki Y. Vasopressin and related disorders. *Intern Med* 1998;37(2):213–215.
2. Robinson AG, Verbalis JG. Diabetes insipidus. *Curr Ther Endocrinol Metab* 1997;6:1–7.
3. Singer I, Oster JR, Fishman LM. The management of diabetes insipidus in adults. *Arch Intern Med* 1997;157(12):1293–1301.
4. Robertson GL. Diabetes insipidus. *Endocrinol Metab Clin North Am* 1995;24(3):549–572.
5. Moses AM, Streeten DH, Disorders of the neurohypophysis in Isselbacher KJ, Braunwald E, Wilson JD, et al. (eds). *Harrison's Principles of Internal Medicine*. 13th ed. New York, McGraw-Hill, 1994, pp. 1921–1928.

55-YEAR-OLD WOMAN WITH A SORE THROAT

A 55-year-old woman with type 2 diabetes mellitus, hypertension, and hypothyroidism presented with a 2-day history of progressive malaise, myalgias, earache, and a severe sore throat. During this time she felt feverish, experienced odynophagia (pain on swallowing), and had high blood sugars despite a decreased appetite. She denied shortness of breath, cough, rhinorrhea, chills, and night sweats. No family members were ill. Her medications included enalapril, Glucotrol, NPH insulin, and levothyroxine. She was married and had two healthy adult children. She did not smoke or drink alcohol and reported no recent travel.

PHYSICAL EXAMINATION

VITAL SIGNS: Temperature, 101.2°F (38.4°C); pulse, 121; respiration, 20; bp, 140/79

GENERAL: Moderately obese, ill-appearing

HEENT: Oropharynx: right posterior pharynx swelling with uvular deviation to the left, exudate with mild erythema; no leukoplakia

NECK: Tender, right anterior cervical lymphadenopathy; no thyromegaly

LUNGS: Clear

CARDIAC: Normal

ABDOMEN: Obese, normoactive bowel sounds, soft, nontender, no hepatosplenomegaly

EXTREMITIES: No edema

SKIN: Warm, no rash

LABORATORY FINDINGS

WBC, 24 K/μL (7% bands, 72% segmented polys, 15% lymphocytes); Hb, 12.9 g/dL (MCV 89 fl); platelets, 373 K/μL; electrolytes, blood urea nitrogen, and creatinine, normal; neck CT scan shown in Fig. 44-1.

What is the likely diagnosis and how should this patient be treated?

This patient has a peritonsillar abscess or quinsy. The neck CT demonstrated a 2-cm abscess adjacent to the right palatine tonsil with narrowing of the airway posterior to the soft palate (see Fig. 44-1). The abscess extended inferiorly along the lateral margin of the pharynx to the piriform sinus.

Acute pharyngitis is one of the most common presenting problems in primary care. Although the vast majority are caused by the common cold, other microorganisms may be responsible. It is important to establish the

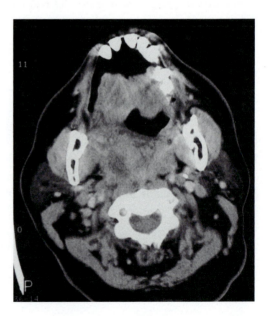

Figure 44-1
CT scan of the neck.

etiology, which guides treatment, uncovers associated diseases such as primary HIV infection or infectious mononucleosis, and portends potential complications such as quinsy or Lemierre's syndrome.

Viral pharyngitis predominates during the winter months when the peak prevalence of adenovirus, influenza, and parainfluenza viruses and coronavirus occur, whereas infection in the fall and spring is more often from rhinovirus. Unlike streptococcal pharyngitis, pharyngeal discomfort with viral infections is usually not the primary complaint, which is usually a constellation of symptoms including myalgias, headache, cough, and rhinorrhea. The virally infected pharynx may appear normal or show only mild edema and erythema. Pharyngeal exudates and painful lymphadenopathy are usually not seen with a common cold. In contrast, Epstein–Barr virus, herpes virus, and adenovirus usually causes a more severe illness with exudative pharyngitis and tender lymphadenopathy. Up to half of those with adenoviral pharyngitis also have conjunctivitis. Viral pharyngitis is thus a diagnosis of exclusion. Its treatment is supportive, except for rare cases of infectious mononucleosis in which airway patency may be threatened, necessitating treatment with systemic glucocorticoids.

Streptococcus pyogenes is the most important bacterial pathogen causing acute pharyngitis, accounting for about 15 percent of all cases. The most important reason for differentiating it from common viral pharyngitis is its response to antibiotics and subsequent prevention of rheumatic fever and suppurative complications. Streptococcal pharyngitis peaks in the late winter and early spring, and is easily transmissible among family members. As with viral pharyngitis, the clinical presentation may vary greatly. In severe cases, patients present with high fever, severe pharyngeal pain, and odynophagia. The pharynx is often severely erythematous with uvular edema and a thick exudate. Tender cervical lymphadenopathy and marked leukocytosis are the rule. Some strains of *S. pyogenes* produce an exotoxin that results in the characteristic diffuse erythematous rash of scarlet fever. In addition, the tongue may become red with swollen papillae (strawberry tongue). Noninvasive pharyngitis owing to *S. pyogenes* has recently been implicated in the streptococcal toxic shock syndrome. The diagnosis of streptococcal pharyngitis is easily established with rapid streptococcal antigen tests. Unfortunately, otherwise healthy streptococcal carriers account for about 20 percent of positive tests and there is no way to distinguish them from patients with active infection. Although the infection is typically self-limited, even in symptomatic patients, the early administration of antibiotics is important to prevent complications and limit transmission of the infection.

Peritonsillar abscess is the most common deep infection of the head and neck. It occurs along a spectrum from acute pharyngitis to follicular tonsillitis to peritonsillar cellulitis and abscess formation. Prompt recognition and treatment are mandatory to prevent spread of the infection to nearby vital structures and the blood stream. Peritonsillar abscess may occur at any age but is most common in young adults. The vast majority of cases are caused by *S. pyogenes*, although a mixture of oral bacteria, particularly anaerobes, contaminates most cultures. Patients typically present with fever, sore throat, pain referred to the ear, and odynophagia. Edema and pain may result in the characteristic muffled or "hot potato" voice. An exudative tender peritonsillar mass with marked edema that displaces the soft palate and the uvula away from the mass and is sometimes associated with trismus may help differentiate an abscess from other retro- and parapharyngeal infections. A CT scan usually helps clarify the diagnosis and guides therapy. The traditional therapy of a peritonsillar abscess has been immediate drainage and antibiotics followed by tonsillectomy 4 to 6 weeks later. More recent studies report up to a 90 percent success rate with needle aspiration and oral antibiotics alone, thereby avoiding hospitalization and an operation. However, the most appropriate management depends on the success rate of needle aspiration and the patient's overall health. Patients who may benefit from an early tonsillectomy are those at greatest risk for recurrence after medical treatment, especially patients under age 40 who have had a history of tonsillar disease. Although penicillin is the drug of choice, extended-spectrum penicillins with penicillinase activity, erythromycin for those who are penicillin allergic, and clindamycin are acceptable alternatives. Ten to 14 days of therapy is best.

Our patient responded well to needle aspiration and parenteral penicillin. She was discharged on the fourth hospital day to complete a 14-day course of antibiotics. She has had no recurrence of infection at last follow-up.

 CLINICAL PEARLS

- The most common cause of acute pharyngitis is the common cold.
- Viral pharyngitis is associated with headache, myalgia, coryza, and rhinorrhea.
- Streptococcal pharyngitis is not typically associated with the symptoms of a cold.

- Peritonsillar abscess is an uncommon but serious complication of streptococcal pharyngitis or tonsillitis.
- Peritonsillar abscess is characterized by fever, sore throat, pain referred to the ear, odynophagia, and a "hot potato" voice.
- Peritonsillar abscess is treated with aspiration or surgical drainage of the abscess and a 10- to 14-day course of antibiotics.
- Tonsillectomy is indicated for patients with a history of recurrent infections, or who are at risk for them.

REFERENCES

1. Epperly TD, Wood TC. New trends in the management of peritonsillar abscess. *Am J Fam Pract* 1990;42:102–112.
2. Parker GS, Tami TA. The management of peritonsillar abscess in the 90's: An update. *Am J Otolaryngol* 1992;13:284–288.
3. Patel KS, Ahmad S, O'Leary G, Michel M. The role of computed tomography in the management of peritonsillar abscess. *Otolaryngol Head Neck Surg* 1992;107:727–731.

39-YEAR-OLD MAN WITH COUGH, WEAKNESS, AND DARK URINE

A 39-year-old man with no previous serious illnesses presented to the emergency department with a 1-week history of malaise, fevers, chills, and cough productive of dark sputum. His symptoms were accompanied by thigh pain that progressed to bilateral lower extremity weakness. He also reported a decreased urine output for 2 to 3 days prior to admission and a dark brown color to his urine. His review of systems was positive for about five loose stools per day for the past several days. He denied recent heavy muscular exertion or loss of consciousness. He was taking no medication and lived alone, having no recent contacts with persons known to be ill. He had a 40-pack year history of tobacco use.

PHYSICAL EXAMINATION

VITAL SIGNS: Temperature, 102.6°F (39.2°C); pulse, 100; respiration, 18; bp, 160/100 mmHg

GENERAL: Ill-appearing, avoiding leg movement

HEENT: Dry mucous membranes, otherwise normal

NECK: No lymphadenopathy or thyromegaly

LUNGS: Diminished breath sounds at bases, egophony, and increased tactile fremitus over right base

CARDIAC: Tachycardic, regular rate, and rhythm without murmurs, rubs, or gallops

ABDOMEN: Normoactive bowel sounds, mild epigastric tenderness, nondistended

EXTREMITIES: No cyanosis or edema, bilateral thigh tenderness on palpation

NEUROLOGIC: Cranial nerves intact; deep tendon reflexes 2+; normal strength and sensation throughout

LABORATORY FINDINGS

WBC, 10.7 K/μL (9% bands, 81% neutrophils, 8% lymphocytes, 2% monocytes); Hb, 15.7 g/dL; platelets, 146 K/μL; electrolytes: sodium, 131 mEq/L; potassium, 3.5 mEq/L; chloride, 94 mEq/L; bicarbonate, 20 mEq/L; bun, 27 mg/dL; creatinine, 2.1 mg/dL; glucose, 137 mg/dL; creatine kinase, 66,296 U/L; quantitative CK-MB, 3.2 ng/mL; urinalysis: pH, 8.0; positive for myoglobin and hemoglobin; no active urine sediment. Arterial blood gas measurements on room air: pH, 7.43; P_{CO_2}, 27 mmHg; P_{O_2}, 67 mmHg; CO_2, 18 mEq/L, O_2 saturation, 93%; ECG, sinus tachycardia; chest x-ray shown in Figure 45-1.

What is the likely diagnosis and how should this patient be treated?

This patient has right lower lobe pneumonia by physical examination, which is confirmed by chest radiogram. He also has rhabdomyolysis and gastrointestinal symptoms, indicating a severe infection. The unifying diagnosis in this case is *Legionnaires' disease.* The severity of untreated infection mandates empirical treatment of legionella in our patient and others hospitalized with community-acquired pneumonia. The gram–negative bacteria are transmitted either by inhalation or aspiration. Characteristic clinical manifestations include pneumonia with headache, gastrointestinal symptoms, and hyponatremia. Rhabdomyolysis with acute renal failure from Legionnaires' disease is uncommon and has a high mortality rate.

Legionnaires' disease was first recognized during an outbreak of pneumonia involving the delegates to the 1976 American Legion convention at a Philadelphia hotel. Full appreciation of its importance other than as an exotic pathogen has only come in the past several years. It is now apparent that legionella is a common cause of community-acquired and nosocomial pneumonia. Studies in which diagnostic tests, especially cul-

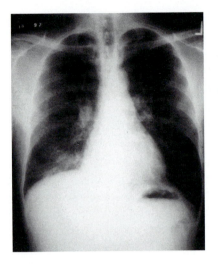

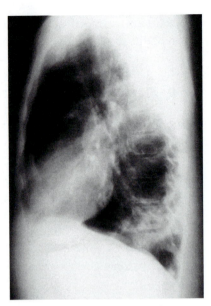

Figure 45-1
PA and lateral chest x-ray.

tures, showed *Legionella pneumophila* to be among the top three or four microbial causes of community-acquired pneumonia. Patients with community-acquired Legionnaires' disease are more likely to have severe pneumonia, as defined by more severely abnormal vital signs, extensive infiltrates on chest radiography, and need for admission to an intensive care unit.

Cigarette smoking, chronic lung disease, and immunosuppression (especially that caused by corticosteroid therapy) have been consistently implicated as risk factors for Legionnaires' disease. Surgery is a major predisposing factor in nosocomial legionella infections, with transplant recipients being at greatest risk. The incidence of Legionnaires' disease in AIDS is low. However, when it occurs the clinical manifestations are more severe and include bacteremia, lung abscesses, and extrapulmonary infections.

Legionnaires' disease can be acquired by the inhalation of aerosols containing legionella or by microaspiration of water contaminated with the organism. Aerosol-generating systems that have been linked to transmission of this disease include cooling towers, respiratory-therapy equipment, and whirlpool baths. One of the more fascinating outbreaks originated from an ultrasonic mist machine in a grocery store. Aspiration, which has not been widely recognized as a mode of transmission, has been clearly documented in cases of legionella pneumonia. *L. pneumophila* generally causes more severe disease than most other bacterial pathogens responsible for community-acquired pneumonia. The various strains of legionella differ in virulence, but *L. pneumophila* is the most pathogenic, accounting for 90 percent of the cases of Legionnaires' disease. Moreover, of the more than 14 serogroups of *L. pneumophila* that have been identified, serogroup 1 accounts for more than 80 percent of the reported cases of Legionnaires' disease.

As Legionnaires' disease has been appreciated with greater frequency, less severely ill patients have been recognized earlier in their course. Pneumonia is the predominant clinical syndrome. The disease presents with a broad spectrum of illness, ranging from a mild cough and low-grade fever to stupor, respiratory failure, and multiorgan failure. Gastrointestinal symptoms are prominent, especially diarrhea, which occurs in up to 40 percent of cases. Hyponatremia (serum sodium concentration <130 mmol/L) occurs more frequently in Legionnaires' disease than in other types of pneumonia. Extrapulmonary legionellosis is rare, but the clinical manifestations are often dramatic. Legionella has been implicated in cases of sinusitis, cellulitis, pancreatitis, peritonitis, and pyelonephritis. Dissemination apparently occurs through bacteremia. The most common extrapulmonary site is the heart, with numerous reports of myocarditis, pericarditis, postcardiotomy syndrome, and prosthetic-valve endocarditis.

Once considered fairly rare, rhabdomyolysis is now recognized as one of the more common conditions encountered in clinical medicine. Indeed, it now seems that almost every serious medical disorder may be associated with various degrees of rhabdomyolysis, which may be life-threatening when extensive. Rhabdomyolysis is defined as an injury to the sarcolemma of skeletal muscle, resulting in leakage of its components into the blood or urine. A major life-threatening complication of acute rhabdomyolysis is hyperkalemia, which may result in cardiac conduction disturbances, arrhythmias, or skeletal muscle paralysis. Metabolic acidosis and hypocalcemia from acute precipitation of calcium carbonate in the injured tissues are other serious complications. Dumping of myoglobin into the renal tubules may result in acute tubular necrosis, intratubular obstruction, and acute oliguric renal failure. Because of these potentially serious events, any patient complaining of weakness, myalgia, muscle tenderness, or swelling, especially with identifiable heme pigment in the urine, should undergo appropriate evaluation to identify rhab-domyolysis and its complications.

The mechanism of sarcolemmal injury may differ with its etiology. For example, strenuous exertion is thought to produce muscle cell hyper-thermia and hypoxia, which activates various enzymes that destroy actin. Drugs such as ethanol and cholesterol-lowering statins (3-hydroxy-3-methylglutaryl coenzyme A [HMG-CoA] reductase inhibitors) cause di-rect sarcolemmal plasma membrane injury. Among various infections that cause rhabdomyolysis, some produce myotoxins (e.g., clostridia), others directly invade skeletal muscle (influenza viruses), and yet others gener-ate cytokines such as tumor necrosis factor-α and interleukin-1 that can cause acute proteolysis within skeletal muscle. Legionella is thought to cause rhabdomyolysis by either a direct toxic effect or an unidentified cir-culating factor that causes muscle cell necrosis.

The specialized laboratory tests that are necessary to diagnose Legion-naires' disease often must be specifically requested because they are not routinely performed. The definitive diagnostic test is culture of the or-ganism. Sputum from patients who are suspected of having Legionnaires' disease should be cultured, regardless of its quality, since it will often yield the organism. A urine test that detects antigens of *L. pneumophila*, which is relatively inexpensive and rapid, has a sensitivity of 70 percent and a specificity of nearly 100 percent. Unlike culture, the urine test remains positive for weeks despite antibiotic therapy. A minor drawback is that it detects only *L. pneumophila* serogroup 1, but this accounts for the major-ity of cases of Legionnaires' disease.

A delay in instituting therapy for legionella pneumonia significantly in-creases its mortality. Therefore, empirical anti-legionella therapy should be included in the treatment of severe community-acquired pneumonia. Erythromycin has historically been the drug of choice, but the newer macrolides, especially azithromycin, have superior in vitro activity and greater intracellular and lung-tissue penetration. Quinolones also have greater in vitro activity and better intracellular penetration than the macrolides. Given the pharmacologic interaction of the macrolides with immunosuppressive medications used after transplantation, quinolones are recommended in transplant recipients with Legionnaires' disease. Ri-fampin is highly active in vitro and in vivo against legionella and is rec-ommended for severely ill patients as part of combination therapy that includes a macrolide or quinolone. Parenteral therapy should be given until there is an objective clinical response, after which oral therapy can be substituted. Ten to 14 days of therapy has been recommended in the past, but recent studies suggest that a 5- to 10-day course of azithromycin is sufficient in uncomplicated disease. However, a 21-day course is recommended for immunosuppressed patients or those with extensive pneumonia on chest radiography.

In our patient, the legionella urinary antigen test was positive, and sputum culture demonstrated heavy growth of *L. pneumophila*, serogroup 1. Treatment with intravenous azithromycin and intravenous alkaline fluids for rhabdomyolysis resulted in resolution of his fevers and cough and his renal function returned to normal. He recovered completely and was discharged from the hospital in good condition.

 CLINICAL PEARLS

- Initial antibiotics for community-acquired pneumonia requiring hospitalization should include coverage for *Legionella pneumophila*.
- Intravenous macrolide or quinolone antibiotics should be started immediately for patients who are severely ill with community-acquired pneumonia, before test results are available.
- Duration of therapy is based on the clinical severity of disease and its response to therapy.
- Cigarette smoking, chronic lung disease, and immunosuppression are associated with increased risk for Legionella pneumonia.
- Gastrointestinal symptoms and hyponatremia in a patient with pneumonia should raise the suspicion for *L. pneumophila*.
- Legionnaires' disease can present with a broad spectrum of problems ranging from cough and fever to severe disease with rhabdomyolysis and renal, respiratory, and multiorgan failure.
- The Legionella urinary antigen test is a rapid and highly specific test for *L. pneumophila* serogroup type 1.

REFERENCES

1. Stout JE, Yu VL. Legionellosis. *N Engl J Med* 1997;337:682–687.
2. Zager RA. Rhabdomyolysis and myohemoglobinuric acute renal failure. *Kidney Int* 1996;49:314–326.
3. Knochel JP. Mechanisms of rhabdomyolysis. *Curr Opin Rheumatol* 1993;5:725–731.

4. Shah A, Check F, Baskin S, Reyman T, Menard R. Legionnaires' disease and acute renal failure: case report and review. *Clin Infect Dis* 1992;14:204–207.

46-YEAR-OLD WOMAN WITH CHRONIC COUGH AND DYSPNEA

A 46-year-old woman presented to the emergency department with a 3-week history of cough, worsening dyspnea, and intermittent hemoptysis. She denied fever or chills, pleuritic chest pain, myalgias, or fatigue. Her symptoms were occasionally worsened by exertion but also occurred at rest. Over the past 2 to 3 years she had experienced similar symptoms and had been treated several times with antibiotics for chronic bronchitis. However, her symptoms never completely resolved and each episode had become progressively worse. She had no serious past medical or surgical illnesses and was on no medication. Family history was unremarkable. She had smoked one-half pack of cigarettes daily for 15 years but had quit 7 years ago. She denied any alcohol or other illicit drug use. She lived at home with her husband and was employed as a secretary.

PHYSICAL EXAMINATION

VITAL SIGNS: Temperature, 98.6°F (36.9°C); pulse, 84; respiration, 18; bp, 110/89 mmHg
GENERAL: Thin woman who did not appear acutely ill
HEENT: Normal
NECK: No lymphadenopathy or thyromegaly
LUNGS: Clear
CARDIAC: Regular rate and rhythm; loud S1 with a normal S2; opening snap heard after S2, no murmurs or rubs appreciated

ABDOMEN: Normoactive bowel sounds; soft, nontender with no hepatosplenomegaly

EXTREMITIES: No edema

INTEGUMENT: Normal

NEUROLOGIC: Cranial nerves intact; deep tendon reflexes 2+; normal strength and sensation throughout

LABORATORY FINDINGS

Complete blood cell count, serum levels of electrolytes, glucose, urea nitrogen, and creatinine, normal; urinalysis, normal; arterial blood gas measurements on room air: pH, 7.4; Pco_2, 38 mmHg; Po_2, 79 mmHg; CO_2, 22 mEq/L; O_2 saturation, 95%; ECG: sinus rhythm, broad P waves in limb lead II and precordial lead V1; chest x-ray shown (Fig. 46-1).

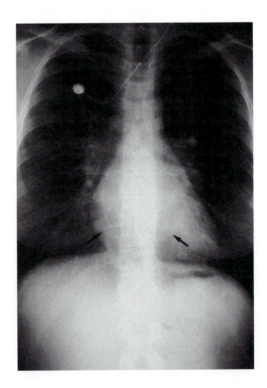

Figure 46-1
PA chest x-ray.

What is the likely diagnosis and how should this patient be treated?

This patient has mitral stenosis. Physical exam revealed an opening snap of mitral stenosis associated with a loud, accentuated first heart sound. The electrocardiogram findings are consistent with left atrial enlargement and the chest x-ray shows the classic finding of left atrial enlargement. As the left atrium enlarges it can often be recognized as a "double density" through the cardiac silhouette (marked by arrows in Fig. 46-1). Subsequent surface echocardiogram confirmed the diagnosis.

Mitral stenosis develops when scarring or other pathologic processes obstruct flow through the mitral valve, eventually leading to left atrial enlargement, episodic pulmonary edema, pulmonary hypertension, and right heart failure. Rheumatic heart disease is still the most common cause of mitral stenosis. Rare causes are congenital mitral stenosis causing a parachute mitral valve deformity, atrial myxoma, thrombus, vegetations, and calcification of the annulus and leaflets. Calcification, which is often seen in elderly patients, is more common in females and is quite common with chronic renal failure. It usually is not functionally important but can produce stenosis and regurgitation.

In rheumatic mitral stenosis the leaflets are scarred and contracted, leading to thickened leaflets and shortening of the chordae tendineae. This results in a funnel-shaped leaflet structure with the inlet at the level of the atrial floor and the narrow apex in the ventricular cavity. The valve leaflet tissues eventually becomes calcified and fragmented and its surface may become covered with thrombi that commonly occur in the atrial appendage and other areas of the atrium. Calcific or thrombotic material may embolize into the arterial circulation.

In the normal adult the mitral orifice area is approximately 4 to 6 cm^2. A decrease in the orifice area causes left atrial hypertension and a diastolic pressure gradient between the left atrium and the left ventricle. When the orifice area exceeds 2 cm^2, the left atrial pressure and the transvalvular pressure gradient are only minimally elevated, and the patient is usually asymptomatic. By contrast, an orifice area of 1 cm^2 is usually associated with a significant pressure gradient across the valve and a pressure overload of the left atrium, pulmonary vasculature, and right ventricle. Although a decrease in the valve area is primarily responsible for left atrial hypertension, the hemodynamics of mitral stenosis are critically dependent on cardiac output and the heart rate. As the heart rate increases, the diastolic filling period decreases and the transvalvular pressure gradient rises. Dynamic exercise, by increasing the transvalvular flow *and* reducing the diastolic filling period, can produce a marked elevation of the left atrial pressure. The development of atrial fibrillation with a rapid ventricular response is thus generally associated with an increase in left atrial pressure and symptoms of pulmonary venous hypertension that can be dramatically improved with reduction of the ventricular rate.

Chronic elevation of left atrial pressure causes structural and functional alterations in the pulmonary vasculature that eventually lead to reduced lung compliance, which increases the work of breathing and causes dyspnea at rest even when the heart rate is well controlled. Hyperplasia and hypertrophy of pulmonary vessels in concert with passive transmission of the increased pulmonary venous pressure to the pulmonary artery and pulmonary vasoconstriction leads to pulmonary hypertension. Because these changes can be reversible, pulmonary hypertension largely resolves following corrective surgery. By contrast, pulmonary hypertension owing to *in situ* thrombosis, chronic pulmonary embolism, or other obliterative changes in the pulmonary vasculature tend to be irreversible.

Accordingly, mitral stenosis causes a variety of changes in right and left ventricular function. Early in the course of the disease, right ventricular function may remain normal, even in the presence of moderate pulmonary hypertension, but eventually the excess afterload on the right ventricle and its decreased contractility lead to right heart failure. At this stage functional tricuspid regurgitation is generally present. Left ventricular size and function remain normal in most patients with pure mitral stenosis, but scarring and thickening of the mitral valve apparatus can produce a regional dysfunction and a decline in the ejection fraction (EF). An overloaded right ventricle may also influence left ventricular size and function and this ventricular interaction is modulated by the pericardium, especially when right heart pressures are elevated.

Most patients with rheumatic mitral stenosis do not recall an episode of acute rheumatic fever. The most frequent and prominent presenting complaint is dyspnea. Conditions that suddenly increase cardiac output and transmitral flow such as physical exertion or fever, emotional upset, and pregnancy can elevate the left atrial and pulmonary venous pressures and produce acute dyspnea or even pulmonary edema. With atrial fibrillation, the loss of atrial contraction and especially the rapid ventricular response that accompany it contribute to dyspnea, palpitations, and fatigue. Hemoptysis, which can occasionally be massive, usually consists merely of pink or blood-tinged sputum caused by pulmonary edema and rupture of capillaries or other thin-walled vessels. Chest pain may be related to pulmonary hypertension and right ventricular ischemia in the absence of coronary disease or thromboemboli. Hoarseness may result from left atrial enlargement that compresses the recurrent laryngeal nerve.

The typical auscultatory findings of mitral stenosis are an accentuated first heart sound, a mitral opening snap, and a low-frequency diastolic murmur (rumble) best heard at the cardiac apex. Although early in its course the apical murmur may not be detected, with more advanced disease its vibrations at the cardiac apex and the first heart sound may be palpable. This is often accompanied by a palpable right ventricular lift—a sign of pulmonary hypertension—along the left sternal border and the patient may display *mitral facies* with a malar flush and peripheral cyanosis. Accentuation of the first heart sound is owing to abrupt cessation of the upward motion of the mitral valve that has been depressed in the left ventricular chamber during diastole. The mobility of the valve leaflets, the diastolic gradient across the valve, and the contractile state of the left ventricle all contribute to the intensity of the first heart sound. The first heart sound diminishes in intensity when mitral valve mobility is restricted by leaflet calcification or when mitral regurgitation is present.

The opening snap is perhaps the most important physical sign of mitral stenosis. It is produced during maximum excursion of the anterior leaflet of the mitral valve. The opening snap occurs 0.03 to 0.14 seconds after the second heart sound. The higher the left atrial pressure the shorter the interval between aortic closure and the opening snap. Opening snaps, however, are not specific for mitral stenosis. They may also be heard in patients with mitral regurgitation, ventricular septal defects, second- and third-degree heart block, tricuspid atresia with a large atrial septal defect, and tetralogy of Fallot after a Blalock-Taussig procedure. Finally, a tricuspid origin should be considered in the differential diagnosis of an opening snap, since these sounds can be generated by the tricuspid valve in tricuspid stenosis, atrial septal defects, or Ebstein's anomaly.

A diastolic rumble may be difficult to detect during the early stages of the disease or may be diminished in the late stage when mitral valve flow decreases. The murmur is low-pitched, best heard with the bell of the stethoscope and becomes accentuated in the latter phase of diastole with atrial contraction. The diastolic murmur may be localized to a small area of the apex and become audible only after the patient exercises. The intensity of the murmur does not necessarily relate to the severity of the mitral stenosis, but severe impairment is suggested by a rumble starting with the opening snap and continuing to the first heart sound. The rumble may diminish or disappear in the late stages of the disease when the cardiac output declines.

The characteristic electrocardiographic finding in mitral stenosis is the broad, notched P wave that is most prominent in lead II and has a negative terminal deflection in lead V1. When pulmonary hypertension develops, a rightward deviation of the mean QRS vector may reflect right ventricular hypertrophy. The radiographic changes of mitral stenosis are produced by left atrial hypertension, which results in left atrial enlargement, alterations in the pulmonary venous pattern, prominence of the pulmonary arteries, and right ventricular enlargement. Since the left atrial appendage occupies a position between the pulmonary artery and the left ventricle, left atrial enlargement appears as a straightening of the left cardiac border on the standard posteroanterior chest film. The left atrium enlarges to the right of the spine and can often be recognized as a larger than normal *double density* through the cardiac silhouette on chest film. The large left atrium may also elevate the left main-stem bronchus on chest film.

Echocardiography is the most useful and reliable noninvasive technique for the detection and evaluation of mitral stenosis. Two-dimensional echocardiography reveals a typical doming and restriction of leaflet motion. The orifice size can be visualized and measured, the extent of disease can be assessed, and an echocardiographic score can be used to select patients for corrective surgery. Doppler echocardiography can be used to evaluate the diastolic pressure gradient and to calculate the mitral valve area. Cardiac catheterization can also be used to determine the pressure gradient across the mitral valve, provide data for calculation of the valve area, measure pulmonary artery pressure, identify other valvular lesions, assess ventricular function, and define anatomy of the coronary arteries prior to corrective surgery.

The prognosis of patients with mitral stenosis depends on the stage of the disease and the severity of symptoms. Rheumatic fever remains the most common cause. The average age at the time of the initial attack is 12 years, but a latent period of about 19 years intervenes before the murmur of mitral stenosis is heard. Cardiac symptoms generally develop in the fourth or fifth decade. Atrial fibrillation, which occurs in at least half the patients with mitral stenosis, may cause systemic embolization, a serious complication with morbid sequelae. Bacterial endocarditis is rare in pure mitral stenosis, but persistent fever, especially in the presence of anemia or other systemic findings, should suggest this diagnosis.

Medical management cannot reduce the mechanical obstruction. Therapy is directed at preventing recurrent rheumatic fever and bacterial endocarditis, and correcting some of the consequences of the obstruction, particularly atrial fibrillation. Digitalis, beta-adrenergic blocking drugs, and calcium antagonists have all been used either alone or in combination to control the ventricular rate in atrial fibrillation. When atrial fibrillation is chronic, no agent is likely to restore sinus rhythm once the left atrial size has reached a critical value and chronic anticoagulation must be instituted.

Percutaneous transvenous valvotomy (catheter balloon valvotomy [CBV]) employs balloon catheters that can be advanced across the atrial septum and across the stenotic mitral valve to enlarge its orifice area. First used for pulmonic stenosis, this procedure has been applied to all four native valves as well as bioprosthetic valves. CBV may be the treatment of choice for many patients with rheumatic mitral stenosis, but the relative merits of CBV versus surgical correction must be considered for each patient. The mechanism providing relief of the stenosis is a simple separation of the fused commissures similar to that produced by closed surgical mitral commissurotomy. Long-term results of this procedure are under study.

The decision to perform open surgical reconstruction (i.e., valvuloplasty) versus a replacement procedure is often made at the time of surgery. A valve without calcification and with adequate subvalvular structures and with fibrosis at both commissures is ideal for conservative reconstruction. Valve replacement is necessary if the leaflets are immobile, heavily calcified, or associated with severe subvalvular scarring, but reconstruction of the valve may be possible when it is partially calcified and can be debrided. The technique of mitral valve replacement has changed considerably over the years and now more hemodynamically efficient low-profile prosthetic valves and bioprosthetic valves are used. A prosthetic valve is generally used if chronic atrial fibrillation that is refractory to cardioversion is present since anticoagulation required for this arrhythmia obviates the advantages of porcine or pericardial valves. Biologic prosthetic valves should be considered when valve replacement is required in women of childbearing age or in the older patient in sinus rhythm because it may be possible to avoid long-term anticoagulation.

Our patient underwent further evaluation by echocardiography and cardiac catheterization. Her mitral valve area was 0.9 cm^2 with a peak transvalvular gradient of 45 mmHg. She underwent surgical correction of her mitral stenosis with placement of a prosthetic mitral valve and recovered uneventfully. Her symptoms improved and she was discharged home.

 # CLINICAL PEARLS

- An accentuated first heart sound, a mitral opening snap, and a low-pitched diastolic rumble are the classic auscultatory findings of mitral stenosis.
- The "double density" sign on chest x-ray can be seen in mitral stenosis and is caused by left atrial enlargement.
- Rheumatic heart disease is the most common cause of mitral stenosis, although most patients do not recall having acute rheumatic fever.
- A mitral valve area of 1 cm^2 or less is usually associated with a significant pressure gradient across the valve, pressure overload of the left atrium, and symptoms of mitral stenosis.
- The loss of atrial contraction, and especially the rapid ventricular response with atrial fibrillation, can cause clinical deterioration in those with mitral stenosis.
- Echocardiography is the most reliable and noninvasive way to detect and evaluate mitral stenosis.
- Medical management of mitral stenosis is directed at preventing its consequences (atrial fibrillation), whereas surgical management is directed at correcting the mechanical obstruction.

REFERENCES

1. Guidelines for the management of patients with valvular heart disease. Executive Summary, ACC/AHA Practice Guidelines. *Circulation* 1998;98:1949–1984.
2. Lawrie GM. Mitral valve repair vs. replacement: Current recommendations and long-term results. *Cardiol Clin* 1998;16(3):437–448.
3. Bruce CJ, Nishimura RA. Newer advances in the diagnosis and treatment of mitral stenosis. *Curr Prob Cardiol* 1998;23(3):125–192.

4. BenFarhat M, Ayari M, Maatouk F. Percutaneous balloon vs. surgi-
    cal closed and open mitral commissurotomy: Seven-year follow-up
    results of a randomized trial. *Circulation* 1998;97(3):245–250.
5. Gaasch WH, O'Rourke RA, Cohn LH, Rackley CE. Mitral valve
    disease, in *Hurst's The Heart*, 8th ed. Schlant RC, Alexander RW
    (eds). McGraw-Hill, New York 1994; pp. 1483–1491.

81-YEAR-OLD WOMAN
WITH INDIGESTION

An 81-year-old woman was admitted to the hospital with a 3-hour history of severe indigestion, which she described as a substernal and epigastric burning that started without provocation. She had some initial relief with antacids, but over the past hour the discomfort had worsened. She denied diaphoresis, palpitations, dizziness, or lightheadedness, but was dyspneic. Her past medical history was significant for essential hypertension but diltiazem was the only medication that she took regularly. There was a family history of hypertension, coronary artery disease, and type II diabetes mellitus. Her social history was positive for smoking one-half pack of cigarettes daily for many years, but she denied any alcohol use. She lived at home with her husband and had no recent ill contacts.

PHYSICAL EXAMINATION

VITAL SIGNS: Temperature, 99.5°F (37.4°C); pulse, 120; respiration, 18; bp, 162/91 mmHg
GENERAL: Somewhat anxious appearing, occasionally taking deep breaths
HEENT: Normal
NECK: No lymphadenopathy or thyromegaly
LUNGS: Scant bi-basilar crackles, otherwise clear
CARDIAC: Tachycardic and regular; S4 gallop, no murmurs or rubs
ABDOMEN: Soft, nontender, normoactive bowel sounds
EXTREMITIES: No clubbing, cyanosis, or edema; 2+ pulses throughout
NEUROLOGIC: Deep tendon reflexes 2+; normal strength and sensation throughout

LABORATORY FINDINGS

WBC, 10.1 K/μL (normal differential); Hb, 13.2 g/dL; platelets, 272 K/μL; electrolytes, glucose, urea nitrogen, creatinine, normal; initial creatine kinase, 210 U/L with CK-MB fraction of 4.5 ng/mL; arterial blood gas measurements on room air: pH, 7.41; P_{CO_2}, 36 mmHg; P_{O_2}, 75 mmHg; CO_2, 24 mEq/L; O_2 saturation, 94%; chest x-ray, unremarkable; ECG: shown in Figure 47-1.

What is the likely diagnosis and how should this patient be treated?

This patient is having an acute myocardial infarction (MI). The patient's history is of concern, suggesting an acute coronary ischemic event. Although the initial set of cardiac enzymes was not diagnostic, her ECG clearly shows a posterior myocardial infarction. The ECG changes of posterior myocardial infarction can be subtle, making this the most com-

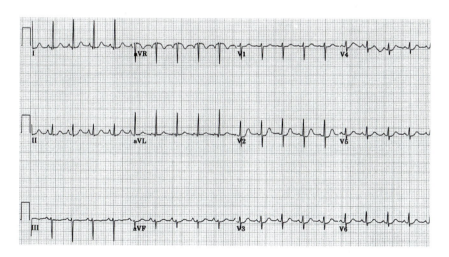

Figure 47-1
Patient's initial electrocardiogram.

monly missed MI. The ECG shown in Figure 47-1 has ST-segment depression throughout the precordial leads that is most pronounced in leads V2 and V3, which may represent either anteroseptal myocardial ischemia or posterior myocardial injury. In V1, V2, and V3 the upright T waves associated with ST-segment depression are diagnostic of posterior myocardial injury. Also, the R to S ratio of the QRS complex in V2 is greater than 1—a finding indicating loss of posterior forces (myocardium)—which is especially apparent on the second ECG that was done after the patient had been treated and her heart rate was slower (Fig. 47-2).

Each year 900,000 people in the United States experience an acute MI. Of these, about 225,000 die, mainly of arrhythmias, including 125,000 who die "in the field" before obtaining medical care. Because early reperfusion improves left ventricular (LV) systolic function and survival with MI, every effort must be made to minimize the prehospital delay. There are ongoing public efforts to promote rapid identification and treatment of patients with acute MI, including patient education about the symptoms of acute MI along with appropriate actions to take, and the dispensation of prompt care by emergency medical squads. In treating the patient with chest pain, emergency medical personnel must act with a sense of urgency.

When the patient with a suspected acute MI reaches the hospital emergency department (ED), the initial evaluation and management should

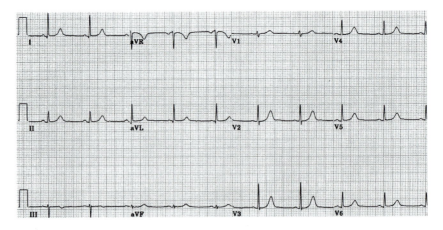

Figure 47-2
Patient's electrocardiogram after treatment.

take place promptly, because the benefit of myocardial reperfusion is greatest if it is initiated early. The initial evaluation ideally should be completed within 10 minutes of arrival in the ED, and certainly not more than 20 minutes should elapse before this is done. The patient should immediately receive (1) oxygen by nasal cannula; (2) sublingual nitroglycerin (unless systolic arterial pressure is <90 mmHg or heart rate is <50 or >100); (3) adequate analgesia (with morphine sulfate or meperidine); and (4) aspirin, 325 mg orally. A 12-lead ECG should be performed. ST-segment elevation of 1 mV or more in contiguous leads on the ECG is strong evidence of thrombotic coronary arterial occlusion, making the patient a candidate for immediate reperfusion therapy either by fibrinolysis or primary percutaneous transluminal coronary angioplasty (PTCA). Symptoms of acute MI associated with a left bundle branch block (LBBB) should be managed as though ST-segment elevations were present. In sharp contrast, the patient *without* ST-segment elevation should receive neither thrombolytic therapy nor primary PTCA because in this case the benefit of such therapy remains uncertain.

In comparison with standard medical therapy, thrombolytic therapy exerts a highly significant 21 percent reduction in 35-day mortality among patients with acute MI and ST elevation, corresponding to 21 lives saved per 1000 patients treated. A powerful impact on mortality—which is a time-dependent effect—has been observed with the administration of thrombolytic agents. The greatest benefit occurs when thrombolysis is initiated within 6 hours of the onset of symptoms, although a definite benefit occurs if it is begun within 12 hours. For example, of the total lives per 1000 saved with thrombolytic therapy, an estimated 35 per 1000 are saved when it is used within the first hour of symptoms compared with 16 saved lives per 1000 when it is given 7 to 12 hours after the onset of symptoms. Thrombolysis given under the proper circumstances benefits all patients, albeit at different rates, regardless of age, gender, or the presence of comorbid conditions such as diabetes mellitus, although there is slight risk of intracranial hemorrhage that usually occurs within the first day of therapy. Variables that predict an increased risk of intracranial hemorrhage are age greater than 65 years, body weight less than 70 kg, systemic arterial hypertension, and the administration of tissue plasminogen activator (tPA).

Primary PTCA is an alternative to thrombolytic therapy, providing it is done in a timely fashion by skilled persons and prompt access to emergency coronary artery bypass graft (CABG) surgery is available.

The patient must be hospitalized when reperfusion therapy is initiated. However, the subsequent short- and long-term management are similar, regardless of the initial ECG and whether or not thrombolytic therapy is given. Once hospitalized, the patient's ECG should be continuously monitored and the diagnosis of MI should be confirmed by serial ECG studies and serum markers of cardiac myocyte necrosis, such as creatine kinase isoenzymes or cardiac specific troponin T or I. The patient should be monitored closely for adverse electrical or mechanical cardiac events, especially within the first 24 hours, when reinfarction and death are most apt to occur. The patient's physical activities should be limited for at least 24 hours, when pain and anxiety should be minimized with appropriate analgesics. Although the use of prophylactic antiarrhythmic agents is not recommended, atropine, lidocaine, transcutaneous pacing patches, or a transvenous pacemaker, a defibrillator, and epinephrine should be immediately available.

Patients who survive a large anterior MI or have a LV mural thrombus (which may be seen on echocardiography) are at high risk of having an embolic stroke, a risk that may be reduced by early administration of intravenous heparin. For those without a large anterior MI or LV thrombus and those who did not receive reperfusion therapy, heparin provides no therapeutic benefit beyond those achieved with aspirin, β-adrenoceptor blocking agents, nitrates, and angiotensin-converting enzyme (ACE) inhibitors. The recommendation for heparin administration after thrombolytic therapy is based more on current practice than on evidence and depends on the specific thrombolytic agent. For example, only limited evidence exist for a beneficial effect of heparin following the use of nonspecific fibrinolytic agents such as streptokinase, anisoylated plasminogen streptokinase activator complex (APSAC), or urokinase. However, when tPA (alteplase) is administered, intravenous heparin is more likely to maintain the patency of an infarct-related vessel, although the clinical outcome may not necessarily be improved. Considering the superior performance of accelerated tPA plus intravenous heparin in the Global Utilization of Streptokinase and TPA for Occluded Arteries (GUSTO) trial, it seems judicious to give heparin intravenously for at least 48 hours after tPA has been given. Newer thrombolytic agents that can be given in bolus fashion (Reteplase [rPA], Lanoteplase [nPA], TNK-tissue plasminogen activator [TNK-tPA]) are actively under investigation with and without concurrent heparin administration.

There is clear evidence that aspirin, 160 to 325 mg daily, should be given to patients with MI and continued indefinitely. Antiplatelet agents are actively under investigation in the treatment of acute coronary syndromes. Antiplatelet agents similar to aspirin (ticlopidine and clopidogrel) as well as platelet receptor blockers (glycoprotein IIb/IIIa receptor blockers) may be particularly efficacious if occlusive thrombus is the main problem. Clinical trials of intravenous as well as oral glycoprotein IIb/IIIa inhibitors are under investigation. The major concern with these agents is bleeding, particularly in patients who are already receiving heparin and aspirin. The precise combination of these agents in the treatment of acute coronary syndromes is yet to be elucidated.

Despite the absence of definitive outcome data, it is reasonable to treat the patient with acute MI—who does not have hypotension, bradycardia, or excessive tachycardia—with intravenous nitroglycerin for 24 to 48 hours after hospitalization. Concern exists about the use of oral nitrate preparations because the dose cannot be titrated in an acutely evolving hemodynamic situation, whereas intravenous infusion can be titrated against frequent measurements of the heart rate and blood pressure. Nitroglycerin should not be used as a substitute for narcotic analgesia.

The patient with an evolving acute MI should promptly receive intravenous β_2-adrenergic blocker therapy, followed by oral therapy, provided that there is no contraindication, regardless of whether reperfusion therapy was given. Several studies in both the prethrombolytic and thrombolytic eras show that β_2-adrenergic blockers diminish morbidity and mortality, whereas calcium channel blockers do not reduce mortality and in certain cases may be harmful. Diltiazem may reduce the incidence of recurrent ischemic events in the patient without ST-segment elevation or LBBB in whom pulmonary congestion is absent, but its benefit beyond that of β_2-adrenergic blockers and aspirin is unclear. Immediate-release dihydropyridine (nifedipine) is contraindicated in the patient with acute MI.

In the patient with an evolving acute MI with ST-segment elevation or LBBB, an ACE inhibitor should be given within hours of hospitalization, provided that the patient does not have hypotension or a contraindication to the drug, and it may be discontinued after 6 weeks. However, it should be continued indefinitely with impaired LV systolic function (ejection fraction <40%) or clinical congestive heart failure.

After the first day in the hospital, the patient with an acute MI should continue aspirin and an β_2-adrenergic blocker indefinitely. Nitroglycerin should be infused intravenously for 24 to 48 hours. Heparin may be continued, depending on the type of reperfusion strategy used. Patients with myocardial ischemia after an acute MI, regardless of whether thrombolytic therapy was given, should undergo elective angiographic evaluation with percutaneous or surgical revascularization as necessary. There is a paucity of data and considerable variability in the use of coronary angiography and catheter-based interventions among survivors of uncomplicated acute MI with preserved LV systolic function. However, studies demonstrate a survival benefit among patients with decreased LV systolic function treated with surgical revascularization.

The patient should be closely observed for complications of an acute MI. Recurrent chest pain in the first few days might be a symptom of myocardial ischemia or post-MI pericarditis. Congestive heart failure may result from a large MI with loss of LV systolic function that elevates the left ventricular filling pressure or it may be owing to acute mitral valve insufficiency from ischemia or a ruptured papillary muscle. Ventricular septal defect and cardiac rupture can also occur during this time. Cardiogenic shock may require management by intra-aortic balloon pump (IABP) and prompt PTCA or CABG. Right ventricular infarction should be treated vigorously with intravascular volume expansion and inotropic agents if hypotension develops. Cardiac arrhythmias (atrial, ventricular, heart block) can all occur, depending on the site of the MI, and may require treatment with antiarrhythmics or cardiac pacing.

Before hospital discharge or shortly thereafter, the patient with recent acute MI should undergo standard exercise testing (submaximal at 4–7 days or symptom limited at 10–14 days). This is done to (1) assess the patient's functional capacity and ability to perform tasks at home and work; (2) evaluate the efficacy of the patient's current medical regimen; and (3) stratify risk for a subsequent cardiac event. Although markers of electrical instability such as abnormal baroreflex stimulation or the presence of late potentials on a signal-averaged ECG are associated with increased risk of death, their positive predictive value is low and the appropriate therapy when these findings are observed is uncertain.

The patient should take aspirin, a β_2-adrenergic blocker and, in some cases, an ACE inhibitor for an indefinite period after an acute MI. The patient should be instructed to achieve an ideal weight and educated about a diet low in saturated fat and cholesterol. Drug therapy should be given, if needed, to lower LDL cholesterol to less than 100 mg/dL. Smoking cessation is essential. Finally, the patient should be encouraged to participate in a formal rehabilitation program and ultimately to engage in 20 minutes of exercise at least three times a week.

Our patient had an acute posterior MI that was treated with thrombolytic therapy, aspirin, β_2-adrenergic blockade, intravenous heparin, and nitroglycerin that resulted in resolution of her discomfort and ECG changes. Cardiac catheterization revealed a high-grade right coronary artery lesion that was treated with PTCA and intracoronary stent placement. She recovered uneventfully from her MI and was discharged home taking aspirin, β_2-adrenergic blockade, an ACE inhibitor, and oral nitrates. A stress test was planned as an outpatient for further stratification.

 ## CLINICAL PEARLS

- Myocardial infarction (MI) affects nearly 1 million people each year, and 25 percent die from it.
- Early use of reperfusion therapy is the most important factor in survival with MI.
- Suspicion of an acute MI should be high in all patients with chest pain, even when serum markers are negative and ECG changes are subtle.
- Thrombolytic therapy confers the greatest survival advantage if given within 6 hours of the onset of symptoms, but is beneficial up to 12 hours.
- Most complications following MI occur within the first 24 to 72 hours.
- Oxygen, aspirin, β_2-adrenergic blockers, and intravenous nitrates (often with intravenous heparin) should be given to all patients with MI.
- Standard exercise testing should be done for further risk stratification after MI, either submaximal testing at 4 to 7 days or symptom-limited at 10 to 14 days.
- All MI patients should be discharged from the hospital on aspirin, β-adrenergic blockade, and an ACE inhibitor unless contraindicated.

REFERENCES

1. Ross AM. New plasminogen activators: A clinical review. *Clin Cardiol* 1999;22:165–171.
2. Ross R. Atherosclerosis—An inflammatory disease. *N Engl J Med* 1999;340(2):115–126.

3. Savonitto S, Ardissino D, Granger CB, et al. Prognostic value of the admission electrocardiogram in acute coronary syndromes. *JAMA* 1999;281(8):707–713.

4. Kullo IJ, Edwards WD, Schwartz RS. Vulnerable plaque: Pathobiology and clinical implications. *Ann Intern Med* 1998;129:1050–1060.

5. Ryan TJ, Anderson JL, Antman EM, et al. ACC/AHA guidelines for the management of patients with acute myocardial infarction: Executive summary. *Circulation* 1996;94:2341–2350.

16-YEAR-OLD BOY WITH HEMATURIA AND JOINT PAIN

A 16-year-old high school student was admitted to the hospital with a 4-day history of bilateral hip pain, severe right knee pain, and dark urine for 2 days, which began after his knees struck the dashboard during a motor vehicle accident. Over the past 4 days his joint symptoms had worsened to the point of immobility and 2 days ago he began noticing dark urine that he described as Coca-Cola colored without dysuria. He had experienced similar symptoms in the past with minor trauma, but they had resolved spontaneously except for persistent knee pain that he attributed to his sport activities. He denied other significant past medical history and had never undergone surgery or invasive dental procedures. He was taking no medication at the time of admission. There was a family history of some type of bleeding problem, but he was unaware of the specific details. Social history was negative for alcohol or tobacco use.

PHYSICAL EXAMINATION

VITAL SIGNS: Temperature. 98.6°F (36.9°C); pulse, 88; respiration, 16; bp, 110/70 mmHg
GENERAL: Thin male who did not appear acutely ill
HEENT: Normal
NECK: No lymphadenopathy or thyromegaly
LUNGS: Clear
CARDIAC: Regular rate and rhythm without murmurs, rubs, or gallops
ABDOMEN: Normoactive bowel sounds; soft, nontender with no hepatosplenomegaly

EXTREMITIES: Pain on abduction and adduction of the hips; right knee warm, slightly swollen, ecchymotic, painful on palpation and with flexion and extension
INTEGUMENT: Normal
NEUROLOGIC: Cranial nerves intact; deep tendon reflexes 2+; normal strength and sensation throughout

LABORATORY FINDINGS

WBC, 10.2 K/μL (normal differential); Hb, 10.7 g/dL; MCV, 88 fl; platelets, 200 K/μL; electrolytes: sodium, 138 mEq/L; potassium, 3.8 mEq/L; chloride, 102 mEq/L; bicarbonate, 24 mEq/L; urea nitrogen, 20 mg/dL; creatinine, 1.4 mg/dL; glucose, 90 mg/dL; prothrombin time (PT), 12 seconds; INR, 1.1; partial thromboplastin time (PTT), 58 seconds (range 20–34 seconds); urinalysis, pH, 8.0; positive for hemoglobin; urine sediment, unremarkable;. Westergren sedimentation rate, 45 mm/h; bilateral hip x-rays, unremarkable; right knee x-rays, decreased joint space at the margins of the joint, small punched-out area of cavitation involving medial femoral condyle.

What is the likely diagnosis and how should this patient be treated?

This patient has factor VIII deficiency or hemophilia A. The history and physical examination are consistent with a plasma coagulation defect causing bleeding into the joint spaces after trauma. His knee x-rays and chronic knee pain and the history of a familial bleeding problem all suggest a congenital coagulation defect.

Patients with congenital plasma coagulation defects characteristically bleed into muscles, joints, and body cavities hours or days after an injury. Most of the *inherited* plasma coagulation disorders are owing to defects in single coagulation proteins. Two X-linked disorders—factors VIII and IX deficiencies—account for the majority of the congenital coagulation disorders. Familial clotting disorders usually prolong either the prothrombin time (PT) or the partial thromboplastin time (PTT), although both may be prolonged. If either is abnormal, quantitative assays of specific coagulation proteins are done using plasma from congenitally deficient individuals as substrate in the PT or PTT. The corrective effect of varying concentrations of patient plasma is measured and expressed as a percentage of normal pooled plasma standard. The interval range for most coagulation factors is from 50 to 150 percent of this average value, although the minimal level needed for adequate hemostasis is 25 percent for most clotting factors.

The antihemophilic factor (AHF) or factor VIII coagulant protein is a large single-chain protein that regulates the activation of factor X by proteases generated in the intrinsic coagulation pathway. Factor VIII is synthesized in liver parenchymal cells and circulates complexed to the von Willebrand protein (vWF). Cloning and sequencing of complementary DNA (cDNA) encoding the factor VIII molecule and mapping its gene on the X chromosome have given a detailed picture of its structure and location, providing improved methods for the detection of asymptomatic carriers and the prenatal diagnosis of hemophilia A.

The genetics of hemophilia A, which is the classic example of an X-linked recessive trait, have been studied intensively. The defective recessive gene located on the X chromosome manifests clinical hemophilia in males who lack a normal allele, but not in females who have a normal allele on the other X chromosome. An affected male does not transmit the disorder to his sons because his Y chromosome is normal, but all his daughters are carriers of the trait because they inherit their father's X chromosome. A female carrier who has a normal X allele from her mother is clinically unaffected but transmits the disorder to half of her sons and the carrier state to half of her daughters. The clinical severity of bleeding—the expression of the genetic defect—varies among kindreds but is relatively constant within kindreds.

Molecular studies have failed to demonstrate a uniform genetic abnormality in hemophilia A, which instead is comprised of deletions, insertions, and mutations throughout the factor VIII gene. However, about 40 percent of severe hemophilia A cases result from a major inversion of the tip of the long arm of the X chromosome, which permits accurate genetic testing of individuals in affected kindreds.

The regularity with which the abnormal gene is suppressed by the normal allele in female carriers of hemophilia varies because of the phenomenon of random X-chromosome inactivation. Although the mean concentration of factor VIII in the plasma of heterozygous female carriers is approximately 50 percent of that in normal women, observed values scatter widely around this mean and often overlap with those found in the normal population. This is a result, in part, of the large error of assay methods and the wide range of factor VIII levels in normal subjects. Although subnormal factor VIII levels strongly suggest a carrier state, the converse—normal levels—do not exclude it. Detecting carriers has been greatly improved by measuring their vWF factor levels by immunoassay—which are normal or increased even when the factor VIII deficiency is mild—and calculating the ratio of VIII to vWF; which separates hemophilia A carriers (0.18:0.9) from normals (0.74:2.2). Testing several serum samples from the same woman improves the accuracy of detecting carriers and may be essential in some cases. Polymorphic DNA probes are capable of detecting 90 percent of affected families and over 96 percent of the carriers, and their use also has been adapted to prenatal diagnosis.

One in 10,000 males is born with a deficiency or dysfunction of factor VIII. This causes hemophilia A, a disorder characterized by bleeding into soft tissues, muscles, and weight-bearing joints. Although normal hemostasis requires factor VIII levels of at least 25 percent, they are usually below 5 percent in symptomatic hemophiliacs and closely correlate with the clinical severity of the disease. Patients with factor VIII activity less than 1 percent have severe disease and bleed frequently without discernible trauma. Those with levels between 1 and 5 percent have moderate disease with less frequent bleeding, whereas patients with levels over 5 percent have mild disease that causes excessive bleeding only with trauma. However, most hemophiliacs have factor VIII levels below 5 percent. Bleeding continues for hours or days after injury if untreated and can involve any organ. The resulting large collections of partially clotted blood exert pressure on adjacent tissues, which may cause muscle necrosis (compartment syndrome), venous congestion (pseudophlebitis), or ischemic nerve damage. Large calcified masses of blood and inflammatory tissue may develop, which are often mistaken for soft tissue sarcomas (pseudotumor syndrome).

Severe hemophilia is usually recognized shortly after birth by extensive cephalhematoma or profuse bleeding after circumcision. However, patients with moderate disease may not bleed until they begin to walk or crawl and mild hemophiliacs may not be diagnosed until adolescence or young adulthood. The hemophiliac typically presents with pain and swelling in one or more weight-bearing joints such as the hip, knee, or ankle. Blood in the joint (hemarthrosis) causes synovial inflammation, and repetitive bleeding erodes the articular cartilage, causing osteoarthritis, articular fibrosis, joint ankylosis, and eventually muscle atrophy. Hematuria, in the absence of any genitourinary pathology, is also common but is usually self-limited and may not require therapy. The most feared complications are oropharyngeal and central nervous system bleeding. The former may require emergency intubation to maintain an adequate airway and the latter may occur without trauma or underlying lesions.

Patients who are suspected of having hemophilia should have a platelet count, bleeding time, PT, and PTT. Typically, the PTT is prolonged and the other tests are normal. Because of the clinical similarity of factor VIII deficiency and factor IX deficiency, any male with a bleeding history and a prolonged PTT should have specific assays for factor VIII and factor IX.

The patient must be alert to early symptoms of bleeding, usually pain, so that treatment can be promptly initiated. Waiting for other signs of bleeding before treating the patient is inappropriate because they may not be apparent for several days after trauma. Early treatment is more effective, less costly, and may be lifesaving. Plasma products enriched in factor VIII have revolutionized treatment, reduced the degree of orthopedic deformity and permitted virtually any form of elective and emergency surgery. However, the widespread use of factor VIII concentrates also has produced serious complications, including viral hepatitis, chronic liver disease, and AIDS.

The standard therapeutic products are cryoprecipitate and factor VIII concentrate. *Cryoprecipitate*, which contains about half the factor VIII activity of fresh frozen plasma in one-tenth the volume, is simple to prepare and is produced in hospital or regional blood banks. It must be stored frozen and is thawed and pooled prior to administration. However, most utilize partially purified *factor VIII concentrate*, which is prepared from multiple donors and supplied as a lyophilized powder that can be refrigerated and reconstituted just prior to use. Recent developments in the preparation of these products and the use of recombinant factor VIII have increased the safety of therapy. Hemophiliacs should receive either monoclonal purified or recombinant factor VIII to minimize viral infections and exposure to other proteins. Each unit of factor VIII infused, defined as the amount present in 1 milliliter of normal plasma, will raise the plasma level of the recipient by 2 percent per kilogram of body weight. Because factor VIII has a half-life of 8 to 12 hours, it must be infused continuously or at least twice daily to sustain the target factor VIII level. With mild disease, desmopressin (DDAVP) is an alternative therapy that transiently increases factor VIII levels two- to threefold.

Uncomplicated soft tissue bleeding or early hemarthrosis can be treated with one infusion of cryoprecipitate or factor VIII concentrate sufficient to raise the factor VIII level to about 15 percent of normal. More extensive hemarthrosis or more complicated bleeding such as retroperitoneal hemorrhage requires twice-daily or continuous infusions in order to keep the factor VIII level between 25 and 50 percent of normal for 72 hours. Life-threatening central nervous system bleeding or major surgery may require therapy that maintains the factor VIII level at a minimum of 50 percent of normal for at least 2 weeks. Prior to surgery, every hemophiliac should be screened for the presence of an inhibitor to factor VIII. Those who do not have an inhibitor should receive factor VIII infusions immediately prior to surgery and require daily monitoring to maintain the factor VIII level above 50 percent of normal for 10 to 14 days after surgery or as long as 3 weeks for major orthopedic surgery. A single infusion of cryoprecipitate or factor VIII concentrate and the administration of 4 to 6 g of E-aminocaproic acid (EACA) four times daily for 72 to 96 hours after a dental procedure is usually appropriate. EACA is a potent antifibrinolytic agent that inhibits plasminogen activators present in oral secretions and stabilizes clot formation in oral tissue. Many centers have home care programs in which patients self-administer factor VIII infusions immediately after the onset of symptoms.

As a result of their frequent use of blood products, most hemophiliacs experience multiple episodes of hepatitis and have elevated hepatocellular enzyme levels and an abnormal liver biopsy. Some develop chronic active or persistent hepatitis or cirrhosis and a few hemophiliacs have undergone liver transplantation, which cures both diseases. Unfortunately, as many as 80 percent of multiply transfused hemophiliacs are HIV-positive and some have clinical AIDS, but advances in factor VIII concentrate technology will hopefully prevent this. Despite frequent bleeding, most of it is internal and severe iron-deficiency anemia is uncommon because iron is effectively recycled.

Following multiple transfusions, between 10 and 20 percent of patients with severe hemophilia develop inhibitors to factor VIII. Usually IgG antibodies, inhibitors rapidly neutralize factor VIII activity and prevent effective transfusion therapy. There are two types of inhibitors. Patients with *type I* inhibitors have a typical anamnestic response that raises their antibody titer after exposure to factor VIII and should not receive factor VIII. In an emergency, they may require plasmapheresis to remove the inhibitor or infusion of prothrombin complex concentrates that contain trace quantities of activated coagulation factors, which can bypass the block in coagulation produced by the inhibitor. Patients with a *type II* inhibitor have a low antibody titer that is not stimulated by factor VIII infusion and may respond to higher than normal doses of factor VIII.

The prognosis in severe hemophilia has improved greatly. With proper treatment using sterile replacement products the crippling sequelae of the disease can be minimized. Our patient had a prolonged PTT and a factor VIII level of 2 percent. The patient was treated with factor VIII concentrate to raise his factor VIII level to approximately 20 percent of normal and slowly improved. Prior to discharge from the hospital, he was educated about his disease, including appropriate prophylaxis and follow-up.

 CLINICAL PEARLS

- Congenital plasma coagulation defects cause bleeding into muscles, joints, and body cavities with or without injury.
- Inherited as defects in single coagulation proteins, most cause factor VIII and IX deficiencies, which are X-linked disorders.
- One in 10,000 males is born with factor VIII deficiency, resulting in hemophilia A.
- Factor VIII levels are usually less than 5 percent of normal in symptomatic hemophilia A.
- Severe hemophilia is usually diagnosed shortly after birth, but when mild may not be apparent until adolescence or young adulthood.
- Treatment of an acute bleeding episode usually consists of factor VIII concentrate infusion to reach the target level of factor VIII activity.
- Up to 20 percent of multiply transfused hemophiliacs develop inhibitors to factor VIII that alter treatment, depending on the type of inhibitor (type I vs. type II).

REFERENCES

1. Sultan S. Acquired hemophilia and its treatment. *Blood Coag Fibrinol* 1997;8(Suppl.1):S15–S18.
2. Mannucci PM. Desmopressin (DDAVP) in the treatment of bleeding disorders: The first 20 years. *Blood* 1997;90(7):2515–2521.
3. Lusher JM. Prophylaxis in children with hemophilia: Is it the optimal treatment?. *Thrombo Hemostas* 1997;78(1):726–729.

4. Rodgers GM, Greenberg CS. Inherited coagulation disorders, in *Wintrobe's Clinical Hematology*, 10th ed. Lee GR, Foerster J, Lukens J. (eds). Baltimore, Lippincott Williams & Wilkins, 1999, 1682–1692.
5. Handin R. Disorders of coagulation and thrombosis, in *Harrison's Principles of Internal Medicine*, 13th ed. Isselbacher KJ, Braunwald E, Wilson JD, et al. (eds). New York, McGraw-Hill, 1994, 1804–1805.

31-YEAR-OLD MAN WITH ABDOMINAL PAIN, ANXIETY, AND DISORIENTATION

A 31-year-old man was admitted to the hospital with a 1- to 2-day history of abdominal pain, nausea, vomiting, and constipation. He described the abdominal pain as crampy in nature and without localization. He denied any recent fever, chills, or diarrhea associated with this abdominal pain. His wife reported that over the preceding 48 hours prior to admission he had developed insomnia, increasing anxiety, disorientation, and what she thought was a visual hallucination. She reported that he had similar episodes in the past; one such episode was associated with seizure activity that required treatment with antiseizure medication. The patient was weak on arrival, requiring a wheelchair to bring him into the emergency department. His past medical history was unremarkable except for previous similar attacks and he was unaware of his family history secondary to being adopted. He denied tobacco use but his wife did admit to a history of alcohol abuse. The patient had been drinking fairly heavily for the week prior to admission with minimal nutritional intake.

PHYSICAL EXAMINATION

VITAL SIGNS: Temperature, 99.6°F (37°C); pulse, 104; respiration, 20; bp, 165/99 mmHg

GENERAL: Thin male who appeared dehydrated, weak, and somewhat malnourished

HEENT: Normal

NECK: No lymphadenopathy or thyromegaly

LUNGS: Clear

CARDIAC: Flat neck veins; tachycardic and regular without murmurs, rubs, or gallops

ABDOMEN: Hypoactive bowel sounds; soft, mild distention, tender to palpation in all quadrants; no hepatosplenomegaly

EXTREMITIES: No clubbing, cyanosis, or peripheral edema

INTEGUMENT: Normal

NEUROLOGIC: Cranial nerves intact; deep tendon reflexes 2+; 3/5 MRC strength in all major muscle groups; normal sensation throughout

LABORATORY FINDINGS

WBC, 8.2 K/μL (normal differential); Hb, 13.6 g/dL; platelets, 330 K/μL; electrolytes: sodium, 127 mEq/L; potassium, 3.6 mEq/L; chloride, 99 mEq/L; bicarbonate, 26 mEq/L; urea nitrogen, 16 mg/dL; creatinine, 1.0 mg/dL; glucose, 90 mg/dL; serum osmolarity, 265 mOsm/L; urinalysis: port-wine color; pH, 8.0; negative for hemoglobin or myoglobin; urine osmolarity, 680 mOsm/L; urine sediment, unremarkable; abdominal x-rays, generalized ileus; ECG, tachycardic, otherwise normal.

What is the likely diagnosis and how should this patient be treated?

This patient has acute intermittent porphyria (AIP). The history and physical exam are one of intermittent episodes of abdominal pain in association with a known trigger (alcohol and lack of nutritional intake); and the laboratory examination revealed hyponatremia and port-wine colored urine—all consistent with AIP.

The porphyrias are inherited or acquired disorders of specific enzymes in the heme biosynthetic pathway. These disorders are classified as either *hepatic* or *erythropoietic*, depending on the primary site of overproduction and accumulation of the porphyrin precursoror or porphyrin, but some have overlapping features (Table 49-1). The major clinical manifestations of the *hepatic porphyrias* are neurologic symptoms, including abdominal

TABLE 49-1   Classification of Porphyrias

Type/ Porphyria	Deficient Enzyme	Photo-sensitivity	Neuro-visceral Symptoms
Heptic Porphyrias			
ALA dehydratase deficiency	ALA dehydratase	−	+
Acute intermittent porphyria (AIP)	HMB synthase	−	+
Hereditary copro-porphyria (HCP)	COPRO oxidase	+	+
Variegate porphyria (VP)	PROTO oxidase	+	+
Porphyria cutanea tarda (PCT)	URO decarboxylase	+	−
Erythropoietic Porphyrias			
X-linked sideroblastic anemia (XLSA)	ALA synthase	−	−
Congenital erythro-poietic porphyria (CEP)	URO synthase	+++	−
Erythropoietic proto-porphyria (EPP)	Ferrochelatase	+	−

ALA = aminolevulinic acid.
HMB = hydroxymethylbilane.
COPRO = coproporphyrin.
PROTO = protoporphyrin.
URO = uroporphyrin.

pain, neuropathy, and mental disturbances, whereas patients with *erythropoietic porphyrias* primarily have cutaneous photosensitivity. The reason for the neurologic involvement in the hepatic porphyrias is poorly understood. Cutaneous sensitivity to sunlight is owing to the fact that excitation of excess porphyrins in the skin by long-wave ultraviolet light leads to cell damage, scarring, and deformation. Steroid hormones, drugs, and nutrition influence the production of porphyrin precursors and porphyrins, thereby precipitating or increasing the severity of some porphyrias.

Many symptoms of the porphyrias are nonspecific, and diagnosis is often delayed. Laboratory testing can confirm or exclude the diagnosis of a porphyria. Table 49-2 summarizes the major metabolites that accumulate in each porphyria. Urinary aminolevulinic acid (ALA) and porphobilinogen (PBG) are easily quantitated and the urinary porphyrin isomers can be separated and quantitated by high-performance liquid chromatography. Fecal porphyrins can also be extracted and analyzed semiquantitatively. Such studies, especially along with symptoms, make it possible to define the diagnostic profile of accumulated precursors or porphyrins in each disorder. However, a definite diagnosis requires demonstration of the specific enzyme deficiency.

Acute intermittent porphyria is a hepatic porphyria inherited as an autosomal dominant condition resulting from partial deficiency of porphobilinogen deaminase (also known as hydroxymethylbilane [HMB] synthase), activity. The disease is widespread but more common in Scandinavia and perhaps Great Britain. The enzyme deficiency can be demonstrated in most heterozygous individuals, but clinical expression of this porphyria is highly variable. Activation of the disease is related to ecogenic factors, such as drugs, diet, and steroid hormones, which can precipitate the disease manifestations. Attacks can be prevented by avoiding known precipitating factors. Most heterozygotes remain clinically asymptomatic (latent) unless exposed to factors that increase the production of porphyrins. Endogenous and exogenous gonadal steroids, porphyrinogenic drugs, and a low-calorie diet are the most common precipitating factors (Table 49-3).

Clinical features of AIP include those mentioned in the preceding with the exception of cutaneous photosensitivity. Signs and symptoms of AIP are entirely systemic, and they may reflect some or many of a wide array of episodic or chronic dysfunctions of the peripheral or central nervous systems. The most common of these complaints is episodic abdominal pain of sufficient severity to mimic causes of an acute surgical abdomen. Nausea and vomiting, constipation, hypertension, and tachycardia often accompany the abdominal pain. Abdominal pain is usually steady and poorly localized but may be cramping in nature. Ileus, abdominal distention, and decreased bowel sounds are common. At such times, the content of porphobilin, an autooxidation product of porphobilinogen, and

TABLE 49-2   MAJOR METABOLITES ACCUMULATED
IN PORPHYRIAS

Type/ Porphyria	Increased Erythrocyte Porphyrins	Porphyrin Excretion	
		Urine	Stool
Hepatic Porphyrias			
ALA dehydratase deficiency	—	ALA, COPRO III	—
Acute intermittent porphyria (AIP)	—	ALA, PBG	—
Hereditary copro- porphyria (HCP)	—	ALA, PBG, COPRO III	COPRO III
Variegate porphyria (VP)	—	ALA, PBG, COPRO III	COPRO III, PROTO IX
Porphyria cutanea tarda (PCT)	—	URO I	ISOCO PRO
Erythropoietic Porphyrias			
X-linked sideroblastic anemia (XLSA)	—	—	—
Congenital erythro- poietic porphyria (CEP)	URO I	URO I	COPRO I
Erythropoietic proto- porphyria (EPP)	PROTO IX	—	PROTO IX

ALA = aminolevulinic acid.
PBG = porphobilinogen.
COPRO I = coproporphyrin I.
COPRO III = coproporphyrin III.
PROTO IX = protoporphyrin IX.
URO I = uroporphyrin I.
ISOCOPRO = isocoproporphyrin.

TABLE 49-3   CATEGORIES OF UNSAFE AND SAFE DRUGS
IN AIP, HCP, AND VP

UNSAFE	SAFE
Barbiturates	Narcotic analgesics
Sulfonamide antibiotics	Aspirin
Meprobamate	Acetaminophen
Glutethimide	Phenothiazines
Methyprylon	Penicillin and derivatives
Succinimides	Streptomycin
Carbamazepine	Glucocorticoids
Phenytoin	Bromides
Valproic acid	Insulin
Pyrazolones	Atropine
Griseofulvin	
Ergots	
Synthetic estrogens and progestogens	
Danazol	
Alcohol	

oxidized porphyrin by-products of the heme synthetic pathway become sufficiently abnormal to tint the urine a *port-wine* color. Paresthesias, seizures, and other peripheral or central neuropathies may complicate the crisis. A history of neurotic or psychotic behavior is not uncommon. Neurovisceral or neuropsychiatric symptoms most often do not become manifest until after puberty; but have occurred in children, most often in the form of a childhood seizure.

The peripheral neuropathy is owing to axonal degeneration and affects primarily motor neurons. Significant neuropathy does not occur with all acute attacks. Motor neuropathy affects the proximal muscles initially, more often in the shoulders and arms, but may be variable. Deep tendon reflexes may be normal or hyperactive but are usually decreased or absent with advanced neuropathy. Motor weakness can be asymmetric and focal and can involve cranial nerves. Progressive muscle weakness leading to respiratory and bulbar paralysis and death may occur when diagnosis and treatment are delayed. Sudden death may result from sympathetic over-activity and cardiac arrhythmia.

Mental symptoms such as anxiety, insomnia, depression, disorientation, hallucinations, and paranoia can accompany acute attacks. Seizures
can be owing to direct neurologic effects or result from hyponatremia.
Treatment of seizures is difficult because virtually all anitseizure drugs
(except bromides) have at least some potential for exacerbating AIP. Hyponatremia results from hypothalamic involvement and inappropriate vasopressin secretion or from electrolyte depletion owing to vomiting, poor
intake, or excess renal sodium loss. When an attack resolves, abdominal
pain may disappear within hours, and paresis begins to improve within
days but may continue to improve over months to years.

Aminolevulinic acid (ALA) and porphobilinogen (PBG) are increased
in plasma and urine during acute attacks. Urinary PBG excretion is usually 220 to 880 μmol/d (normal, 0–18 μmol/d), and urinary ALA is 150
to 760 μmol/d (normal, 8–53 μmol/d). The excretion of these com-
pounds generally decreases with clinical improvement, particularly after
hematin infusions (see the following). A normal urinary PBG level effectively excludes AIP as a cause for current symptoms. Fecal porphyrins are
usually normal or minimally increased in AIP, in contrast to other forms
of porphyria. Most asymptomatic (latent) heterozygotes with AIP have
normal urinary excretion of ALA and PBG. Therefore, measurement of
HMB synthase (PBG deaminase) in erythrocytes is useful to confirm the
diagnosis and to screen asymptomatic family members.

The enzyme deficiency is detectable in erythrocytes from most AIP
heterozygotes (*classic AIP*); however, the activity is higher in young erythrocytes and may increase into the normal range in an AIP patient with
increased erythropoiesis owing to a concurrent condition. The erythroid
and housekeeping forms of HMB synthase are encoded by a single gene.
Several deletions and over 20 different point mutations in the coding region of the gene have been found in unrelated AIP families. Heterozygotes can be identified by RFLP studies in informative families using
various polymorphic sites in the HMB synthase gene. Efforts are now un-
derway to identify the specific mutations in the HMB synthase gene in
all AIP families; this information will make possible the accurate identification of heterozygotes. Identified heterozygotes can be advised to avoid
factors known to cause acute attacks, and this technology can also lead to
prenatal diagnosis of a fetus at risk.

During acute attacks, narcotic analgesics may be required for abdominal pain, and phenothiazines are useful for nausea, vomiting, anxiety, and
restlessness. Benzodiazepines in low doses are probably safe if a minor
sedative is required. Although intravenous glucose was recommended in

the past for acute attacks, a more complete parenteral nutritional regimen may be beneficial if oral feeding is not possible for a prolonged period. However, intravenous heme is more effective than glucose in reducing porphyrin precursor excretion and probably leads to more rapid recovery. The response to heme therapy is reduced if therapy is delayed. Therefore, 3 to 4 mg heme, in the form of hematin, heme albumin, or heme arginate, may be infused daily for 4 days beginning as soon as possible after onset of an attack. Heme arginate and heme albumin are chemically stable and less likely than hematin to produce phlebitis or an anticoagulant effect. The rate of recovery from an acute attack depends on the degree of neuronal damage and may be rapid (1–2 days) with prompt therapy. Recovery from severe motor neuropathy may continue for months or years. Identification of and avoidance of inciting factors can hasten recovery from an attack and prevent future attacks.

Our patient was treated with daily infusions of hematin as well as nutritional support with total parenteral nutrition (TPN). His abdominal pain and mental status symptoms improved rapidly over the next 24 to 48 hours. On discharge from the hospital, he still had mild proximal muscle weakness that was slowly improving. He was educated about his disease, including avoidance of alcohol and other potential inciting factors.

 CLINICAL PEARLS

- Porphyrias are inherited or acquired disorders of specific enzymes in the heme biosynthetic pathway.
- Porphyrias are classified as either hepatic or erythropoietic depending on the primary site of overproduction.
- Symptoms of hepatic porphyrias include neurologic changes, abdominal pain, and mental disturbances; whereas erythropoietic porphyrias have primarily cutaneous photosensitivity.
- Acute intermittent porphyria (AIP) is a hepatic porphyria inherited as an autosomal dominant disorder owing to HMB synthase deficiency.
- The most common symptom of AIP is episodic abdominal pain that may mimic an acute surgical process in the abdomen.
- *Port-wine* colored urine is owing to porphobilinogen and prophyrin by-products in the urine and should suggest porphyria.
- Treatment of an acute attack consists of analgesia, sedation if needed, and heme infusions to decrease porphyrin precursor excretion and prevent neuronal damage.

REFERENCES

1. Poh–Fitzpatrick MB. Clinical features of the porphyrias. *Clin Dermatol* 1998;16:251–264.
2. Suarez JI, Cohen ML, Larkin J, et al. Acute intermittent porphyria: Clinicopathologic correlation. *Neurology* 1997;48:1678–1683.
3. McDonagh AF, Bissell DM. Porphyria and porphyrinology: The past fifteen years. *Semin Liver Dis* 1998;18(1):3–15.
4. Grandchamp B. Acute intermittent porphyria. *Semin Liver Dis* 1998; 18(1):17–24.
5. Elder GH, Hift RJ, Meissner PN. The acute porphyrias. *Lancet* 1997;349:1613–1617.

23-YEAR-OLD WOMAN WITH EASY FATIGABILITY

A 23-year-old female Asian postgraduate student presented with a several week history of easy fatigability while playing intramural hockey and soccer. She described dyspnea with extreme exertion and fatigue that occurred earlier than her peers. She was otherwise healthy and denied complaints of chest pain, wheezing, palpitations, presyncope, syncope, or weight loss. Her menses were regular without excessive bleeding. The family history was notable only for adult-onset diabetes in her maternal grandmother. She was single and enrolled in school full-time. She did not smoke or drink alcohol and reported no recent exposures or travel.

PHYSICAL EXAMINATION

VITAL SIGNS: Temperature, 98.2°F (36.7°C); pulse, 68; respiration, 18; bp, 100/70

GENERAL: Age-appropriate female in no acute distress

NECK: No thyromegaly

LUNGS: Clear

CARDIAC: Regular rate and rhythm, S1 normal, fixed split S2; grade II/VI systolic murmur over the left upper sternal border, grade II/VI diastolic rumble over the left lower sternal border; right ventricular heave; borderline elevated jugular venous pulse

ABDOMEN: Normal bowel sounds, soft, nontender, no hepatosplenomegaly

EXTREMITIES: No edema

LABORATORY FINDINGS

WBC, 8.3 K/μL (normal differential); Hb, 12.5 g/dL (MCV 89 fl); platelet count, 283 K/μL; electrolytes, urea nitrogen, and creatinine, were normal; chest x-ray demonstrated focal right ventricular enlargement with mildly enlarged pulmonary arteries; electrocardiogram is shown in Figure 50-1.

What is the likely diagnosis and how should this patient be treated?

This patient has an ostium secundum type atrial septal defect. The electrocardiogram reveals first-degree AV block, right axis deviation, and an incomplete right bundle branch block. Together, the history, physical examination, chest x-ray, and electrocardiogram strongly suggest the diagnosis, which was confirmed by a 2-D echocardiogram.

Atrial septal defect (ASD) is the second most common congenital cardiac anomaly presenting in adulthood (proceeded only by bicuspid aortic valve). It frequently goes undiagnosed until adulthood because of the lack of symptoms. ASD usually occurs sporadically as an isolated cardiac

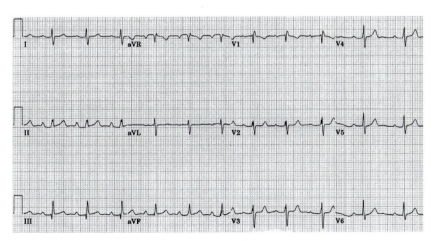

Figure 50-1
Patient's electrocardiogram.

anomaly, but may be a familial disorder or may occur with other congenital cardiac anomalies. The Holt-Oram syndrome, probably the best-known familial cause of atrial septal defect, is associated with congenital deformity of the upper limbs (absent or hypoplastic radii) and electrocardiographic abnormalities (right bundle branch block or first-degree atrioventricular block).

ASD is anatomically classified into one of three types. *Sinus venosus ASD* is located superior and posterior in the atrial septum, near the entry of the superior vena cava, and accounts for up to 10 percent of ASDs. *Ostium primum ASD* is located in the inferior atrial septum, as a result of a deficiency in endocardial cushion tissue—sometimes referred to as a partial atrioventricular septal defect—and accounts for up to 10 percent of ASDs. Ostium secundum ASD occurs in the mid-atrial septum as either a single large defect or several small ones (fenestrations). It is the most common type of ASD, comprising 80 percent of ASDs and occurring twice as often in females.

The physiologic consequence of an ASD is a left-to-right shunt, the magnitude of which is dependent not on the size of the defect but rather on the relative compliance of the ventricles. With significant left-to-right shunting (pulmonary to systemic shunt ratio >2:1) pulmonary blood flow increases, which leads to volume overload of the right ventricle. This is initially so well tolerated that normal intracardiac pressures are maintained. By about the second decade of life, however, the shunt becomes manifest in some patients by exercise intolerance, easy fatigability, and exertional dyspnea. As the left-to-right shunting increases with age, it produces congestive heart failure and atrial arrhythmias, which largely account for the disorder's morbidity and mortality. Right-sided pressures increase over time, amplifying the right-to-left shunting, which sometimes results in cyanosis. Less commonly, progressive pulmonary vascular disease develops that leads to right-to-left shunting, especially in females.

The classic auscultatory finding—wide and fixed splitting of the second heart sound—is thought to occur from increased volume across the pulmonic valve, delaying its closure (P2), irrespective of the phase of respiration. A pulmonary systolic ejection murmur arising from exaggerated flow across the pulmonic valve can also be appreciated. In addition, an early to mid-diastolic murmur along the left sternal border results from high flow across the tricuspid valve, particularly when the left-to-right shunt is greater than 2 to 1. As the right-sided pressures increase during the later stages and the left-to-right shunt decreases, the physical findings may resolve, leaving only accentuation of the pulmonic valve closure sound (P2).

The electrocardiogram with a secundum ASD, which reflects the increased right heart volume, typically shows right-axis deviation, right ventricular hypertrophy, and incomplete right bundle branch block. The PR interval may be prolonged by the right atrial enlargement and impaired internodal conduction that are caused by the defect. The chest x-ray often demonstrates right atrial and right ventricular enlargement and an enlarged main pulmonary artery segment with prominent pulmonary vascular markings.

The diagnosis is usually confirmed by Doppler-echocardiography, which allows visualization of the ASD on two-dimensional imaging, supplemented by color flow Doppler, or agitated-saline contrast echocardiography. In addition, pulsed Doppler measurements can quantify the pulmonary-to-systemic blood flow ratio or shunt calculation. Transesophageal echocardiographic (TEE) imaging provides an excellent diagnostic alternative when the surface images are inadequate. Cardiac catheterization is unnecessary when the diagnosis has been established by noninvasive means, except if pulmonary vascular disease is suspected and measurement of pulmonary vascular resistance is necessary.

Unlike a true defect in the atrial septum (ASD), a patent foramen ovale (PFO) represents a persistence or re-opening of the normal fetal circulation "flap valve" between the right and left atrium—it can be detected in up to 30 percent of adults. In this setting, although minimal left-to-right shunting can occur, right atrial pressure commonly increases sufficiently during respiratory excursions, even in normal individuals, to cause transient right-to-left shunting through the PFO. This may provide access for blood clots from a deep venous thrombosis to embolize across the atrial septum into the systemic circulation (paradoxical embolus), leading to a potentially devastating embolic event—a cerebrovascular accident.

It is generally recommended that a secundum ASD be electively closed during childhood when it is associated with a large left-to-right shunt (pulmonary to systemic shunt ratio >2:1), cardiac symptoms, or ventricular enlargement. This is supported by the results of a long-term follow-up study that found a dramatic increase in survival with surgical repair before the age of 25 years. Because the risk of surgical repair is substantially higher with pulmonary hypertension, the decision for repair is more difficult and must be individualized. Percutaneous catheter-based occlusion devices that have been recently introduced may provide an alternative to surgical closure in selected patients.

 # CLINICAL PEARLS

- ASD is the second most common congenital cardiac anomaly presenting in adulthood.
- ASD is anatomically classified into one of three types: sinus venosus, ostium primum, and ostium secundum.
- Ostium secundum is the most common type of ASD, accounting for 80 percent of ASDs and occurring twice as often in females.
- The classic auscultatory finding is wide and fixed splitting of the second heart sound.
- The diagnosis of ASD is usually confirmed by Doppler-echocardiography.
- A patent foramen ovale (PFO) can be detected in up to 30 percent of adults.
- Early closure of an ASD is suggested in patients with a large left-to-right shunt, ventricular enlargement, or cardiac symptoms.

REFERENCES

1. Vick III GW. Defects of the atrial septum including atriventricular septal defects, in *The Science and Practice of Pediatric Cardiology*, 2nd ed. Garson Jr. A, Bricker JT, Fisher DJ, Neish SR (eds). Baltimore, Williams & Wilkins, 1998.
2. Auslender M, Beekman III RH, Lloyd TR. Transcatheter closure of atrial septal defects. *J Interven Cardiol* 1995;8:533–542.
3. Murphy JG, Gersh BJ, McGoon MD, et al. Long-term outcome after surgical repair of isolated atrial septal defect. Follow-up at 27 to 32 years. *N Engl J Med* 1990;323:1645–1650.

INDEX

ISBN 0-07-006692-2

90000